Second Edition

DISEASE

Identification, Prevention, and Control

Second Edition

DISEASE
Identification, Prevention, and Control

Barbara P. Hamann, Ph.D.
University of Wisconsin-Superior

Boston   Burr Ridge, IL   Dubuque, IA   Madison, WI   New York   San Francisco   St. Louis
Bangkok   Bogotá   Caracas   Lisbon   London   Madrid
Mexico City   Milan   New Delhi   Seoul   Singapore   Sydney   Taipei   Toronto

McGraw-Hill Higher Education

A Division of The **McGraw-Hill** *Companies*

DISEASE: IDENTIFICATION, PREVENTION, AND CONTROL
SECOND EDITION

Published by McGraw-Hill, an imprint of The McGraw-Hill Companies, Inc., 1221 Avenue of the Americas, New York, NY 10020. Copyright © 2001, 1994 by The McGraw-Hill Companies, Inc. All rights reserved. No part of this publication may be reproduced or distributed in any form or by any means, or stored in a database or retrieval system, without the prior written consent of The McGraw-Hill Companies, Inc., including, but not limited to, in any network or other electronic storage or transmission, or broadcast for distance learning.

Some ancillaries, including electronic and print components, may not be available to customers outside the United States.

 This book is printed on recycled, acid-free paper containing 10% postconsumer waste.

1 2 3 4 5 6 7 8 9 0 QPD/QPD 0 9 8 7 6 5 4 3 2 1 0

ISBN   0–8151–2847–9

Vice president and editor-in-chief: *Kevin T. Kane*
Executive editor: *Vicki Malinee*
Developmental editor: *Carlotta Seely*
Senior marketing manager: *Pamela S. Cooper*
Project manager: *Joyce M. Berendes*
Associate producer: *Judi David*
Production supervisor: *Kara Kudronowicz*
Coordinator of freelance design: *Rick D. Noel*
Cover designer: *Kristyn A. Kalnes*
Cover image: *© Tony Stone Images, image by David Becker*
Photo research coordinator: *John C. Leland*
Compositor: *Precision Graphics*
Typeface: *10/12 Times Roman*
Printer: *Quebecor Printing Book Group/Dubuque, IA*

The credits section for this book begins on page 441 and is considered an extension of the copyright page.

Library of Congress Cataloging-in-Publication Data

Hamann, Barbara P.
   Disease : identification, prevention, and control / Barbara Hamann. —2nd ed.
      p.   cm.
   Includes bibliographical references and index.
   ISBN 0–8151–2847–9 (alk. paper)
      1. Diseases.   I. Title.
   [DNLM: 1. Disease. 2. Diagnosis. 3. Preventive Medicine. QZ 40 H198d 2001]

RC46 .H225   2001
616—dc21   00–037253
                                                                      CIP

www.mhhe.com

CONTENTS

PREFACE

For the past twenty-five years I have taught introductory and community health courses about disease to health education students. During that time, the field of health education has steadily grown. Today, with the burgeoning interest in holistic health and fitness, it is expanding even more rapidly, and the need for a course in disease designed for health educators has become urgent. National certification in health has become an important career goal for health educators working in schools, corporations, and communities. Certification guidelines for such organizations as The National Commission for Health Education Credentialing (NCHEC) and The American College of Sport Medicine (ACSM) either imply or require knowledge of diseases. The ACSM's emphasis on the need for knowledge of noninfectious diseases such as heart disease and arthritis suggests a need for knowledge about infectious diseases, such as Lyme disease or strep throat, that can lead to chronic disease in later life.

When I began teaching a course specifically concerned with disease ten years ago, my research revealed that no appropriate text existed for my class. The texts available were written for pre-med students, nurses, and allied health personnel. These texts were more technical and clinical than necessary for preparing students who will be health educators in schools, corporations, or community agencies. This text has been written for these students, although it could also serve as an introductory course in disease for those entering allied health fields. The text assumes that students have had a class or classes in anatomy and physiology.

ORGANIZATION

Unit I of the text presents a brief history of disease (Chapter 1), discusses the principles of disease occurrence (Chapter 2), and explains the body's defenses (Chapter 3).

Unit II of the text organizes infectious diseases in a somewhat different format than other texts. Diseases are grouped by disease agent, rather than by body system; this has the advantage of keeping information on a specific agent in one chapter, rather than scattered among several different chapters. In each chapter, general characteristics, transmission, symptoms, treatment, prevention, and control are discussed for each disease covered. Time and space did not allow for coverage of all infectious diseases; discussed in this text are infectious diseases common in the United States and some (such as smallpox and leprosy) that have historical significance.

Unit III begins by discussing the two major noninfectious diseases: cardiovascular disease (Chapter 12) and cancer (Chapters 13 and 14), followed by other noninfectious diseases (Chapters 15 to 17). (In this text, the word *chronic* will be used as an adjective meaning long-lasting; it may be used for either infectious or noninfectious disease.) In each of these chapters, general characteristics, predisposing factors, symptoms, prevention, and treatment of selected diseases are discussed. Again, diseases discussed are those prevalent in the United States. The final chapter of this part, Chapter 18, deals with genetic and pediatric diseases.

PEDAGOGY

The new edition continues with its unique approach to exploring diseases. In this textbook you will find

- Brief opening discussions for each part that are designed to arouse interest in what is ahead.
- Case studies integrated throughout the text that highlight client-related examples, as well as educational settings. Topics include: Legionnaires' disease, salmonellosis, meningitis, plague, varicella, herpes simplex virus Type I, histoplasmosis, cryptosporidiosis, heart disease, prostate cancer, esophageal cancer, emphysema, fibromyalgia, multiple sclerosis, and Huntington's disease.
- Behavior objectives and an outline at the beginning of each chapter that will prepare the reader for an organized approach to the chapter's content.

- A summary table of diseases at the end of the chapter that discusses and reviews the content covered.
- Each chapter concludes with up-to-date suggestions for further reading.

ILLUSTRATION PROGRAM

Time lines in the opening chapter put the history of disease and the accomplishments of the last two centuries into perspective for the student. Throughout, illustrations (both line drawings and photographs) have been chosen or created for their effectiveness in depicting relevant disease states or explaining disease processes.

ACKNOWLEDGMENTS

I would like to thank the following reviewers for their input on the revision of this textbook:

Nina Beaman-Blodgett, RNC, CMA
    Commonwealth College
Richard Bynum, Ed.D.   *Moorhead State University*
Gerald C. Hyner, Ph.D.   *Purdue University*
Alice Prince, Ph.D.   *Southern Illinois University—Edwardsville*

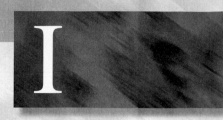
Introduction

Some of the earliest traces of community life have included signs of disease (see Figure 1-1). The efforts of early people to understand why disease happened and then to prevent it met with little success. In fact, not until the revolutionary scientific discoveries of the nineteenth and twentieth centuries could humanity begin to make significant progress against one of its oldest enemies. However, the benefits of those discoveries have not yet reached many of the people in the developing countries.

The heartrending picture of a young boy, squatting on stick-thin legs and too weak to use his equally thin arms to brush away the flies and other insects surrounding him, has been used in televised appeals for help for children in developing countries. This boy shows the effects of too little food, little or no medical treatment, and other factors, such as

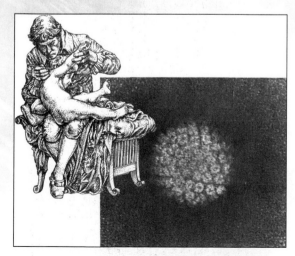

Statuo of Edward Jenner inoculating his son against cowpox.

Human papillomavirus (right). Electron micrograph of a negatively stained papillomavirus that occurs in human warts. Warts on the hands and feet have never been known to progress to cancer, however, cervical warts can go on after many years to become cancerous (×240,000).

poverty and poor sanitation. These factors combine to make such children, as well as their elders, vulnerable to the attacks of disease.

Poverty, ignorance, and often politics have kept information on human anatomy and physiology, infectious and noninfectious disease, drugs, and treatment procedures from many in the developing countries. Defense against disease in these countries often is limited to folk medicine, religious ritual, and cultural practices.

In an attempt to change conditions in developing nations and globally, the World Health Organization (WHO) developed "A Global Strategy for Health for All." Among the strategies intended to prevent disease and promote health are safe water and adequate sanitary facilities within homes or no more than fifteen minutes' walking distance away; adequate nutrition for children; medically trained personnel to assist with pregnancy, childbirth, and care of the newborn; local health care; availability of at least twenty essential drugs within one hour's travel; and immunization against many infectious diseases.

In the developed countries, the discoveries of the last 200 years have led to an understanding of the necessity for clean water supplies and sanitation, a decrease in the incidence of most infectious diseases, lower disease and death rates, and (in the last thirty years) emphasis on preventive medicine.

Ironically, however, progress against infectious disease means that more people are living longer and are suffering from more chronic noninfectious diseases. The effects of industrialization, urbanization and lifestyle have been a blessing in some ways but people now fall ill from the hazards accompanying modernization.

The eradication of smallpox through WHO's efforts, along with the understanding of how to prevent or control most other infectious diseases, was a great accomplishment. However, acquired immune deficiency syndrome (AIDS), Ebola fever, and other emerging diseases; the resistance of microorganisms to antibiotics; continuing problems involved in establishing and delivering adequate health care to all and the need to convince all the world's people to take responsibility for their own health pose a continuing challenge.

Chapter 1, The History of Disease, is a look backward in time, a brief review of humanity's triumphs and failures in the ongoing fight against disease. Chapter 2 explains the epidemiologic model of disease, now used by public health workers as they study the causes of disease. This model proposes the interaction of disease agents, host characteristics, and environmental factors as the key to disease occurrence. The chain of infection, or means of disease transmission, and the stages of disease are also discussed in this chapter.

The final chapter in this part of the text deals with the body's defenses against disease, and a few of the disorders that occur because, at times, these defenses are mistakenly turned inward.

The History of Disease

O B J E C T I V E S

1. *State important events in the understanding and treatment of disease through the ages.*
2. *Explain the major theories that have been held concerning the cause of disease from the earliest times to the present.*
3. *Identify the contributions of key individuals to advances in medicine through the ages.*
4. *Identify highlights in the history of disease prevention and control.*
5. *Describe the development of the major methods used to prevent and control infectious and noninfectious diseases today.*

6. *Explain the reasons for the change in focus from prevention and control of disease to health promotion.*
7. *Explain the concept of emerging and reemerging diseases.*
8. *State ten examples of diseases that have emerged in the past twenty years.*
9. *List the ways that CDC and WHO are addressing the problem of emerging disease.*
10. *Identify new technologies and techniques used to diagnose and treat disease today.*

The Prehistory of Disease

The seeds of disease were present long before recorded history began. Bacteria were among the earliest forms of plant life on earth, and evidence of their ability to infect humans and animals has been found in fossils from prehistoric times. These fossil remains show signs of a number of diseases, including osteomyelitis, tuberculosis, arthritis, rickets, and bone tumors. The well-preserved remains of Egyptian mummies, along with the papyri upon which the Egyptians inscribed case histories of polio, tuberculosis, pneumonia, leprosy, and kidney stones, provide additional evidence of assaults

osteomyelitis   os-te-o-my-e-LI-tis

3

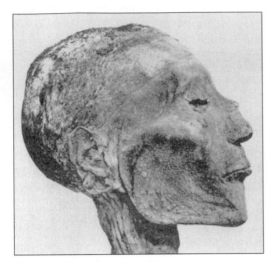

Figure 1-1

Mummified head of Pharaoh Ramses V, showing small-pox lesions.

upon the body by disease agents. Lesions on the head of the mummy shown in Figure 1-1 indicate that smallpox may also have been present in early times. Physical discomfort, sickness, and death from "unnatural" causes have been unwanted companions of the human race since its beginning. The information in this chapter will give you a brief glimpse of the progress made in identifying and learning to prevent and control disease from the time of the early Egyptians to the present. The time line beginning on page 8 shows this progress.

ANCIENT CIVILIZATIONS: THEORIES OF DISEASE CAUSATION

Egyptian Medicine

The early Egyptians (4000–1000 B.C.) had many remedies for illness. Spells, incantations, and magic were integral parts of their medicine. Among early races, illness and death were attributed to actions of the gods and demonic possession. (The concept is present today among some isolated races and individuals.) Despite the Egyptians' lack of scientific knowledge, some of the treatments they used were

effective and are still used, and the Egyptians are recognized as the first to treat disease systematically.

Egyptian physicians recognized that weather and the ingestion of "noxious" substances affected the body. They used drugs such as castor oil, olive oil, opium, and saffron. Pulses were taken, body temperature noted, the heart was regarded as the vital organ, and respiration was considered the most important function. There were severe penalties for letting a patient die, and for this reason no one was accepted for treatment who appeared to have a fatal condition. Unfortunately, one of the conditions looked upon as fatal was a compound fracture. Egypt was regarded as the medical center of the ancient world, and Egyptian physicians were sought after by foreign rulers. Prescriptions for diet and cleanliness were part of the religion. Records also indicate that physicians specialized. Some treated only diseases of the eye, others diseases of the head, others diseases of the intestines, and so on.

The treatments the early Egyptian doctors used were based on what they perceived as the cause of the disease, and medical science still uses this principle today.

Chinese Medicine

Chinese medicine of the same period also contributed to the remedies in use today. An early Chinese emperor is credited with identifying over 100 herbal remedies and also inventing the technique of acupuncture. As with the Egyptians, magic and superstition played a part in the development of medicine in China, yet some Chinese prescriptions were effective also. Among these were the use of iron to treat anemia and the use of opium as a narcotic to reduce pain.

chi out of balance

The Bible and Medicine

In biblical times and earlier, treatments that were effective in helping people with disease were developed and used without any understanding on the part of the practitioners as to why they worked. And we have no indication that there was any concerted effort to discover the cause of most diseases, probably because disease was generally thought of as coming from gods who controlled human events. But glimmerings of the understanding of disease can be found in the Bible. For example, the story of plague among the Philistines in the Old Testament indicates recognition of a relationship between rats and the disease, and the segregation of lepers indicates some understanding of preventive medicine. The Mosaic law or code, in addition to providing for the segregation of lepers, also prescribed the control of communicable diseases, fumigation, decontamination of buildings, protection of water supplies, disposal of wastes, protection of food, and sanitation of campsites.

GREECE: THE TEACHINGS OF HIPPOCRATES

The writings of Hippocrates (460–377 B.C.) show that by his time interest in determining the cause of and treatment for disease was widespread. Hippocrates, known as the Father of Medicine, believed that each individual contained four *humors,* or fluids: blood, phlegm, yellow bile, and black bile. Disease occurred when these humors were not in balance and could be treated by removing any excess. The practice of bloodletting (Figure 1-2), which persisted well into the nineteenth century, was based on this theory.

Hippocrates also believed in the healing power of nature, taught that disease developed from natural causes, and prescribed diets, rest, fresh air, massage, and baths as treatments. Although it would be centuries before the first pathogenic organism was identified, Hippocrates's logical approach to disease and clinical observation were first steps on the way to the prevention and control of disease.

We are not sure how many of the books credited to Hippocrates were actually written by him, but we do know that the ideas those books contained were revolutionary in the practice of medicine. Among them was the first known work on physiotherapy; a description of the symptoms that precede death; and forty-two case histories presented in a style close to modern scientific form for case histories.

wrote more than 100 books

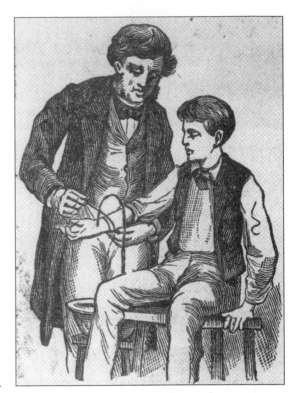

Figure 1-2 *→ uses leaches*
Bloodletting, a practice that derived from the concept of humors in the body, which must be kept in balance to prevent disease. This practice continued into the early nineteenth century.
— theory lasted for 1000 yrs.

ROME: THE CONCEPT OF PUBLIC HEALTH

Roman civilization adopted many Greek ideals, including respect for the search for scientific knowledge and an appreciation of physical health and beauty. As Roman power grew, public health measures were adopted. Aqueducts were built to carry pure water to the cities (Figure 1-3). Sewers prevented the spread of epidemics, and street cleaning was required. Public and private baths were available everywhere. Physicians were educated at public expense, and their services were made available to the poor. One Roman, Marcus Terentius Varro (116–21 B.C.), described "small creatures, invisible to the eye." These creatures, according to Varro, filled

green

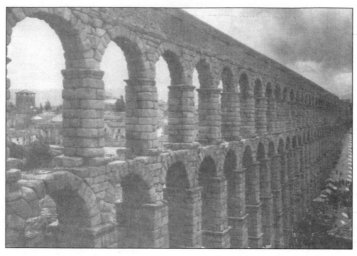

Figure 1-3
A Roman aqueduct at Pont du Gard, Nimes, in France.

the air, were breathed in, and caused dangerous diseases. How this early scientist arrived at this conclusion is a mystery because the microscope, enabling researchers to actually see pathogenic organisms, would not be invented for hundreds of years.

THE TEACHINGS OF GALEN

Galen (A.D. 130–200), a native of Asia Minor, was the imperial physician of the Roman Empire. Regarded as the founder of experimental physiology, he dissected animals and wrote extensively on the anatomy of the brain and other organs. However, the religious beliefs of the time forbade human dissection. This limited Galen's investigations, and he reached some incorrect conclusions about the structure and function of the human body. Because of his position, he was accepted as the final authority by the early church. His influence persisted for centuries, delaying advances in understanding the human body.

THE MIDDLE AGES: WAR, RELIGION, AND DISEASE

After the fall of Rome (A.D. 476) political chaos and the rise of new religions affected the search for scientific knowledge. Those same factors also influenced the spread of disease. The collapse of centralized government led to the collapse of the Romans' aqueducts and sewer systems. New cities arose, but the kind of public engineering known under the Romans had been lost.

Christianity, Islam, and Contagion

In Europe, early Christians reacted against the Greco-Roman emphasis on physical health and beauty. This seemed to them to glorify the body at the expense of the spirit. A healthy mind in a healthy body was no longer the ideal. The body became something shameful, to be ignored in the pursuit of spiritual perfection. This reaction softened somewhat as the Middle Ages progressed, but the Greco-Roman ideal was lost.

The rise of another religion, Islam, in the seventh century also contributed to the spread of disease. Followers of Islam, called Moslems, were required to make a pilgrimage to the holy city of Mecca in what is now Saudi Arabia. Because this faith had spread from southern Europe to India, large numbers of pilgrims traveled long distances to reach Mecca, carrying and transmitting infectious diseases as they went. Among these diseases was cholera, which became pandemic after each *hajj,* or pilgrimage.

[Handwritten notes at top:]
Dead rats burned - thousands - people worry
Plague spread by fleas, insects, travel
  looked black - internal bleeding - discolored
Jew's - poisoning the wells

Christian reaction to Islam also contributed to the spread of disease. From the eleventh to the thirteenth centuries, crusades against the "infidels," as Moslems were called, swept thousands of Europeans into the Middle East. Returning crusaders sometimes brought back treasures; they also brought back diseases. Cholera was one of these diseases; leprosy was probably another.

The most deadly of all pandemics, however, were the waves of disease caused by bubonic plague (the "Black Death"). Figure 1-4 shows the protective clothing worn to treat victims of this deadly disease. Twenty percent of the population of Europe perished from a combination of the plague and pulmonary anthrax. In England, two million died, approximately half of the population. London alone had

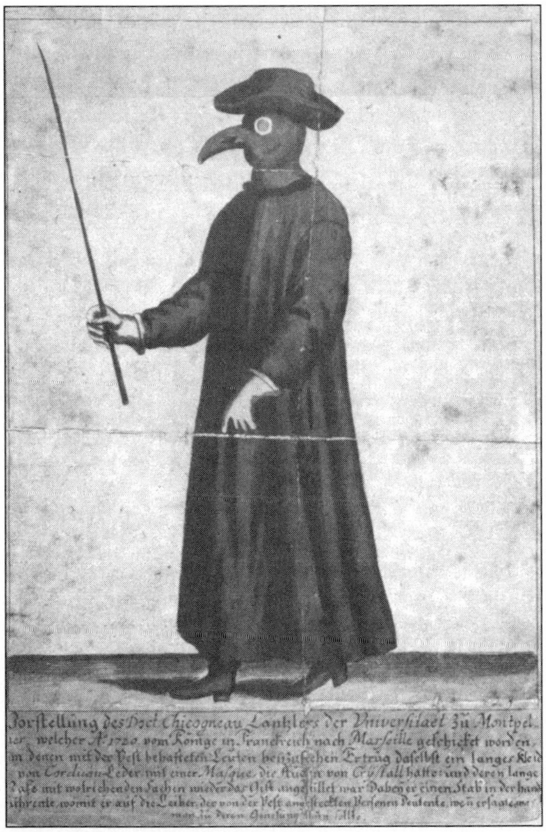

[Handwritten margin note:] 25 mill ← ¼ Europe population

100,000 of these deaths. Another deadly disease, syphilis, spread rapidly throughout Europe and the Near East shortly after the return of Columbus from America. It is thought to have been carried back to Europe by Columbus and his men. Other diseases known to exist during this period, although little mention of them is made in history books, include typhoid, typhus, diphtheria, streptococcal infections, and dysenteries. During all this time there was little understanding of the ways by which disease was spread. Isolation and quarantine, as with lepers, were the only control methods, and they were practiced unevenly, depending upon the recognition of symptoms that were thought to be dangerous.

THE RENAISSANCE: DA VINCI, VESALIUS, GALILEO, AND THE MICROSCOPE

[Handwritten notes:] = re-birth — allowed to have ideas, study, think

It took the intellectual revolution and stimulation of the Renaissance to release once more the spirit of scientific inquiry. As this "rebirth" swept through all areas of human knowledge, among those who contributed to advances in medicine were Leonardo da Vinci (1452–1519) and Andreas Vesalius (1514–1564). Each produced anatomical works based on dissection of the human body that were to show Galen's mistakes and become the foundation for modern anatomy. Figure 1-5 shows an illustration from a page from one of Vesalius's works. As was mentioned earlier, syphilis appeared in Europe in 1495. It was named by Girolamo Fracastoro (1483–1553), who also recognized typhus and the contagious nature of tuberculosis. In his writings, he spoke of "the existence of invisible seeds of infection which multiply and penetrate the organism." Fracastoro's book, *De contagione,* was convincing enough that the humoral doctrine of disease, taught by Hippocrates almost a thousand years earlier, was replaced by the idea of specific causes for specific diseases.

[Handwritten margin note:] founder of modern Anatomy

One of the most significant inventions of the sixteenth century was the microscope. Although the ability to magnify objects with spherical pieces of glass had been known to the ancients, it was not until the late sixteenth century that microscopes

Figure 1-4
Protective clothing worn by physicians when treating plague victims.

were used in scientific investigations. It is not known who first used magnifying lenses in researching disease, but Galileo (1564–1642) is given credit for actually placing a tube between

two lenses to examine a specimen some time after he had constructed his first telescope in 1608.

THE SEVENTEENTH CENTURY: ADVANCES IN UNDERSTANDING DISEASE

In the seventeenth century, inductive reasoning emphasized by Francis Bacon (1561–1626) and the philosophical writings of René Descartes (1596–1650), which encouraged questioning of any former "truths," opened the way for the development of the scientific method. William Harvey described his experiments, which demonstrated the circulation of blood. It was not long before Anton van Leeuwenhoek described red blood cells. Van Leeuwenhoek constructed more than 200 microscopes and was the first to identify bacteria, although he did not connect them to disease. Athanasius Kircher was the first to connect the live microorganisms in the blood with disease. As more scientists were able to use the microscope—and with more understanding of human anatomy and physiology—advances in the knowledge of disease accelerated.

Advances in Diagnosis

The vitamin deficiency diseases rickets and beriberi were described, the difference between diabetes mellitus and diabetes insipidus was discovered, and

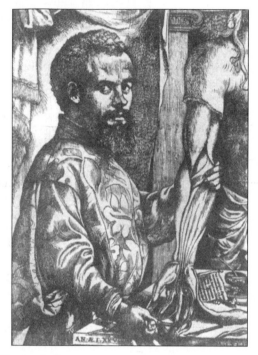

Figure 1-5

Page from the treatise of Andreas Vesalius on anatomy, showing the author.

HIGHLIGHTS IN DISEASE IDENTIFICATION, PREVENTION, AND CONTROL

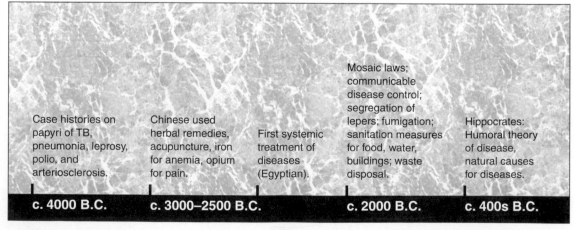

Case histories on papyri of TB, pneumonia, leprosy, polio, and arteriosclerosis.	Chinese used herbal remedies, acupuncture, iron for anemia, opium for pain.	First systemic treatment of diseases (Egyptian).	Mosaic laws; communicable disease control; segregation of lepers; fumigation; sanitation measures for food, water, buildings; waste disposal.	Hippocrates: Humoral theory of disease, natural causes for diseases.
c. 4000 B.C.	**c. 3000–2500 B.C.**		**c. 2000 B.C.**	**c. 400s B.C.**

the possibility of a nonvenereal route for syphilitic infection was demonstrated. Physicians learned to count the pulse with a watch. Thomas Sydenham was responsible for many advances, including differentiation between acute rheumatism and gout and between scarlet fever and measles. But it was to take more than 100 years before scientists would begin to identify the organisms and causes for most diseases.

THE EIGHTEENTH CENTURY: VACCINATION

The eighteenth century was a time for nurturing the new scientific spirit that had begun in the Renaissance. Progress in the search for answers about disease continued amid the remnants of earlier times. It was a century of paradoxes: an age of enlightenment, an age of quackery; an age of rationalism, yet an age of superstition. Toward the end of this century, Edward Jenner, an English country doctor, made a discovery that was to open the doors for the relief of untold suffering and death.

Jenner's Milestone

Smallpox had killed millions, and there was no indication that the number of cases was decreasing. Jenner overheard a dairymaid say that she could not catch smallpox because she had already had cowpox. Knowing that cowpox was a mild disease, he decided to experiment and vaccinated a small boy with pus from a cowpox lesion. Eight weeks later, the boy was inoculated with smallpox but did not get the disease. Jenner published his findings in 1798. Although Jenner was greeted with some skepticism at first, it was not long before the incidence of smallpox was greatly reduced in developed countries all over the world.

THE NINETEENTH CENTURY: PASTEUR, LISTER, KOCH, AND THE GERM THEORY

Jenner's discovery of the benefits of vaccination was just the beginning of a great cascade of scientific breakthroughs in the nineteenth century. Scientists in different laboratories all over the world identified many microorganisms and the diseases they caused at such great speed that following each new discovery is beyond the scope of this text. The time line on pages 12–13 shows the fast pace of progress against disease in the latter half of the nineteenth century.

Many individuals made contributions to the prevention and control of disease in the nineteenth century. Claude Bernard (1813–1878), Louis Pasteur (1822–1895), and Robert Koch (1843–1910) were research scientists whose work brought attention to

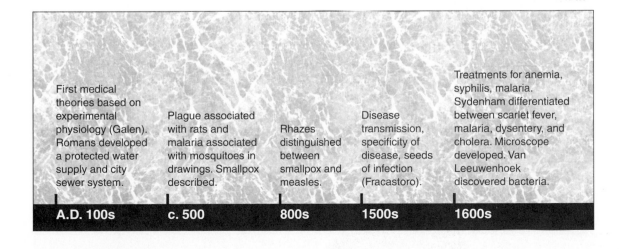

First medical theories based on experimental physiology (Galen). Romans developed a protected water supply and city sewer system.

Plague associated with rats and malaria associated with mosquitoes in drawings. Smallpox described.

Rhazes distinguished between smallpox and measles.

Disease transmission, specificity of disease, seeds of infection (Fracastoro).

Treatments for anemia, syphilis, malaria. Sydenham differentiated between scarlet fever, malaria, dysentery, and cholera. Microscope developed. Van Leeuwenhoek discovered bacteria.

A.D. 100s   **c. 500**   **800s**   **1500s**   **1600s**

the value of laboratory research in addition to clinical observations.

The understanding of the human body was enhanced by Bernard, who demonstrated that digestion took place in the small intestine as well as in the stomach, discovered glycogen and its manufacture by the liver, unfolded some of the mysteries of the endocrine system, and formulated the basic principles of research and experiment. Louis Pasteur was the first to show without question that microorganisms could be pathogenic to humans. He also continued Jenner's work in immunology with the development of vaccines for anthrax and rabies. His procedure for destroying pathogenic organisms in milk and other liquids, pasteurization, is well known.

Building on the work of Louis Pasteur, Joseph Lister (1827–1912) applied antiseptics to surgical wounds and thus made surgery a hundred times safer. Koch developed postulates concerning disease that stated that, for an organism to be identified as the cause of a specific disease, it must (1) always be present in the disease, (2) be capable of growth in pure culture in the laboratory, (3) cause the disease when injected into a susceptible healthy animal, and (4) be recovered from the experimental animal. These postulates clearly established the germ theory of disease and are still used today. Among Koch's many other contribu-

tions was the discovery of the bacilli for anthrax, cholera, and tuberculosis.

Progress in Public Health

During this century there was rapid population growth in major cities in Europe and America. Little was then known about the connection between sanitation and disease, and piles of garbage and waste accumulated because of lack of community organizations to deal with the problem. In response to this, Edwin Chadwick published a report in England (1842) concerning the poor state of health and the deplorable sanitary conditions. England then passed the British Public Health Act of 1848.

Soon after the passage of this act in England, an American, Lemuel Shattuck, published a report (1850) that was to be a guide in the field of health for many years. Shattuck (1792–1859) was chairman of the newly appointed Sanitary Commission of Massachusetts. Although many of his recommendations (Box 1-1) have not yet been fulfilled, the report provided the impetus for a concerted public effort in the struggle to identify, prevent, and control disease.

At the time of these reports, the miasma theory of disease was popular. This theory ascribed disease to bad air (the term *miasma* means noxious

HIGHLIGHTS IN DISEASE IDENTIFICATION, PREVENTION, AND CONTROL *(continued)*

Miasma theory. First officially recognized smallpox vaccination (Jenner). Circulation of blood (Harvey).

Shattuck's sanitary report. Milk inspection. Pathogenic nature of bacteria. Rabies and anthrax vaccines (Pasteur). Antisepsis (Lister). Germ theory of disease (Pasteur and Koch). Identification of pathogens for many diseases. Rabies treatment. X rays and radium (Curie). Vaccines and antitoxins developed for many diseases. First successful removal of part of the stomach for cancer. Water treatment plant (Massachusetts).

Vitamin hypothesis confirmed. Diphtheria skin test (Schick). Insulin for diabetes. Chemotherapy (Ehrlich). Penicillin discovered (Fleming). Sulfa drugs found useful for streptococcal infection. Improved anesthesia. Partial and complete removal of the lung for cancer. U.S. Public Health Service established. Pure Food and Drug Act. Chlorination of water supply (New Jersey).

1700s   **1800s**   **Early 1900s**

air or vapor), and thus efforts to prevent disease were aimed at reducing the bad odors in the air.

Toward the end of the nineteenth century, the earlier work initiated by Pasteur, Koch, and other bacteriologists led to the acceptance of the germ theory of disease. One of the most important discoveries at this time was the protozoan malarial parasite in human blood and its carrier, the *Anopheles* mosquito. This discovery marked the beginning of the conquest of a tropical disease that had been responsible for the decline and devitalization of many civilizations for centuries. Malaria could finally be controlled by systematic destruction of the mosquito larvae.

In addition to the progress made in the area of infectious disease, new procedures were being developed that would help prevent and control

anopheles a-NOF e-leez

Box 1-1

Lemuel Shattuck's Recommendations for Public Health (1850)

Establishment of state and local boards of health

    Hiring of sanitary inspectors
    Keeping of vital statistic records
    Establishment of systems for data exchange
    Studies of schoolchildren's health
    Establishment of sanitations programs for towns
    Studies of tuberculosis
    Supervision of the mentally ill
    Study of immigrants' problems
    Building of model tenements

Establishment of public bathhouses and washhouses

    Control of smoke nuisances
    Control of food adulteration
    Exposure of quack medicines
    Preaching of health in the churches
    Establishment of training schools for nurses
    Teaching of sanitary science in medical schools
    Inclusion of preventive medicine in clinical practice (routine physical examination, keeping records of family illnesses)

From Pickett and Hanlon. 1990. *Public health: Administration and practice,* 9th ed. Mosby, St. Louis.

Electron microscope. Streptomycin used for TB. Viruses for polio, measles, and influenza A identified. Vaccines for polio (Salk), measles, mumps, and rubella. First successful organ transplant (kidney). Open heart surgery. Surgeon General's report on smoking and lung cancer. Risk factors for cancer and heart disease identified. Test for cervical cancer (Papanicolaou). WHO founded. Most vitamins synthesized.

CT scan. Test for breast cancer (mammogram) and colorectal cancer. Cancer research intensified seeking possible viral cause. National high blood pressure education and screening. Official eradication of smallpox worldwide.

MRI. Objectives for the Nation in disease prevention and health promotion. Block grants. First permanent artificial heart implanted. AIDS first reported. Drug for treating AIDS. Warning labels on cigarettes. Federal support for disease prevention and health promotion.

First trials for an AIDS vaccine.

Mid 1900s   **1970s**   **1980s**   **1990s**

noninfectious disease. Blood pressure readings were begun in the 1860s; inspection of the throat, especially the larynx and vocal cords, was facilitated by the construction of the laryngoscope; visualization of the esophagus was accomplished; and the bladder could be observed with a cystoscope. Roentgen discovered the X ray, and Marie and Pierre Curie discovered radium, both useful in diagnosing and treating cancer and other diseases.

The nineteenth century, which began with more quackery and superstition than scientific knowledge, ended with an outstanding record of discoveries and achievements in the prevention and control of communicable disease. A longer, comparatively disease-free life at last seemed possible.

THE TWENTIETH CENTURY: "WONDER" DRUGS AND NEW EPIDEMICS; TECHNOLOGY AND TECHNIQUES

In the twentieth century, studies continued with infectious diseases, and effective serums were developed for diphtheria, meningococcus meningitis, and pneumococcal pneumonia. But the most dramatic discoveries in the control and treatment of infectious diseases came with the discovery of the sulfa drugs, penicillin, and other antibiotics.

Paul Ehrlich was the first to use a specific chemical agent against a specific organism. In 1907 he used a compound called arsphenamine, or "606," to cure syphilis. A scientist in France learned how to produce sulfanilamide in 1936, and soon after, sulfathiazole was produced and is still one of the best cures for meningococcus meningitis. But the most dramatic breakthrough in chemotherapy came with the discovery of penicillin by Alexander Fleming in 1928. Although it was to be more than ten years before the drug was ready for public use, it soon became the treatment of choice to cure many bacterial infections.

Antibiotic Breakthroughs

Streptomycin, the first antibiotic that helped in the treatment and cure of tuberculosis, was isolated in 1943 and soon joined by two other drugs, para-aminosalicylic acid and isoniazid. The discovery of these three drugs led to cooperative efforts of many government agencies and other groups to determine the safety and effectiveness of administering them at the same time. Instead of individuals working alone as they had in the nineteenth century, joint efforts now became common in the fight against disease.

PROGRESS IN DISEASE IDENTIFICATION, PREVENTION, AND CONTROL 1855–1899

Rudolf Virchow (1821–1902) established the cell as center of pathological processes. Louis Pasteur (1822–1895) realized and demonstrated pathogenic nature of bacteria. Anthrax and rabies vaccines developed.	Germ theory of disease became the dominant theory through efforts of Pasteur, Lister, and Koch.	Leprosy bacillus identified.	Gonococcus identified.	Typhoid bacillus, pneumo-coccus, and malaria plasmodium identified.	Robert Koch (1843–1910) developed his Four Postulates.	Tuberculosis bacillus identified.
1855	**1873**	**1874**	**1879**	**1880**	**1881**	**1882**

Vitamin-Deficiency Diseases

Another great advance in treating disease occurred in the early years of the twentieth century with the discovery of the cause for a number of disorders, now known as vitamin-deficiency diseases, which had afflicted humans for centuries. For years physicians had treated pellagra, rickets, and beriberi with lime juice because it seemed to help. After the germ theory of disease was accepted in the nineteenth century, most scientists believed that these diseases were due to bacteria and toxins. But evidence was gradually accumulating that some "accessory substance" to the known nutrients was necessary for health and growth.

In 1912, the experiments of an English biologist left no doubt that there were other elements vital to good nutrition, and Casimir Funk, a Polish biochemist, suggested the name "vitamine." Later, when it was realized that these substances were not amines, the name was changed to vitamin. Vitamin A was the first to actually be identified (1915), followed by vitamin D (1918), and thiamine (vitamin B_1) in 1921. By 1946 all but one of the vitamins that are known today had been identified and synthesized. Cobalamin (B_{12}) was not discovered until 1948 and was synthesized in 1973 (Table 1-1).

The availability of vitamins led to spectacular cures for the deficiency diseases and commercial mass production of vitamins as the public began using them prophylactically, often in much larger quantities than necessary and in some cases (particularly with vitamin A) with dangerous side effects.

Antiviral Vaccines

Although researchers had known since the nineteenth century that there existed disease-causing agents so small that they passed through filters capable of catching bacteria, it was not until the invention of the electron microscope in 1930 that viruses could be seen and studied. In 1955, Jonas Salk introduced a killed-virus vaccine for poliomyelitis, one of the most feared diseases of the time because of its potential for permanent crippling and disability, if not death. Soon after, in 1956, the field test was made for a live-virus vaccine developed by Albert B. Sabin, which was so successful that it is now used most of the time for protection from polio. Vaccines are now available

arsphenamine	ars-FEN-a-mean
isoniazid	i-so-NI-a-zid
laryngoscope	la-RING go-scope
sulfanilamide	sul-fa-NIL a-mide
sulfathiazole	sul-fa-THI a-zol

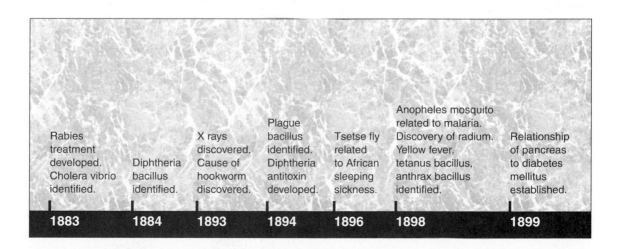

1883	1884	1893	1894	1896	1898	1899
Rabies treatment developed. Cholera vibrio identified.	Diphtheria bacillus identified.	X rays discovered. Cause of hookworm discovered.	Plague bacillus identified. Diphtheria antitoxin developed.	Tsetse fly related to African sleeping sickness.	Anopheles mosquito related to malaria. Discovery of radium. Yellow fever, tetanus bacillus, anthrax bacillus identified.	Relationship of pancreas to diabetes mellitus established.

TABLE 1-1	Discovery, Isolation, and Synthesis of Vitamins		
	Discovery	**Isolation**	**Synthesis**
FAT-SOLUBLE VITAMINS			
Vitamin A	1915	1937	1946
Vitamin D	1918	1930	1936
Vitamin E	1922	1936	1937
Vitamin K	1934	1939	1939
WATER-SOLUBLE VITAMINS			
Thiamine (B_1)	1921	1926	1936
Ascorbic acid (C)	1932	1932	1933
Riboflavin (B_2)	1932	1933	1935
Pantothenic acid	1933	1938	1940
Biotin	—	1935	1942
Pyridoxine (B_6)	1934	1938	1939
Niacin (B_3)	1936	1936	1936
Folacin	1945	1945	1945
Cobalamin (B_{12})	1948	1948	1973

for all of the "childhood" diseases but the greatest challenge for researchers is ahead as AIDS and other emerging diseases present new puzzles for them to solve.

Emerging Infectious Diseases

Throughout the history of disease, new infections have suddenly appeared. Beginning in the latter part of the twentieth century, there was a proliferation of new and reemerging infections coupled with drug-resistant strains of bacteria for diseases that were thought to have been controlled.

Legionnaires' disease was first documented in a 1957 outbreak. The disease had probably been around for some time but not reported because its symptoms could be so mild. However, at an American Legion convention in Philadelphia in 1976, it was the cause of 29 deaths and 182 hospitalizations. Once the disease agent was identified as a bacterium, antibiotics were found to treat it.

It was another story when the first cases of AIDS were reported in 1981. Since then, this devastating infection has been found to be caused by a virus that attacks the core of the body's defense system. More than ten years after the appearance of AIDS there is no known cure for the immune deficiency it causes. Recently, there has been some success in treating the disease with a "cocktail" of drugs that stops the replication of human immunodeficiency virus (HIV). No one knows how long the effect will last. And HIV keeps mutating, causing some scientists to wonder if a vaccine will ever be developed that is safe and effective. New, reemerging, and drug-resistant infectious diseases have appeared all over the world since the early 1970s. Tables 1-2, 1-3 and 1-4 provide information about some of these diseases and factors in their emergence.

A CHANGING FOCUS

While the hope for prevention and control of infectious disease was growing in the twentieth century, a new trend in disease became apparent. Death and suffering from infectious disease were on a downward trend, but the second decade saw a rise in noninfectious disease. By 1930, deaths

TABLE 1-2	Factors in Emergence
Categories	**Specific Examples**
Societal events	Economic impoverishment; war or civil conflict; population growth and migration; urban decay
Health care	New medical devices; organ or tissue transplantation; drugs causing immunosuppression; widespread use of antibiotics
Food production	Globalization of food supplies; changes in food processing and packaging
Human behavior	Sexual behavior; drug use; travel; diet; outdoor recreation; use of child care facilities
Environmental changes	Deforestation/reforestation; changes in water ecosystems; flood/drought; famine; global warming
Public health infrastructure	Curtailment or reduction in prevention programs; inadequate communicable disease surveillance; lack of trained personnel (epidemiologists, laboratory scientists, vector and rodent control specialists)
Microbial adaptation and change	Changes in virulence and toxin production; development of drug resistance; microbes as cofactors in chronic diseases

From CDC. 1994. *Addressing emerging infectious disease threats: A prevention strategy for the United States.* Atlanta, Georgia: U.S. Dept. of Health and Human Services.

from noninfectious disease had surpassed those from infectious disease in the United States and other developed countries.

A number of factors led to this change and, ironically, the ability to prevent and control many infectious diseases was one of them. In countries where people were escaping death from infectious disease, they were living longer and becoming more susceptible to diseases that took a longer life span to emerge. In addition, because most noninfectious diseases do not attack with the dramatic symptoms of infectious diseases, not as much attention was given to their prevention and control until the soaring death rates from heart disease and cancer were evident. In the United States and other developed nations, changing lifestyles and environmental influences were also involved as the accumulation of great wealth, or at least enough for a comfortable living, led to excesses in eating and drinking, a decrease in exercise, and increased physical, mental, and emotional stressors, all now known as factors in the development of noninfectious disease. Table 1-5 indicates the percentage contribution of lifestyle and three other factors to

the ten leading causes of death in the United States.

Although there is much concern over the emerging infectious diseases, projections to the year 2020 by WHO show noncommunicable diseases accounting for seven out of every ten deaths in developing regions. Today these diseases account for less than half these deaths. The age-adjusted death rates for the fifteen leading causes of death in the United States are found in Figure 1-6. As can be seen even with HIV, noninfectious disease is still responsible for causing over half of the fatalities in the United States.

Some scientists believe that the developed nations are pouring too much money into research on AIDS and other infectious diseases and too little into research on noninfectious disease. Even with the emerging diseases, the trend for deaths as a result of infectious disease is still going down worldwide while deaths caused by noninfectious disease are rising. Ways to help people change lifestyles that predispose to heart disease, cancer, and most other noninfectious disease should be at the forefront now so the dire predictions for 2020 will not come true.

TABLE 1-3	Some Emerging Infectious Diseases with Year of Identification, Disease Agent, and Possible Enabling Factors		
Year	**Disease**	**Disease Agent**	**Enabling Factors***
1973	Infantile diarrhea	Rotavirus	Human behavior/day care
1976	Ebola hemorrhagic fever	*Ebola virus*	Environmental change
1976	Acute and chronic diarrhea	*Cryptosporidium parvum*	Human behavior/public health infrastructure
1976	Legionnaires' disease	*Legionella pneumophila*	Public health infrastructure
1982	Toxic shock syndrome	*Staphylococcus aureus*	Human behavior
1982	Hemorrhagic colitis; hemolytic uremic syndrome	*Escherichia coli 0157:H7*	Public health infrastructure
1982	Lyme disease	*Borrelia bergdorferi*	Human behavior
1983	Acquired immune deficiency syndrome	Human immunodeficiency virus	Human behavior
1983	Peptic ulcer disease	*Helicobacter pylori*	Recently recognized
1988	Non-A, non-B hepatitis (enterically transferred)	Hepatitis E	Public health infrastructure
1989	Human ehrlichiosis	*Ehrlichia chafeensis*	Human behavior
1989	Non-A, non-B Hepatitis (parenterally transmitted)	Hepatitis C	Human behavior
1992	Cholera (new strain)	*Vibrio cholerae O139*	Societal events
1993	Adult respiratory distress syndrome	Sin nombre virus (hantavirus)	Societal events

*There are multiple factors involved in the emergence or reemergence of any disease—the ones listed here are some of the most evident.

Note: More information on these diseases will be included in the text in the chapters that deal with them.

Technologic Advances

Frederick Banting and Charles Best succeeded in producing insulin in 1922, and from their discovery came the ability to control diabetes. Cardiac catheterization, open-heart surgery, and replacement of clogged blood vessels were among the first techniques to aid in diagnosis and repair of damaged hearts. New radiologic diagnostic modalities such as computed axial tomography (CAT) scanning, magnetic resonance imaging (MRI), and positive emission tomography (PET) scanning have increased diagnostic potential.

The use of lasers for surgery has made eye surgery and some other surgeries office procedures. New types of anesthetic reduce pain and discomfort of surgery. Some of these advances and others will be mentioned under the disease processes for which they are used, later in the text.

Transplants and Cancer

The ability to transplant hearts, kidneys, and other organs has alleviated suffering and extended life for some, but the progress in fighting the second

TABLE 1-4 Examples of Reemerging Infections in the 1990s and Enabling Factors

Year	Place	Reemerging Infections	Enabling Factors*
1997	Los Angeles County	Plague	Human behavior
1997	Ghana; Australia	Anthrax	Public health infrastructure
1997	Cook Islands; Cuba	Dengue hemorrhagic fever	Demographics; international travel; ineffective control of mosquitos
1996	United States	Cyclosporiasis	Human behavior
1996	Japan; USA; Scotland	*E. coli 0157:H7*	Human behavior
1996	Sierra Leone	Lassa fever	Environmental change
1996	England	Bovine spongiform encephalopathy	Food production
1995	Zaire	Ebola hemorrhagic fever	Environmental
1994	India	Plague	Demographics, behavior
1994–96	Oregon	Meningococcal disease	Microbial evolution; increased travel; crowded living space
1993	Wisconsin	Cryptosporidiosis	Public health infrastructure
1993	United States	Hantavirus	Weather—hot, dry, arid; poor living conditions
1993	Ohio	Pertussis (whooping cough)	Economics—lack of vaccination
1993	Oregon; Washington	*E. coli 0157:H7*	Public health infrastructure
1992	California	Coccidioidomycosis	Climatic, demographics
1992–96	United States	Vancomycin-resistant enterococci infections	Microbial evolution
1993–96	United States	Penicillin-resistant pneumococcal infections	Microbial evolution
1990	New York	Multidrug-resistant tuberculosis	Microbial evolution
1990	Russia	Diphtheria	Human behavior

*There are multiple factors involved in the emergence or reemergence of any disease—the ones listed here are some of the most evident.

Note: More information on these diseases will be included in the text in the chapters that deal with them.

TABLE 1-5 The Importance of Lifestyle in Good Health: Estimated Contribution of Four Factors to Ten Leading Causes of Death (Expressed in Percent)

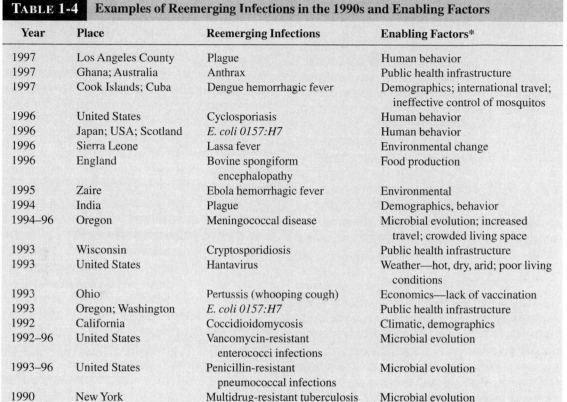

Causes of Death	Factors			
	Lifestyle	Environment	Genetics	Health Care Services
Heart disease	54	9	25	12
Cancer	37	24	29	10
Stroke	50	22	21	7
COPD *=chronic obstructive pulmonary disease*	80	5	6	9
Unintentional injuries	73	18	1	8
Influenza/pneumonia	23	20	39	18
Diabetes	34	0	60	6
AIDS	85	5	5	5
Suicide	60	35	2	3
Liver disease	70	9	18	3
All ten causes	56	15	21	8

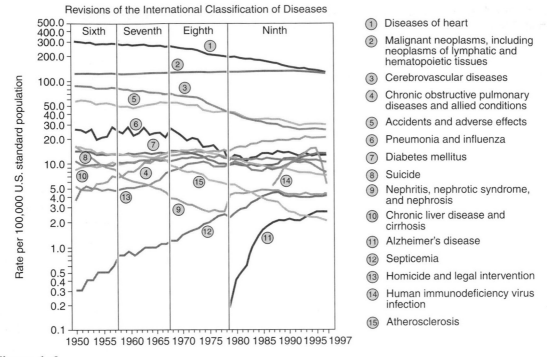

Figure 1-6

Age-adjusted death rates for the fifteen leading causes of death: United States, 1950–97.

leading cause of death, cancer, has been disap-pointing, despite much time, effort, and money spent in seeking answers.

Research is continuing to determine the origin, development, and metabolism of cancer cells, and new information is leading to new possibilities for prevention and treatment of this often fatal disease. The cure rate for cancer has risen from one-third to one-half in the past ten years, but for lung cancer and some others, chances of survival are much less. The Papanicolaou test (Pap smear) for cervical cancer has led to earlier diagnosis and improved survival rates. Chances of surviving breast and colorectal cancer have also improved with earlier detection by the use of mammography and proctoscopy.

For cancer, as for other noninfectious diseases, the greatest hope for prevention seems to lie in changing lifestyles. Elimination of smoking and excesses in drinking and eating, diets that meet the nutritional requirements of the body, exercise on a regular basis, and stress management are all known to be important in sustaining the resistance to disease with which everyone is born.

Disease Prevention and Health Promotion

By the mid-1970s, a new interest in health promotion, not just disease prevention and control, was stirring among the people of the United States and other developed nations. In the United States, reports from task forces, committees, and, finally, the Surgeon General were indicative of the new focus. The Surgeon General's report on health promotion and disease prevention was in two volumes, *Healthy People* (1979) and *Promoting Health, Preventing Disease: Objectives for the Nation* (1980). These objectives were adopted as policy for the nation in 1981. Objectives for 1990 and 2000 were also developed, and now there are objectives for the year 2010 (*Healthy People 2010*). Two worldwide targets were identified: (1) the provision of a safe drinking water supply for everyone and (2) the immunization of all children in the world against major childhood infectious diseases.

Not all of the objectives for 2000 were met, nor is it probable that all of the 467 objectives for 2010 will be met. Yet progress has been made, and it is hoped that all nations and peoples will at least be able to have safe drinking water and immunizations for their children by 2010.

Scientists and physicians have achieved much in helping us survive the attacks of invading microorganisms by repairing the damage done by disease processes and easing pain and suffering. However, many diseases have regressed and even disappeared without medical intervention.

McKeown has stated, "We can attribute the modern improvement in health to food, hygiene and medical intervention in that order of time and importance—but we must recognize that it is to a modification of behavior that we owe the permanence of this improvement."[*]

If we are to succeed in preventing and controlling disease in the twenty-first century, all men, women, and children will have to accept the responsibility for their own health and pursue lifestyles that will enable them to present the strongest possible resistance to disease. Scientists and physicians can show us the way, but only individuals can choose which behaviors they will follow.

*Philip R. Lee and Carroll L. Estes, *The Nation's Health* (Boston: Jones and Bartlett Publishers, 1990), 11.

SUMMARY

From ancient times there has been evidence of devastation of human life by disease. Although a few treatments used by early physicians are still used, no real progress was made against infectious disease until the late seventeenth century. Then the newly discovered microscope opened up new worlds of swarming microorganisms to scientists and physicians, and in the late eighteenth century Jenner discovered the vaccination for smallpox. These two milestone discoveries opened the way for an avalanche of identification of diseases and disease agents in the nineteenth century. With the discovery of penicillin and other "wonder drugs" in the twentieth century, more progress was made in the control of infectious disease.

Attention turned to the control of noninfectious disease. Although advances were made in understanding the human body, an intensive effort to deal with cardiovascular disease, cancer, diabetes, and other life-threatening noninfectious diseases did not begin in earnest until the late nineteenth and early twentieth centuries when the leading cause of fatal disease changed from infectious agents to noninfectious origins. The recognition of the effect of lifestyle upon the development of noninfectious diseases brought about a new focus for the twentieth century and the years beyond. But the microbes with whom we share the planet once again became the focus of attention as new diseases emerged, old diseases returned, and the organisms developed resistance to antibiotics. The emergence of new, devastatingly destructive, and frequently fatal infectious diseases including AIDS and Ebola fever and new strains of antibiotic-resistant bacteria for tuberculosis and other diseases reminded all those involved in the struggle that success in preventing and controlling disease is an elusive goal, not soon to be achieved.

QUESTIONS FOR REVIEW

1. Starting with the Egyptians, what have been the highlights in disease prevention and control?

2. What different theories have been held concerning the cause of disease from early times to the present?

3. What prescriptions used by Chinese doctors in early times are still used?

4. What kind of measures were taken to guard the health of the community in early times?

5. Why were Galen's writings on anatomy flawed, and why was he believed?

6. How were the ideas about disease affected in the Middle Ages?

7. How are the terms *pandemic* and *hajj* connected in discussions about disease?

8. Where and when in history were the Black Death and pulmonary anthrax connected?

9. What developments in the seventeenth century led to an acceleration in the knowledge of disease in the nineteenth century?

10. How did Vesalius, da Vinci, and Fracastoro contribute to advances in medicine during the Renaissance?

11. What individuals are thought to be responsible for the arrival of syphilis in Europe?

12. What were some of Thomas Sydenham's accomplishments?

13. What eighteenth-century event led to the eradication of smallpox in the twentieth century?

14. What contributions were made by Bernard, Pasteur, and Lister in the nineteenth century?

15. What report was Edwin Chadwick responsible for?

16. Who was Lemuel Shattuck, and how was he important in the prevention and control of disease?

17. What new diagnostic tools were used in the nineteenth century?

18. What are Koch's postulates?

19. What important advances in the knowledge of disease were made in the nineteenth century?

20. When did chemotherapy begin, and what was one of the most dramatic discoveries in the field?

21. When were vitamins discovered? Why was this important?

22. What twentieth-century invention led to the vaccines for polio?

23. What newly discovered infectious diseases caused death in the twentieth century?

24. What change in focus concerning disease occurred in the 1970s? Why?

25. What new technologies and techniques are used to diagnose, treat, and control disease today?

FURTHER READING

Bartlett, John G., M.D. 1997. Infectious diseases. *Journal of the American Medical Association* 277:1865.

Bockler, Donald. 1998. Let's play doctor: medical rounds in ancient Greece. *The American Biology Teacher* 60:106.

Carmichael, Ann G. 1991. Contagion theory and contagion practice in fifteenth-century Milan. *Renaissance Quarterly* 44:213.

Chaiken, Miriam S. 1998. Primary health care initiatives in colonial Kenya. *World Development* 26:170.

Cole, Thomas B. 1996. Eighteenth century medical institution renews its educational and scientific mission. *The Journal of the American Medical Association* 276:9.

Dalen, James F. 2000. A second century for the archives of internal medicine. *Archives of Internal Medicine* 160:5.

Dawbarn, Frances. 1998. Learned physicians, medical heterodoxy and court patronage: conflict in early modern England. *Endeavor* 22:98.

Dobson, Andrew P. and E. Robin Carper. 1996. Infectious diseases and human population history: Throughout history the establishment of disease has been a side effect of the growth of civilization. *BioScience* 46:115.

Etiology of malaria. *The Journal of the American Medical Association.* 282:1312b, 1999.

Kiple, Kenneth E., and Virginia H. Kiple. 1977. Black tongue and black men: pellagra and slavery in the antebellum South. *The Journal of Southern History* 43:411.

Lorber, B. 1996. Are all diseases infectious? *Annals of Internal Medicine* 125:844.

Maddocks, Ian. 1999. Medicine and palliative care. *The Medical Journal of Australia* 171:63.

Martensen, Robert L. 1997. Medicine, surgery, and gastric cancer in 1900: debating when to go 'radical.' *The Journal of the American Medical Association* 277:1495.

Martensen, Robert L., and David S. Jones. 1997. Searching for medical certainty: medical chemistry to molecular medicine. *The Journal of the American Medical Association* 278:609.

Moberg, Carol L. 1999. Rene Dubos, a harbinger of microbial resistance to antibodies. *Perspective in Biology and Medicine* 42:559.

Numbers, Ronald L. 1982. The history of American medicine: a field in ferment. *Reviews in American History* 10:245.

Pound, Pandora, et al. 1997. From apoplexy to stroke. *Age and Aging* 26:331.

Powers, Ramon S., and Gene Younger. 1975. Cholera and the army in the west: treatment and control in 1866 and 1867. *Military Affairs* 39:49.

Progress in medical knowledge is never straightforward. *The Lancet.* 353:1279, 1999.

Riley, James C. 1986. Insects and the European mortality decline. *The American Historical Review* 91:833.

Shattuck, Lemuel, et al. 1850. *Report of the Sanitary Commission of Massachusetts.* Cambridge, Mass: Harvard University Press (originally published by Dutton and Wentworth in 1850).

Shortridge, Kennedy F. 1999. The 1918 `Spanish' flu: pearls from swine? *Nature Medicine* 5:384.

Smith, C.E. 1982. The Broad Street pump revisited. *International Journal of Epidemiology* 11:99.

Snow, J. 1936. On the mode of communication of cholera. In *Snow on cholera.* New York: The Commonwealth Fund.

Stanton, Judith Anne. 1999. Aesculapius: a modern tale. *The Journal of the American Medical Association* 281:476.

Straus, Robert. 1999. Medical sociology: a personal fifty-year perspective. *The Journal of Health and Social Behavior* 40:103.

Sturdy, Steve, and Roger Cooter. 1998. Science, scientific management, and the transformation of medicine in Britain c.1870–1950. *History of Science* 36:421.

Tipton, Charles M. 1997. Sports medicine: a century of progress. *The Journal of Nutrition* 127:878.

Waitzkin, Howard. 1998. Is our work dangerous? *The Journal of Health and Social Behavior* 39:7.

DID YOU KNOW?

Beginning of School and Community Health Education

In 1842, eight years before Lemuel Shattuck made his report, Horace Mann advocated health education in the schools. With Shattuck's report the value of health education for adequate human functioning was reemphasized. In a way, health education had been present since the time when a mother cleaned her children after they played in the mud or a father restricted play in favor of a good night's sleep. But formalized health education in the schools developed only bit by bit after Shattuck's report.

In 1872, the first medical inspector was employed by the New York Board of Education to control the smallpox epidemic. In 1875, because of the influence of the Women's Christian Temperance Union, thirty-eight states passed legislation requiring alcohol education in the schools. From that time until the present, state after state has passed requirements for health education. Slowly but surely, it has been recognized that a comprehensive health education program is needed in the schools.

Shattuck's report had its greatest effect on the development of official community health agencies in the United States. Sadly, Lemuel Shattuck (1793–1859) did not live to see the results of his efforts, for it was 1869 before a state board of health was established in Massachusetts, exactly as Shattuck had recommended in 1842. Today there are official public health agencies on four levels, local, state, national, and international. These health agencies provide health care services for mothers and children who would otherwise have none. They provide (infectious and noninfectious) disease control and medical rehabilitation services. They are also active in educating the public and provide environmental and mental health services.

2

PRINCIPLES OF DISEASE OCCURRENCE

O B J E C T I V E S

1. *Name and explain four theories of disease causation.*
2. *Explain the classic* epidemiologic *model of disease causation.*
3. *Discuss the foundations of epidemiology.*
4. *Describe the disease agents for infectious and noninfectious disease.*
5. *Discuss diseases and symptoms caused by deficiency and excess of nutrients.*
6. *Explain how host resistance may be increased or decreased.*
7. *Identify biologic, physical, and social factors in the environment that influence the occurrence of disease.*
8. *State the significance of the chain of infection.*
9. *Discuss disease transmission.*
10. *List occurrences during the five stages of disease.*

THEORIES OF DISEASE CAUSATION

In Chapter 1, various ideas about the cause of disease were mentioned. The oldest theory of causation, dating from prehistoric times, holds that evil spirits or supernatural beings are responsible for disease. *The sick were thought to be possessed by demons.* The isolation of lepers (based on biblical teachings) led to a decrease in leprosy, and the practice of quarantine arose, based on the idea that isolation might be effective against other diseases also. This second theory of causation, the theory of contagion, soon gained acceptance. Hippocrates introduced the idea of a natural rather than supernatural explanation for disease occurrence in the fourth century B.C., and the humoral theory of disease, but it took hundreds of years for people to recognize that some diseases were contagious and could be transmitted from person to person as well as in other ways. It took even more time to identify the disease agents that were being transmitted.

The development of the third theory of disease causation, the germ theory (explained in Chapter 1) in the 1860s and 1870s, marked the beginning of the conquest of infectious diseases. The germ theory of disease causation was accepted for many years and brought great progress in the understanding of disease, but as infectious disease began to decline and noninfectious diseases began to increase, it became evident that the idea of one cause for one disease did not answer such questions as: Why is it that some people who are exposed to a disease do not get sick? and, How can we carry disease agents on our skin and in our body without getting sick? It was also recognized that more than one factor was responsible for the development of each noninfectious disease. Thus, to explain disease occurrence in both infectious and noninfectious diseases, epidemiologists (those who study the occurrence of disease in populations) developed the modern theory of multiple causation. In this theory, the definition of disease agent is expanded to denote any factor that needs to be present (or absent) for disease to occur. A model of the disease theory of multiple-causation can be seen in Box 2-1.

FOUNDATIONS OF EPIDEMIOLOGY

The more extensive a man's knowledge of what has been done, the greater will be his power to do it.

Benjamin Disraeli

Over 2000 years ago Hippocrates (460–377 B.C.) tried to find the cause of sickness and death in his patients. The "Father of Medicine" is also considered to be the first epidemiologist because he recorded his observations about the spread of disease in populations. Since that time, many scientists including Fracastoro, Kircher, van Leeuwenhoek, and others have contributed their efforts and research regarding the cause of disease

to the fledgling science. As understanding of disease and the identification of disease agents grew, so did the science of epidemiology, until today, the "disease detectives" are the first to be summoned when an outbreak of disease occurs with an unknown cause.

Epidemiologists seek to discover the cause of a disease, establish patterns of disease occurrence, and recommend measures so that diseases can be prevented, controlled, and/or eliminated. They deal with disease all over the world whether it is endemic, epidemic, or pandemic. *Endemic* refers to the constant presence of a disease in a population. An *epidemic* is defined as an outbreak of one specific disease in excess of what would normally be expected, and a *pandemic* is an epidemic that is widespread over a country, continent, or worldwide. AIDS is pandemic.

TERMINOLOGY TO DESCRIBE DISEASE OCCURRENCE

It is not possible in a text on infectious and noninfectious disease to include all epidemiologic and public health concepts. However, for better understanding of the material in this text, a few of the terms that are commonly used to describe disease occurrence will be identified.

Rates of Disease Occurrence

Two terms that have a special meaning for epidemiologists and others dealing with disease are *prevalence rate* and *incidence rate.* Prevalence rate indicates the number of cases of a particular disease in a community at a specified time. It is determined by dividing the number of existing cases by the total population under study. The resulting figure is then multiplied by a power of 10. For prevalence and incidence rates, this number is usually 1000. The formula for prevalence rates follows.

---

epidemiologic ep-i-dee-mee OL-o-jic

BOX 2-1

An Epidemiologic Model of Disease with Examples of Disease Agents, Host, and Environmental Factors

DISEASE AGENTS (CAUSATIVE FACTORS)	HOST (INTRINSIC FACTORS)	ENVIRONMENT (EXTRINSIC FACTORS)
Infectious Agents	**Age**	**Physical Environment**
		Climate
Nutrition	**Sex**	Geology
Excesses		
Deficiencies	**Race**	**Biologic Environment**
		Population
Chemical Agents	**Genetic**	Density
Poisons		Flora
Drugs	**Physiologic State**	Food Sources
Allergens	Inactivity	Fauna
Ragweed	Fatigue	Arthropod vectors
Antibiotics	Pregnancy	Food sources
	Nutrition	Sanitary measures
Physical Agents	Stress	
Ionizing Radiation	Drug use	**Socioeconomic Environment**
		Tensions, pressures, crowding
Sedentary Living	**Immunity**	Occupation
	Passive	Exposure to chemicals
	Active	Urbanization and economic
		development
	Preexisting Disease	Disruptions
		Wars, natural disasters
	Human Behavior	
	Personal hygiene	
	Food handling	
	Diet	
	Occupation	
	Use of health resources	
	Recreation	
	Interpersonal contact	

Prevalence

$$= \frac{\text{Number of cases of disease present in the population at a specified time}}{\text{Number of persons in population at that specified time}}$$
$$\times 1000$$

EXAMPLE: In a college with 2569 students, 18 missed classes on October 1 because of influenza. These students did not all become ill at the same time, but all were ill on the day in question.

$$\frac{18 \text{ (existing cases)}}{2569 \text{ (total school population)}}$$

$$= .0070 \times 1000 = 7.0$$

The prevalence rate for influenza at this college on October 1 was 7.0 (per thousand students).

Incidence rate is the number of *new* cases occurring during a specific time. It is determined by dividing the number of new cases of a disease at a specific time by the population at risk. The formula for incidence rate is:

$$\frac{\text{Number of new cases}}{\text{during a specified time}} \times 1000$$
$$\frac{}{\text{Population at risk}} \times 1000$$
for the disease

EXAMPLE: If we return to the same college and find that 8 of the flu cases actually began on October 1, then the incidence for October 1 would be 3.0. (per thousand students)

$$\frac{8 \text{ (new cases)}}{2569 \text{ (population at risk)}} = .003 \times 1000 = 3.0$$

Prevalence rate and incidence rate are other ways to talk about how widespread an illness is. In other words, incidence rate tells us how many new cases occurred at a given time. Prevalence rate tells us the ongoing level of disease in a population at a given time. The formulas are used to get away from having to deal with decimals (which we would have if simple percentages were used) when writing and talking about disease trends.

Levels of Prevention

The prevention of disease can be described in three levels. *Primary prevention* refers to measures taken before the disease occurs to reduce susceptibility. Vaccinations are an example of primary prevention. *Secondary prevention* refers to measures taken to diagnose a disease that is already present. The Pap smear for cervical cancer is an example of secondary prevention. **Tertiary** *prevention* involves all the measures taken to return the individual to a "normal" state of health or to keep the person alive. Physical therapy for polio victims is a type of tertiary prevention. This text will be concerned mostly with primary and secondary prevention.

EPIDEMIOLOGIC THEORY OF DISEASE OCCURRENCE

Classic epidemiologic theory states that whether anyone gets a disease depends on the relationship among three factors: the *disease agent*, the *host*, and the *environment*. This model was developed for infectious disease, but it also fits noninfectious disease, as can be seen in Box 2-1.

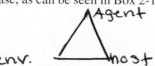

Although a disease agent is necessary for disease to occur, a disease agent can also be present without the occurrence of disease. Many pathogenic organisms are present on and in our bodies all the time, but if the three elements (of the epidemiologic model) are in equilibrium, that is, if the disease agent is not too virulent (powerful), if the resistance of the host is strong, and if the environment is favorable to the host, then the disease agent will not be able to cause an infection (disease), and the host will remain well. But if the disease agent becomes more virulent and/or the resistance of the host is lowered and/or the environment is unfavorable, then the host may become sick.

A vivid example of this process is found in the infection of many people with HIV, which is responsible for AIDS. A person can be infected with HIV for months or years before any symptoms of AIDS occur.

DISEASE AGENTS FOR INFECTIOUS DISEASES

The disease agents for infectious diseases are pathogenic organisms (*Table 2-1*) and range in size from the submicroscopic virus, composed simply of nucleic acid, to the metazoa, which are complex and sometimes grow very large, for example, intestinal worms. Pathogenic organisms can be divided into the following broad categories.

Viruses

The smallest of the disease-causing organisms are viruses. These minute particles could not be detected until the early 1930s, when the electron microscope was first used. Viruses are composed of nucleic acids and protein. They are made up of **deoxyribonucleic** acid (DNA) or ribonucleic acid (RNA) but not both. They are not technically alive by themselves but are able to penetrate cells and

---

tertiary TER-she-ar-e
deoxyribonucleic dee-oksa-ribo-nu-KLA-ik

TABLE 2-1	Pathogens and Common Communicable Diseases		
	Pathogen	**Description**	**Representative Diseases**
DNA	Viruses	Smallest common pathogens; nonliving particles of DNA surrounded by a protein coat. Require a host's living cells for growth and replication.	Red measles, mumps, chickenpox, rubella, influenza, warts, colds, oral and genital herpes, shingles, AIDS, genital warts, pneumonia
Bacilli / Cocci / Spirilla / Rickettsia	Bacteria	One-celled microorganisms with sturdy, well-defined cell walls; three distinctive forms are: spherical (cocci), rod-shaped (bacilli), and spiral-shaped (spirilla). Rickettsia: Require a host's living cells for growth and replication—otherwise, like bacteria	Tetanus, strep throat, gonorrhea, syphilis, chlamydia, toxic shock syndrome, Legionnaires' disease, meningitis, food poisoning, pneumonia Rocky Mountain spotted fever, Rickettsial pox, typhus
Mold / Yeast	Fungi	Plantlike microorganisms; molds and yeasts	Athlete's foot, ringworm, histoplasmosis, candidiasis, coccidioidomycoses, pneumonia
Amoeba	Protozoa	Simplest animal form; generally one-celled organisms	Malaria, amebic dysentery, trichomoniasis, vaginitis, pneumonia (pneumocystis carinii)
Parasitic worms	Parasitic worms (Metazoa)	Multicellular organisms; represented by tapeworms, leeches, pin worms, and round worms	Effects include: abdominal pain, anemia, lymphatic vessel blockage, lowered antibody response, respiratory and circulatory complications

use the cell's nucleic acid to produce more viruses. This process may take place without any change in cell structure or function. The virus may just borrow part of the cell's machinery to synthesize new viruses without disturbing the cell.

A human-virus peaceful coexistence may continue indefinitely. Thus the host is *infected* with the virus but does not have a *disease*. At some later time, an outside factor such as inactivity, poor nutrition, stress, hormonal imbalance, or bacterial or other infection may activate the virus so that it takes over all of the cell's machinery and rapidly produces more viruses. These viruses may burst out of the cell, destroying it, or the cell may simply degenerate until it can no longer function and the viruses are released as the cell dies. Then viral *disease* is present. *Viral infection* is much more common than *viral disease* (Figure 2-1).

DID YOU KNOW?

The scientific community is now investigating another type of pathogenic agent and an American, Dr. Stanley B. Prusiner, has won a Nobel prize for discovering this "new genre of disease-causing agents." This agent is a **prion.** Although prions are known to be a factor in animal diseases (including mad cow disease or spongiform encephalopathy), they are abnormally folded protein and not thought to be transmissible to humans because they have no DNA or RNA to enable them to reproduce. In March of 1996, headlines all over the world announced a "new variant" of Creutzfeldt-Jacob disease (a rare fatal disease of the nervous system), which is thought to have resulted from the ingestion of bovine **spongiform encephalopathy** prions. Controversies have broken out among researchers who are trying to explain if and how prions can transmit disease. Some believe that a yet undiscovered pathogen may accompany the prion in causing disease.

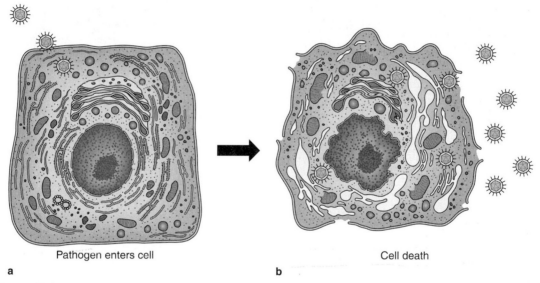

Pathogen enters cell   Cell death

a   b

Figure 2-1

A, A virus invading a body cell. It may coexist with the cell for an indefinite time until it is "triggered" by some outside factor, takes over the cell's machinery, and reproduces. **B,** At some point, the cell becomes engorged and the newly made viruses break out, causing cell death.

Bacteria

Bacteria are single-celled, plantlike organisms that are abundant in our environment—internal and external. Most bacteria are harmless and some beneficial, but we are concerned with those that are capable of causing disease. Although disease-causing bacteria are in the minority, there are still many different kinds that secrete toxins or enzymes that destroy cells or interfere with their function, thus causing disease in the human body.

There are three common groups of bacteria: rod-shaped or *bacilli,* round or *cocci,* and spiral or *spirilla.* For example, tuberculosis is caused by a bacillus, pneumonia by a coccus, and syphilis by a spirillum (see Table 2-1). Many bacteria and other pathogens "live" on the skin and in the intestinal

prion PREE-on
spongiform encephalopathy SPUN-ji-form en-sef-a-LOP-a-thee

TABLE 2-2	Some Pathogenic Inhabitants (Normal Flora) of the Human Body	
Pathogen	**Location**	**Common Diseases**
Staphylococci (*S. aureus, S. epidermidis*)	Skin, nose, mouth, throat, vagina	Impetigo, boils, toxic shock syndrome (TSS), pneumonia, endocarditis, osteomyelitis
Streptococci (*S. pyogenes*)	Mouth, throat, urethra, vagina	Strep, sore throat, tonsillitis, scarlet fever, meningitis, pneumonia
Cornybacteria	Skin, conjunctiva, nose, throat	Diphtheria, conjunctivitis (pink eye)
Enterococci	Skin, genital tract, gastro-intestinal tract	Endocarditis, septicemia
E. coli	Skin, intestines (adults)	Food poisoning, diarrhea, pneumonia
Fungi	Skin, mouth, nose, throat, large intestine, vagina	Tinea: capitis, cruris, corporis, pedis, ungium; candidiasis: vulvovaginitis, thrush
Spirochetes	Mouth, genital tract	Syphilis
Protozoa	Genital tract, intestines	Trichomoniasis, giardiasis, toxoplasmosis, amebiasis

tract of humans (Table 2-2). They do so benignly unless something reduces the immune response of the host or their ecosystem is disrupted.

Rickettsiae

Rickettsiae are now considered to be small bacteria, although, like viruses, they are intracellular parasites (see Table 2-1). Rickettsiae are more like bacteria than like viruses, but with one exception: they are always transported by insects and other **arthropod vectors.** In the United States, Rocky Mountain spotted fever is the most common rickettsial disease.

Fungi

Mushrooms, antibiotics, and ringworm of the scalp, groin, and feet all owe their existence to single-celled or multicelled plantlike organisms referred to as fungi (see Table 2-1). These organisms release enzymes that digest cells. Because of their constant presence in the air, they may find a favorable climate for reproduction on food or any-

where that there is high humidity, warmth, and oxygen supply (such as between human toes not adequately dried after a shower). The use of antibiotics, which destroy some of the friendly bacteria that normally restrain fungal growth, has caused an increase in fungal infections.

Protozoa

These microscopic single-celled parasitic animals are responsible for some of the most important diseases of humanity. They are common in temperate and tropical climates. Like bacteria, protozoa release toxins and enzymes that destroy cells or interfere with their functions. Malaria, amebic dysentery, and African sleeping sickness are all caused by protozoa.

Metazoa

Metazoa are multicellular parasitic animals (worms) that can be divided into three categories: tapeworms, roundworms, and flukes. They can infest any compartment in the body and can travel across various tissue barriers from organ to bloodstream and to another organ. They will lodge in various parts of the body and may block the digestive tract, blood, and lymph vessels as they compete for the body's food. Three diseases caused by metazoa are pinworm, trichinosis, and tapeworm.

DISEASE AGENTS FOR NONINFECTIOUS DISEASE

The disease agents for noninfectious disease can be placed in the following categories.

Nutrients—Deficiency and Excess

When we think of diseases related to nutrition, we usually think of deficiency diseases. However, some of the factors that have been identified as risks for noninfectious disease are due to an excess of nutrients. Table 2-3 summarizes the importance and the results of deficiency and excess for the major nutrients. For instance, scurvy is a vitamin-deficiency disease caused by insufficient vitamin C and a deficiency of protein and has been identified as the cause of **kwashiorkor,** a disease prevalent in children in third-world nations. On the other hand, too much sodium may be an agent of high blood pressure for some, whereas high fat intake has been implicated in heart disease and some cancer. Malnutrition also lowers resistance to infectious disease. Examination of Table 2-3 will help you to understand the significance of ingesting either too much or too little of any one nutrient.

Other Chemical Substances

The nutrients are all made of chemicals, chemicals that the body needs for survival. Alcohol, the chemicals in cigarette smoke, and illicit drugs are not necessary for survival. They alter body processes in unnatural ways and in doing so produce conditions that may lead to disease and disorders. Alcoholism not only predisposes the body to noninfectious diseases such as cirrhosis of the liver but also lowers resistance to infectious dis-

ease. Other **exogenous** chemicals can also produce disease. And there are **endogenous** chemicals, chemicals within our own bodies, that cause noninfectious disease.

The agents for alcoholism, tobacco addiction, or addiction to marijuana, cocaine, and other illicit drugs are easily identified. It is not always easy to track down the agent for illness that is produced by something in the environment. A number of substances are known to be disease agents. A few of the most common are lead, particularly in old paint, radon gas in our homes, asbestos in schools and other buildings, and sulfur dioxide in the air. We are just beginning to recognize how dangerous many of the chemicals in our environment are and to take measures to eliminate the danger.

Just as with nutritional deficiencies or excesses, a deficiency or excess of a normal body product can lead to disease. Everyone is familiar with the difference that steroids can make in the structure of the human body from the use of them by athletes. When the body secretes too much growth hormone, disorders such as *giantism* in children and **acromegaly** (parts of the body resume growth and become greatly enlarged) in adults appear. Too little of the same hormone in childhood leads to *dwarfism* (Figure 2-2). A form of arthritis, *gout,* is caused by excess secretion of uric acid. In fact the most prevalent theory concerning rheumatoid arthritis is an unnecessary secretion (excess) of body chemicals that attack the joint. Many other chronic diseases and disorders can be traced to endogenous factors such as these.

Heredity

As has been stated before, scientific research is identifying more and more disease states that are "in the genes." Genetic research is proceeding at

rickettsiae	ri-KET-see-i
kwashiorkor	kwash-i-OR-kor
exogenous	eks-OJ-e-nus
endogenous	en-DOJ-e-nus
acromegaly	ak-ro-MEG-a-lee

TABLE 2-3	Diseases and Symptoms of Nutrient Deficiency or Excess		
		Disease and/or Symptoms Caused by	
Nutrient	**Importance**	**Deficiency**	**Excess**
CARBOHYDRATES			
Sugar and starch	Quick energy source	None	Obesity, dental caries
Fiber	Protects against appendicitis, hemorrhoids, diverticulosis, colon cancer; Aids control of blood lipids, diabetes II, weight	May be a factor in the development of appendicitis, hemorrhoids, diverticulosis, colon cancer	Limits absorption of minerals and may limit absorption of vitamins
FAT	Energy supply; protection of body organs; helps maintain structure and health of cells	Eczema, skin disorders, retarded growth	Contributes to obesity, diabetes, cancer, hypertension, atherosclerosis
PROTEIN	Growth and development; formation of hormones; enzymes; antibodies; maintains acid-alkali balance; source of heat and energy	Kwashiorkor Marasmas Fatigue; loss of appetite; diarrhea; vomiting; stunted growth; edema	Difficulty in maintaining ideal weight; possible hypertrophy of liver and kidneys; contributes to obesity
WATER-SOLUBLE VITAMINS			
Thiamine (B_1)	Aids in energy metabolism; supports normal appetite and nervous system function	Beriberi Symptoms include edema; abnormal heart rhythms; painful calf muscles; mental confusion	Rapid pulse; weakness; headaches; insomnia; irritability
Riboflavin (B_2)	Energy metabolism; supports normal vision and normal skin	Ariboflavinosis symptoms: cracks at comers of mouth; magenta tongue	Interferes with anticancer medication
Niacin (B_3)	Energy metabolism; supports health of skin, nervous system, and digestive system	Pellagra Symptoms include diarrhea, irritability, loss of appetite, weakness, mental confusion progressing to psychosis; dermatitis	Symptoms include diarrhea, nausea, vomiting; skin flush and rash; abnormal liver function; low blood pressure

TABLE 2-3	*Continued*		

		Disease and/or Symptoms Caused by	
Nutrient	Importance	Deficiency	Excess

WATER-SOLUBLE VITAMINS—CONT'D

Nutrient	Importance	Deficiency	Excess
B_6	Aid in amino acid and fatty acid metabolism; helps convert tryptophan to niacin; helps to make red blood cells	Symptoms include anemia, cracked corners of mouth, irritability, muscle twitching, dermatitis, kidney stones	Symptoms include bloating, headaches, fatigue, depression; damage to nerves leading to loss of reflexes and sensation; difficulty walking
Folic Acid	Used in new cell synthesis	Symptoms include anemia; heartburn; diarrhea; constipation; suppression of immune system; frequent infections; mental confusion; faint; fatigue; smooth, red tongue	Symptoms include: diarrhea, insomnia, irritability, masking of vitamin B_6 deficiency symptoms
B_{12}	Used in new cell synthesis; helps maintain nerve cells	Pernicious anemia Symptoms include smooth tongue; fatigue; degeneration of peripheral nerves, progressing to paralysis; hypersensitivity of the skin	None known
Biotin	Energy metabolism, fat synthesis, amino acid metabolism, and glycogen	Abnormal heart action, loss of appetite, nausea, depression, muscle pain, weakness, fatigue; drying, scaly dermatitis	None known
Pantothenic acid	Energy metabolism	Vomiting, intestinal distress, insomnia, fatigue	Occasional diarrhea, possible water retention
C	Collagen synthesis, antioxidant, thyroxin synthesis, amino acid metabolism; strengthens resistance to infection; helps in absorption of iron	Scurvy Symptoms include anemia, atherosclerotic plaques, pinpoint hemorrhages, depression, frequent infections, bleeding gums, loosened teeth, muscle and joint pain, failure of wounds to heal	Symptoms include nausea, abdominal cramps, diarrhea, headache, insomnia, fatigue, hot flashes, rashes, kidney stones

TABLE 2-3	*Continued*		
		Disease and/or Symptoms caused by	
Nutrient	**Importance**	**Deficiency**	**Excess**
FAT-SOLUBLE VITAMINS			
A	Vision; epithelial cells, mucous membranes, skin; bone and tooth growth; reproduction; hormone synthesis and regulation; cancer protection	Hypovitaminosis A Deficiency of vitamin A causes disorders in almost every organ system in the body. A few of them are night blindness; rough, dry scaly skin; increased susceptibility to infections; frequent fatigue; loss of smell and appetite; anemia; vomiting; abdominal pain; jaundice; and enlargement of liver and spleen	Hypervitaminosis A An excess of vitamin A produces symptoms in all the body systems that are affected by a deficiency. If excessive amounts continue to be ingested, death can occur
D	Improves absorption and utilization of calcium and phosphorus required for bone formation	Rickets Osteomalacia Symptoms include misshapen bones and teeth, retarded growth	Hypervitaminosis D Symptoms include loss of appetite, headache, weakness, fatigue, irritability, kidney stones, irreversible renal damage; death can occur
E	Antioxident stabilization of cell membranes, regulation of oxidation reactions	Anemia, weakness, difficulty in walking; severe muscular wasting; fibrocystic breast disease	Headache, dizziness, fatigue; visual problems; digestive discomfort
K	Synthesis of blood-clotting proteins and a blood protein that regulates blood calcium	Hemorrhaging	Possible jaundice
MAJOR MINERALS			
Sodium	Maintains normal extra-cellular fluid balance and acid-base balance; aids in nerve impulse transmission	Muscle cramps, mental apathy, loss of appetite	Hypertension
Chloride	Maintains fluid and acid-base balance; aids in digestion	Muscle cramps, mental apathy, loss of appetite, lack of growth in children	Vomiting, muscular weakness

TABLE 2-3	*Continued*		

		Disease and/or Symptoms caused by	
Nutrient	**Importance**	**Deficiency**	**Excess**
MAJOR MINERALS—CONT'D			
Potassium	Assists in many reactions, including the making of protein; cell integrity; transmission of nerve impulses; contraction of muscles, including heart	Muscular weakness, paralysis, confusion	Vomiting, muscular weakness
Calcium	Principal mineral of bones and teeth; normal muscle contraction and relaxation, including heart muscle; nerve function, blood clotting; blood pressure; immune defenses	Osteoporosis, stunted growth in children	None (Excess calcium is excreted)
Phosphorus	Part of bones, teeth, and cells; necessary in genetic material, energy transfer, and maintenance of acid-base balance	Unknown	May draw calcium out of body
Magnesium	Necessary for bones, building of protein, enzyme action, muscular contraction, transmission of nerve impulses, and teeth	Symptoms include depressed hormone secretion from pancreas, weakness, confusion	Unknown
Sulfur	Necessary for protein structure, part of biotin, thiamine, and insulin; aids in body's detoxification process	Unknown	Depressed growth

an accelerated pace, with new findings published almost weekly. A gene or combination of genes is known to be responsible for some diseases such as cystic fibrosis or sickle cell anemia, whereas the absence or addition of a chromosome is the agent for others, such as Down syndrome. Heredity also affects the host's resistance to disease and will be discussed later in the chapter.

Psychosomatic Factors

To many people, even some doctors, the term *psychosomatic* means an imaginary illness. This is a false impression, because by definition, *psychosomatic* means a disease or disorder influenced or caused by a person's mind. People who have imaginary illnesses are correctly referred to as

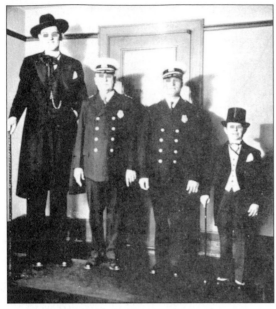

Figure 2-2
This photograph shows the effects of an excess of growth hormone (left) and a deficiency in growth hormone (right) compared with individuals of average stature.

hypochondriacs. Individuals who have a psychosomatic illness have an actual physiological disease or disorder that can be diagnosed by tests, and their mind has played a critical role in the occurrence of the disease. Studies have demonstrated that mental and emotional *stress* can depress the immune system. And some research has indicated that learning to manage stress can be effective in increasing resistance to disease. Evidence continues to accumulate from research and clinical observations of the ability of the mind not only to cause disease but even to assist in, or actually bring about, a cure.

It has long been known that some individuals can learn to control their blood pressure and heartbeat through a technique called *biofeedback,* which trains them to control *autonomic* processes. There are even indications that by certain thought processes we can enhance our immune response.

Evidence of success in this area has increased to the degree that a new field of specialization, **psychoneuroimmunology,** has emerged. All doctors have witnessed the difference that attitude and outlook can have on a patient's response to treatment. And most would agree that learning to manage stress, physical as well as mental, and a positive attitude, can increase the chances of prevention of, and recovery from, many diseases.

Physical Forces

Some of the most common physical forces that act as agents of disease or disorder are mechanical forces, high or low temperatures, and radiation. The best example of a disease caused by mechanical force is **osteomyelitis,** an acute inflammation of bone and bone marrow resulting from pathogenic organisms but occurring at the site of traumatic injury. Most of us have experienced the effects of high temperature by burning ourselves. Burns may be minor or life threatening, depending on their degree of severity. Low temperatures can lead to frostbite and possible loss of fingers or toes. *Hypothermia* (significant loss of body heat) has been the cause of death for older individuals who cannot afford to heat their homes in winter and for those who have no homes.

A physical force that has been the cause of great concern in the years since the development of atomic power is *radiation*. We know that the ultraviolet rays of the sun can be **carcinogenic,** as can X rays used in diagnosis of illness. The ability to control radiation has led to the ability to diagnose and, in the case of cancer, treat disease, although radiation can also cause disease. Individuals who receive therapeutic doses of radiation may develop radiation sickness, and those exposed to radiation fallout develop acute radiation syndrome, which can lead to death, depending on the degree of exposure. The accident at the nuclear power plant at Chernobyl in the former Soviet Union is the fulfillment of our worst nightmares, and it will be years before the full toll on life and the environment is known.

HOST RESISTANCE TO INFECTIOUS DISEASE

The host defenses against infectious disease will be discussed in Chapter 3. It has been known for some time that the ability to resist any particular infectious disease varies with the individual. That is, each person is born with resistance to disease that is more or less effective than the resistance other individuals have. This is why some people never get colds; why some people who have inhaled the tuberculosis bacillus never get the disease; why some people do not become sick in the midst of an epidemic; why some people who smoke get lung cancer and others don't. The list could go on and on. Scientists are still trying to determine the exact cause for this difference in resistance to disease. Some of it seems to be present from birth, and it remains to be determined how much of our resistance to disease is inherited and how much is determined by environmental factors. It is known that the immune response can be slow or ineffective in the elderly, malnourished, seriously ill, debilitated, cancer afflicted, and AIDS afflicted.

HOST RESISTANCE TO NONINFECTIOUS DISEASE

As has already been stated, noninfectious diseases cannot be identified by a pathogenic organism. The etiology of noninfectious diseases lies in many different factors that are related to heredity and/or lifestyle. These are referred to as risk factors or predisposing factors, and for most noninfectious diseases, one or more of these factors has been identified. Unlike the risk factors shown in Table 2-4, there are risk factors that cannot be changed, such as race, heredity, sex, and age. Prevention and control for noninfectious diseases is aimed at reduction and/or elimination of as many of the risk factors as possible.

Through research and study of the causes of noninfectious disease, it has become apparent that the lifestyles of individuals play a major part in determining whether they will have certain noninfectious diseases. We suspect a relationship between the way we live and many diseases and disorders. We are *certain* there is a relationship between the way we live and our susceptibility to cardiovascular disease and some forms of cancer.

Nutrition, Weight, and Health

Nutrition plays an important part in everyone's health. We have only begun to discover many of the adverse effects of poor diets. Americans have become used to too much fat, too much salt, too much sugar, and too little of the whole-grain foods and fruits and vegetables. And one of the worst problems is overnutrition, which leads to obesity. In a survey of some of the growing number of citizens reaching 100 and more years of age, it was found that one of the things they had in common was that none of them had ever been extremely obese.

Recent research has shown that many individuals inherit traits that give them a higher potential for gaining weight, and, for them, losing weight is much more difficult. Americans have typically admired the "chubby" baby as being well fed, but we now know that fat cells added by overfeeding babies and young children do not go away.

Mothers need to help their children learn wise ways to eat. Trying to lose weight by cutting calories has a very low rate of success. Over 90% of those who are able to lose weight on a diet regain what they have lost in a short time. It is now known that the only way to lose weight and keep it off is through a lifetime commitment to changed eating habits and regular exercise.

psychoneuroimmunology syko-neuro-im-mun-OL-o-gee
osteomyelitis os-te-o-mi-el-I-tis
carcinogenic kar-si-no-JEN-ik

TABLE 2-4	Risk Factors Associated with Five Leading Causes of Death (United States)
Cause of Death	**Risk Factors**
Cardiovascular disease	Tobacco use
	Elevated serum cholesterol
	Hypertension
	Obesity
	Diabetes
	Sedentary lifestyle
Cancer	Tobacco use
	Improper diet
	Alcohol
	Sexual and reproductive practices
	Occupational exposure (carcinogens)
	Environmental exposure (carcinogens)
Cerebrovascular disease	Hypertension
	Tobacco use
	Elevated serum cholesterol
Accidental injury	Nonuse of seat belts
	Alcohol or substance abuse
	Reckless driving
	Occupational hazards
	Stress/fatigue
Chronic lung disease	Tobacco use
	Occupational

Sleep

Getting adequate amounts of *sleep* is another factor in being able to resist disease. Individuals who get too much or too little sleep on a regular basis are more susceptible to disease. The amount of sleep necessary for good health varies among individuals, but seven to eight hours a night seems to be what is required for most people. Many studies have shown that more people report coming down with colds and missing work on Monday than any other day of the week, and this has been associated with lack of sleep and a break in regular routines over the weekend.

Exercise and Health

Our society is in the midst of a fitness revolution, and basic to this is the emphasis on getting enough

exercise and the right kind for cardiovascular and respiratory benefits to occur. Many studies in the United States and other countries have proved the benefits of adequate exercise as far as disease prevention and longevity are concerned. One long-term study done more than twenty-five years ago traced fifty pairs of identical twin brothers born in Ireland. In each pair, one brother stayed in Ireland and the other moved to the United States. The incidence of heart disease in the American brothers was significantly higher than in the Irish brothers. When their lifestyles were studied, only two differences were found consistently: the Irish brothers ate more potatoes and less meat and walked everywhere, whereas the American brothers ate fewer potatoes, more meat, and rode everywhere.

Even though most Americans know how important exercise is, many of those who have taken up walking or jogging still try to get the closest parking place available, take elevators or escalators instead of stairs, and ride when they could walk. The rest make no effort at all to increase their activity level. If exercise is going to improve the chances of resisting disease, then each individual needs to get the optimum amount. The majority of Americans fall far short of this goal.

Smoking and Alcohol

The elimination of *smoking,* which has been proved to cause lung cancer and other diseases of the lung, and to have an adverse effect on the heart, and moderation in *drinking* or no drinking at all, are two behaviors that would lead to the prevention of untold physical and mental suffering and disease. Smoking and drinking to excess, cause disease and suffering not only in the individual who uses these substances but in anyone else who is involved. Laws have been enacted to protect innocent bystanders from passive smoke, but we have a long way to go before these two factors, which so obviously lower the resistance of the host, are eliminated or controlled.

Stress Management

The benefits of *stress management* have been discussed. It is not possible to live a life free of stressors. Mental and physical stressors that cannot be eliminated are present in everyone's life. Learning to manage stress can be one of the most effective single steps in preventing disease.

The optimum level of resistance to disease will occur in individuals as they strive to achieve a lifestyle that includes wise eating habits, adequate sleep, regular exercise, elimination of unnecessary drugs, and effective stress management.

ENVIRONMENT AND DISEASE

Environmental factors can be thought of in three categories, biologic, physical, and social. In developed nations, the control of *biologic* environmental factors by sanitary measures to ensure clean water, air, food, adequate disposal of waste prod-

ucts, and pest control has erased the threat of many infectious diseases. During times of disaster when sanitation measures are overwhelmed or in third-world countries where they are still inadequate, the flourishing of infectious diseases that were once rare reminds us of our vulnerability and the need for continual vigilance in maintaining a safe environment.

Physical factors such as climate and geography can also have an effect on disease. Some diseases flourish in warm, tropical climates, and others occur mainly in temperate climates. Geographical features such as low, swampy lands that provide ideal breeding grounds for insect vectors are conducive to disease.

The institutions, cultural norms, and economic features of a *society* can include patterns of hygiene, sanitation, and personal relations that produce an environment that is more favorable to disease. The Japanese practice of eating raw fish (which may be contaminated), the use of "earth" toilet facilities in undeveloped nations, rubbing noses among the Eskimos, and many other societal customs and conditions provide environmental factors that can unbalance the equilibrium between disease agent, host, and environment, providing the conditions for disease to take place.

CHAIN OF INFECTION

As part of the foundation for studying the individual infectious diseases, it is important to look at the chain of infection by which pathogenic organisms are able to continue to exist in the environment.

Infectious agents are all "hitchhikers." They have to find a way to get from one host to another, from one place to another, from their *reservoir* (people, animals, soil, or water) to a susceptible host. They have to find a way to escape their host, or a *portal of exit.* Their transportation is referred to as a *means of transmission.* They also need to find a way to get into their new host, a *portal of entry.*

The "chain of infection" is shown in Figure 2-3. Our success in preventing and controlling infectious

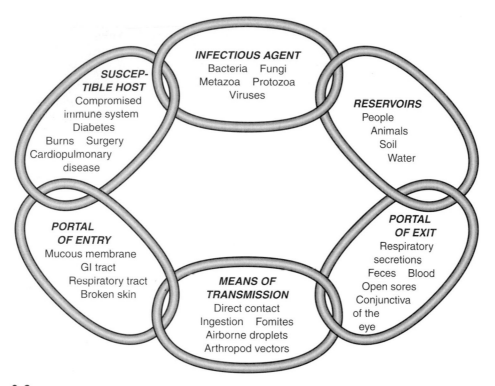

Figure 2-3
The chain of infection.

diseases has come through being able to break one or more of the "links" in the chain.

Transmission may be by *direct* or *indirect* contact. Direct contact would be by skin or mucous membrane: by kissing or sexual intercourse; through droplet infection in the spray of a sneeze or a cough; or through blood transfusion. Indirect contact can be made by using, touching, or ingesting any object or food that has been contaminated with the pathogenic organisms. Pathogens may be carried in the air in evaporated residue of human discharges and in dust arising from contaminated bedding or soil. Insects, sometimes borne by animals and sometimes flying or crawling, may harbor a pathogen and transmit it through a bite or by depositing it on some animal, human, or object. Some examples of disease transmission can be seen in Table 2-5.

STAGES OF DISEASE

A knowledge of the progression of an infection once a pathogenic agent enters the body will also help you to understand infectious diseases. The stages of a disease are divided as shown in Figure 2-4. Although the divisions between these stages are not always apparent, most individuals follow the general pattern.

1. Incubation—Occurs between the time when the agent enters the body and the first symptoms.
2. Prodrome—General symptoms occur: headache, fever, nausea, irritability, and runny nose. The disease is already highly communicable.
3. Clinical—Characteristic symptoms appear. This is the peak or most intense stage of the

TABLE 2-5	Transmission of Selected Diseases		
Portal of Exit	**Means of Transmission**	**Portal of Entry**	**Diseases**
Respiratory secretions	Airborne droplets, particles	Respiratory tract	Common cold, measles, influenza
Feces	Water, food, particles, flies	Mouth	Hepatitis A, poliomyelitis
Open sores	Direct contact, sexual intercourse	Skin, mucous membrane	Boils, chlamydia, AIDS
Conjunctiva of eye	Flies, hands	Ocular mucous membrane	Common cold, trachoma
Blood	Insect vectors, needles, sexual intercourse	Broken skin	Malaria, yellow fever, AIDS

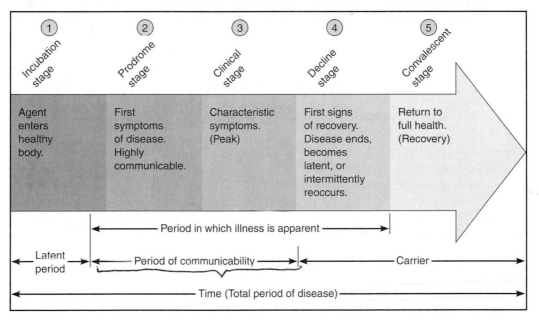

Figure 2-4

Stages of disease.

disease. Communicability of disease organisms is most probable at this time.

4. Decline—Symptoms begin to fade and recovery begins. Relapses may occur if too much is attempted too soon.

5. Convalescent—Rebuilding of the body occurs. The host is immune to the disease, but the agent may still be transmitted if a carrier state exists.

SUMMARY

Ancient peoples attributed disease to gods or to evil spirits. The theory of contagion did not develop until biblical times, when isolation of lepers led to a decrease in leprosy. In the nineteenth century, the discovery of microorganisms and their relation to infection led to the germ theory of disease. Finally, the modern theory of multiple causation evolved. The classic epidemiologic model of disease is based on the need for a balance between the virulence of the disease agent, the resistance of the host, and factors in the biologic, physical, and social environment. Pathogenic organisms can be identified for most infectious diseases, but there are many different causes for noninfectious diseases. These are malnutrition or overnutrition, chemical substances, inherited susceptibility, psychosomatic factors, and physical forces. Some causes of noninfectious disease also play a role in infectious disease because they lower the resistance of the host. The lifestyles of individuals determine their ability to resist infection and also play a major part in determining whether they contract some noninfectious diseases. The important lifestyle factors are nutrition, sleep, exercise, drug use, and stress management. Biologic, physical, and social factors in the environment also affect the occurrence of disease. The chain of infection, methods of disease transmission, and stages of infectious disease are also important concepts in disease occurrence.

QUESTIONS FOR REVIEW

1. What theories of disease causation have human beings believed in through the ages (in chronologic order)?

2. Why was it necessary to develop the theory of multiple causation?

3. What is meant by prevalence rate and incidence rate?

4. What are the differences among the primary, secondary, and tertiary levels of disease prevention?

5. How does the classic epidemiologic theory of disease apply to infectious and noninfectious disease?

6. What do epidemiologists do?

7. What are six broad categories for classifying pathogenic agents?

8. How does a virus cause disease?

9. What is the difference between viral infection and viral disease?

10. How is it possible to get a bacterial disease without being exposed to someone who carries the disease agent?

11. How are rickettsiae like or different from bacteria?

12. How do protozoa and metazoa cause disease?

13. What are the "disease agents" for noninfectious disease?

14. What is the difference between having a psychosomatic disease and being a hypochondriac?

15. What physical forces play a part in disease occurrence?

16. What factors affect the resistance of the host to infectious and noninfectious disease?

17. What is the chain of infection, and why is it important?

18. What are the stages of disease, and what occurs to the victim during each stage?

FURTHER READING

Ader, Robert, Nicholas Cohen, and David Felten. 1995. Psychoneuroimmunology: Interactions between the nervous system and the immune system. *The Lancet* 345:99.

Adler, Nancy, and Karen Matthews. Health psychology: why do some people get sick and some stay well? *Annual Review of Psychology.* 45:229–259.

Aguzzi, Adriano. 1997. Neuro-immune connection in spread of prions in the body? *The Lancet* 349:742.

Arcury, Thomas A., and Sara A. Quandt. 1998. Chronic agricultural chemical exposure among migrant and seasonal farmworkers. *Society and Natural Resources* 11:829.

Brudnjak, Z. 1997. Prions and prion diseases. *Acta Med Croatica* 51:123.

Cohen, Sheldon, and Tracy B. Herbert. 1996. Health psychology: Psychological factors and physical disease from the perspective of human psychoneuroimmunology. *Annual Review of Psychology* 47:113.

Epidemiology in action. 1999. *The Journal of the American Medical Association.* 282:1222.

Epidemiology: what is it and what are its goals? 1999. *Contemporary OB/GYN.* 44:92.

Gordon, John Steele. The passion of Typhoid Mary; Mary Mallon could do one thing very well, and all she wanted was to be left to it. *American Heritage.* May–June '94, 45:118–121.

Jenks, Peter. 1998. Microbial genome sequencing—beyond the double helix. *British Medical Journal* 7171:1562.

Keeling, M.J., and B.T. Grenfell. 1997. Disease extinction and community size: Modeling the persistence of measles. *Science* 275: 65.

Kuhn, John E. 1997. A statistics primer: Prevalence, incidence, relative risks, and odds ratios, some epidemiologic concepts in the sports medicine literature. *American Journal of Sports Medicine* 25:414.

The Lancet. 1997. Putting public health back into epidemiology (editorial). 350:229.

Little, Miles. 1998. Assignments of meaning in epidemiology. *Social Science and Medicine* 47:1135.

McMichael, Anthony J., et al. 1990. Globalization and the sustainability of human health. *Bioscience* 49:205.

Norris, V., D. Cellier, J. Caston, et al. 1997. Hypothesis: The meeting place model for prion disease. *Comptes Rendus De Le Academie Des Sciences* 320:393.

Pennisi, Elizabeth. 1997. Tracing molecules that make the brain-body connection: Neuroimmunology. *Science* 275:930.

Szabo, Gyongyi. 1999. Consequences of alcohol consumption on host defense. *Alcohol and Alcoholism* 34:830.

Vegni, F.E. 1997. What relevance do advances in molecular biology and genetics have for epidemiology: High tech needle and thread to sew the web of causation. *Annali Di Igiene* 9:273.

Von Hertzen, L., et al. 1999. Asthma, atopy and chlamydia pneumoniae antibodies in adults. *Clinical and Experimental Allergy* 29:522.

Weng, Nan-ping. 1999. Telomeres, telomerase, and lymphocyte replicative life span. *Clinical Immunology* 92:1.

Yang, J., et al. 1999. Human endothelial cell life extension by telomerase expression. *Journal of Biological Chemistry* 274:26141.

Yap, Y.G., and A. J. Camm. 1999. The current cardiac safety situation with antihistamines. *Clinical and Experimental Allergy* 29:15.

3

CELLS, AGING, AND THE IMMUNE SYSTEM

OBJECTIVES

1. *Summarize the parts and organelles of the human cell.*
2. *Explain the two major groupings for theories of aging.*
3. *Evaluate the telomerase theory of aging.*
4. *Analyze the free radical theory of aging.*
5. *Describe the role that the external barriers play in protecting us from disease.*
6. *Differentiate between nonspecific and specific natural immunity.*
7. *Relate what happens in the combined immune response.*
8. *Explain the four types of acquired immunity.*

9. *Outline the processes that occur in the acute inflammatory response.*
10. *Distinguish between resolution, regeneration, and repair.*
11. *Discuss the factors that may hasten or delay healing.*
12. *Explain the terms* **autoimmune** *and* **hypersensitivity.**
13. *State and describe the cause(s), symptoms, prevention, and treatment for the following:*
    Allergic rhinitis
    Urticaria and angioedema
    Asthma
    Rheumatoid arthritis
    Lupus erythematosus

THE CELL

Structure and Function

Cells are the basic structural unit of all life—plant or animal. The body's resistance to infectious disease depends upon specialized cells in the blood and lymphatic system. The onset of arthritis and other noninfectious diseases can be the result of death or inappropriate activity of these specialized cells.

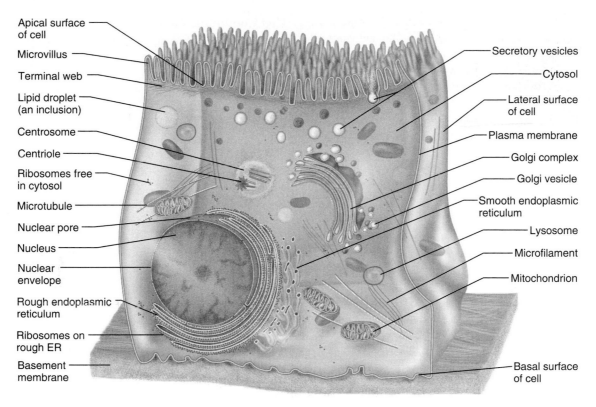

Apical surface
of cell

Microvillus

Terminal web

Lipid droplet
(an inclusion)

Centrosome

Centriole

Ribosomes free
in cytosol

Microtubule

Nuclear pore

Nucleus

Nuclear
envelope

Rough endoplasmic
reticulum

Ribosomes on
rough ER

Basement
membrane

Secretory vesicles

Cytosol

Lateral surface
of cell

Plasma membrane

Golgi complex

Golgi vesicle

Smooth endoplasmic
reticulum

Lysosome

Microfilament

Mitochondrion

Basal surface
of cell

Figure 3-1
Structure of a representative cell.

Human cells vary greatly in size, shape, and function but each one has a nucleus or nuclear material and organelles (Figure 3-1). Following is a brief summary of some of the parts and organelles that are common to human cells.

The **cell membrane** serves as a barrier, allowing very few molecules to enter the cell, and containing those parts necessary to the life of the cell. Raw materials necessary for the cell to live are allowed to enter and waste materials that would kill the cell are allowed to leave.

Scientists originally thought that all of the parts of the cell were suspended in the **cytoplasm,** the jellylike interior of the cell. But, with the advances in electron microscopy, a network of fibers can be seen running through the cytoplasm. This **cytoskeleton** forms a framework that gives mechanical support to the cell and helps maintain

its shape. Many nutrients are stored in the cytoplasm also.

The **nucleus** is the "mastermind" of the cell and is surrounded by two membranes that separate it from other cell components. Pores through both membranes act like small channels, opening and closing to allow selected molecules, most importantly, messenger ribonucleic acid (mRNA), in and out of the nucleus.

Within the nucleus are the chromosomes that contain the genes made of deoxyribonucleic acid (DNA). The genes contain the master plan with directions for everything the cell is and will be. Protein production begins in the nucleus when mRNA is produced from DNA instructions. It carries a coded message for a protein and passes through the nuclear pores into the cytoplasm. There, the mRNA attaches to **ribosomes.** Another kind of RNA, transfer RNA (tRNA) brings the correct amino acids to the ribosome and when all of the amino acids for a protein are joined, the chain (protein) is released.

Mitochondria are the energy producers of the cell. They contain some DNA and other materials for protein synthesis.

The **endomembrane system** refers to the membranes of the cell that are interrelated, directly through physical contact, or indirectly through tiny vesicles that pinch off and travel from one membrane site to another. The following organelles are included in the endomembrane system.

The **endoplasmic reticulum** (ER) is a network within the cytoplasm. There are two distinct forms that differ in structure and function. The smooth ER is involved in the synthesis of fatty acids and membrane components. It also participates in carbohydrate metabolism, detoxifies drugs and poisons, and stores calcium ions necessary for muscle contraction. The rough ER is covered with ribosomes and ribonucleoprotein particles that cling to it, thus giving it the rough appearance. Proteins are synthesized by the ribosomes and stay in the ER or are used to construct the membranes of other organelles.

The **Golgi apparatus** consists of flattened membrane sacs that modify, store, and route products of the endoplasmic reticulum.

Lysosomes are organelles that are active in intracellular digestion, recycling of the cell's own organic material, and programmed cell destruction. Some inherited diseases have been found to be a result of impaired lysosomal function or the lack of a specific lysosomal enzyme.

Perioxisomes contain enzymes that can catalyze hydrogen peroxide to water and oxygen. Their other functions are not yet fully understood.

Vacuoles are various membranous sacs that store and excrete substances within the cytoplasm.

Cell Communication and Metabolism

Communication between cells is vital for proper body functioning.

This is sometimes referred to as "cell talk" and can occur through protein channels to adjacent cells, direct contact, and the secretion of chemicals. If communication is interrupted or compromised in some way, disease can occur.

Cells maintain their functions by *cellular metabolism.* This involves the use (anabolism) and release (catabolism) of energy. Cells take in the substances they need for growth and survival and export the products of metabolism and lysosomal digestion.

Most cells are able to reproduce, and in almost all cases the new cells are created as fast as old ones die. The exception is nerve cells. Their number is set at birth and they are not replaceable.

Cell Adaptation, Injury, and Death

Cells adapt to the stresses and strains of their environment. Common changes are: atrophy (decreased size), hypertrophy (increased size), and hyperplasia (increase in numbers). Sometimes these adaptations are constructive—helping the cells and tissue to survive. But other times, the response may lead to too much or too little change, resulting in disease and/or death. When cells die because of injury, they deteriorate and eventually digest themselves (**autolysis**). This process is referred to as **necrosis.** Another term, **apoptosis,** is used to refer to a different kind of cell death that occurs to both normal and diseased cells because of genetic programming.

There are many factors that can lead to cell injury and death, including the causative factors covered in the epidemiologic model in Chapter 2: infectious agents, nutritional imbalance, chemical agents, and physical agents. Although this model is directed at what happens to the individual subjected to these agents, the amount of damage that occurs on the cellular level determines not only whether the cells will survive but also the survival of the individual. When enough cells die, the tissue of which they are a part will die. When enough

---

BOX 3-1

PROGRAMMED THEORIES

Programmed Senescence Aging is the result of the sequential switching on and off of certain genes, with senescence being defined as the time when age-associated deficits are manifested.

Endocrine Theory Biologic clocks act through hormones to control the pace of aging.

Immunologic Theory A programmed decline in immune system functions leads to an increased vulnerability to infectious disease and thus aging and death.

ERROR THEORIES

Wear and Tear Cells and tissues have vital parts that wear out.

Rate of Living The greater an organism's rate of oxygen basal metabolism, the shorter its life span.

Crosslinking An accumulation of crosslinked proteins damages cells and tissues, slowing down bodily processes.

Free Radicals Accumulated damage caused by oxygen radicals causes cells and eventually organs to stop functioning.

Error Catastrophe Damage to mechanisms that synthesize proteins results in faulty proteins that accumulate to a level that causes catastrophic damage to cells, tissues, and organs.

Somatic Mutation Genetic mutations occur and accumulate with increasing age, causing cells to deteriorate and malfunction.

---

tissue dies the organ it is a part of will die, and when vital organs die, the body dies. This is referred to as *somatic death.*

Aging

Many of the "symptoms" of old age occur because of the damage to and death of cells. Theories of aging can be divided into two groups. The "programmed" theories posit that aging follows a biologic timetable. The other group, "error" theories emphasize environmental factors that affect our systems and gradually cause things to go wrong. A brief and very simplified listing of the major theories developed by the National Institute of Aging can be seen in Box 3-1. This list was part of a report entitled *In Search of the Secrets of Aging,* which was released in 1993. Since that time, research evidence has been accumulating regarding another theory of aging. This theory of aging first emerged in 1986 when Howard Cooke noticed that the ends of human chromosomes, known as *telomeres*, were becoming shorter each time the cells divided. Eventually, the telomeres became so short that the cell could no longer func-

tion. It was proposed that telomere shortening was the "clock" that triggered **senescence** (old age). This new theory was controversial but researchers began testing the theory and in January, 1998 the University of Texas's South Western Medical Center announced that it had found a way to extend the life of human cells indefinitely by using an enzyme, telomerase. Their research was carried out in vitro (in a petri dish in the lab), but it was evidence for a causal relation between telomere shortening and senescence. Many of the conditions in the elderly are due to cellular senescence such as changes in the skin, macular degeneration (of the eye), atherosclerosis, and osteoarthritis. It

---

lysosomes   LI-so-soms
perioxisomes   per-e-OX-i-soms
vacuoles   VAK-u-oles
autolysis   aw-TOL-i-sis
necrosis   ne-KRO-sis
apoptosis   a-pop-TO-sis
telomere   TEL-o-mere
senescence   se-NES-ens

---

cancer patients may have too much telomeres speeding up cell division

is possible that telomerase could be produced for human use (in vivo) and reset the cell's "aging" clock.

With the understanding of the role of telomerase in maintaining the length of the telomeres, came the realization that this could be a significant finding for cancer research. Cancer cells continue to grow into ever larger tumors. The researchers found that instead of having too little telomerase, cancer cells produce it constantly, allowing the cancer cells to grow indefinitely. So, in a healthy person, providing more telomerase for the telomeres could extend life, whereas decreasing or eliminating the amount of telomerase in a person with cancer could possibly cause the cancer cells to die. This may sound simple but it will take years of research before it could become a reality, if at all.

In addition to the telomerase theory, which would fit in with the programmed theories, the theory of free radicals is receiving intense interest from scientists and others. Free radicals are molecules of oxygen that are a by-product of cellular metabolism. They have an unpaired electron and move around the cell seeking an attachment for their single electron and in the process damage proteins, membranes, and nucleic acids such as DNA. Fortunately, the cells have a built-in defense against free radicals in vitamins A, C, and E. There are also enzymes that can break down the free radicals. Unfortunately, not all free radicals are neutralized before causing damage. And as people get older, the defenses get weaker and our cells become more susceptible to the damage that the free radicals can cause. But, scientists have been able to show that some of the aging processes in animals can be prevented or reversed. And, a diet of fresh fruit and vegetables can also reverse some of the changes that come with aging. These are exciting discoveries but it is likely that no one theory will explain the aging process. It is too complicated, involving genes, hormones, molecules, the responses of the immune system, and many other factors.

Lengthening life may not be desirable if it means lengthening the pain and suffering that someone with a chronic disease must endure. And

no one yet knows how to keep people from losing their sight, hearing, and other senses that decline in all humans at some age. Scientists are much more interested in improving and maintaining the quality of life. Until people are able and willing to do this, the lengthening of life only ensures that more will spend those additional years in a total care facility.

The Immune Response

Cells in the blood and lymphoid systems participate in the immune response. White blood cells, or leukocytes, including neutrophils, eosinophils, basophils, phagocytes, and lymphocytes, are essential in the protection of the body from foreign invaders. But the body first wards off bacteria and other disease-causing agents with a natural nonspecific response that will be discussed next.

NATURAL NONSPECIFIC IMMUNE RESPONSE

External Barriers

External barriers are the body's first line of defense against invaders (Figure 3-2). The skin provides a natural barrier to most pathogenic (disease-causing) agents. In addition to being a mechanical barrier, the skin also keeps most bacteria from surviving because of the lactic acid and fatty acids in *sweat* and the low pH generated by **sebaceous** *secretions*.

Another effective defense mechanism is the *mucus* secreted by the membranes lining the inner surfaces of the body. The mucus serves to keep bacteria from attaching to the surfaces, and pathogens and other foreign particles are trapped in the mucus and removed from the body by mechanical means such as the action of the *cilia, sneezing,* and *coughing*.

Body fluid secretions also protect epithelial surfaces by mechanical and chemical means. The washing action of *tears, saliva,* and *urine* removes bacteria and foreign particles from the body, and body fluids such as *tears, gastric juice, semen,*

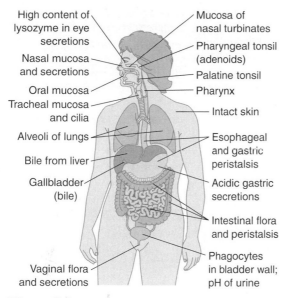

Figure 3-2

First line of defense.

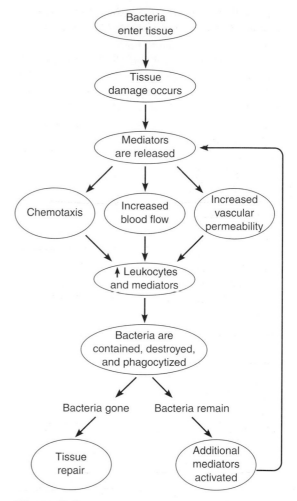

Figure 3-3

The inflammatory response.

nasal secretions, and *saliva* contain bacteriocidal components that destroy pathogens before they can infect the body.

A very different protective function is fulfilled by *"friendly" bacteria,* which naturally inhabit various parts of the body and suppress the growth of pathogenic organisms. For instance, there are bacteria in the vagina that produce lactic acid and metabolize glycogen secreted by the vaginal epithelium. When enough of these nonpathogenic bacteria are destroyed by antibiotic use, the resulting increase in glycogen allows the yeast *Candida albicans* to grow, which can result in candidiasis, a yeast infection.

Inflammation

When pathogenic agents penetrate external barriers, the first reaction of the body is the inflammatory response. Infection is just one cause of inflammation, which can also occur as the result of a simple blow, exposure to the sun, contact with certain chemicals, and in many other ways. Any time the cells or tissues of the body are injured,

internally or on the surface, by whatever agent, the inflammatory response occurs. An inflammatory response (produced by bacterial penetration) is diagramed in Figure 3-3.

Although inflammation may not seem like a desirable thing to have at the time you are injured, it

eosinophils	e-o-SIN-o-fils
sebaceous	se-BA-shus
Candida albicans	KAN-di-da AL-bi-kanz
candidiasis	kan-di-DI-a-sis

is actually the necessary response of the body for the healing process to begin. Everyone experiences inflammation from time to time. The signs are redness, warmth, pain, swelling, and loss of function. Sometimes inflammation is a mild reaction to a slight injury, but at other times it may be a strong reaction to a severe injury, and at some point can become chronic. Comprehension of the inflammatory process is basic to the understanding of disease.

Acute Inflammatory Response

The acute or immediate inflammatory response occurs in the blood vessels in the area of the injury (Figure 3-4). At first there is a brief period when the blood vessels constrict; then they dilate, resulting in an increased flow of blood to the area and an increased amount of fluid leaving the vessels for tissue spaces. At the same time, the **permeability** (ease of penetration) of the blood vessels increases, allowing the passage of plasma proteins, as well as fluid, into the tissue spaces. The blood remaining in the venules becomes thicker and slows down, thus permitting a process called **pavementing,** in which the leukocytes (white blood cells), which are normally traveling in the mainstream of the blood, form a layer covering the endothelium (lining) of the venules.

The leukocytes then move along the endothelium in an amoeba-like fashion, to a point where they can leave the blood vessel. This process is called **diapedesis** or **emigration.**

Once the leukocytes have left the blood vessel, they travel toward the site of injury through another process, **chemotaxis.** Chemotaxis is the movement of an organism or cells in response to a chemical attractant. In the inflammatory response, chemicals called **mediators** lure the leukocytes to the inflammatory site, where they release enzymes (proteins that act as catalysts) and begin the process of **phagocytosis** (engulfing and destroying foreign particles or organisms).

Chemical Mediators of Inflammation

Histamine was the first chemical identified as a mediator of the inflammatory response. As scien-

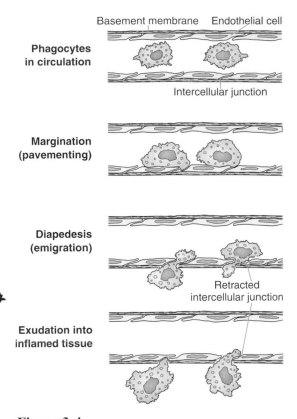

Figure 3-4
Acute inflammatory response

tists realized that more than one chemical must be involved, the search for others got under way. Now many chemicals are thought to take part in the inflammatory response. These mediators come from the plasma, cells, or possibly from damaged tissue. Histamine, **bradykinin,** complement, **prostaglandins, leukotrienes,** lysosomal enzymes, oxygen metabolites, platelet activating factor (PAF), interleukin-1 (IL-1), and tumor necrosis factor (TNF) are considered the principal mediators.

When the leukocytes reach the site of injury, some of them, the neutrophils and the monocytes (which become macrophages), perform phagocytic action, while the others, basophils, mast cells, and **eosinophils,** release chemicals. If the cell injury is due to viral infection, **interferon,** a protein that protects the body against viral infection and possibly some forms of cancer, is released. It is nonspecific in that it protects against many different viruses, and infection by one virus can produce protection against other kinds of viruses. Viruses stimulate cells to produce interferon, and interferon in turn produces antiviral proteins that disrupt viral reproduction.

When interferon was discovered in 1957, great hopes existed for its use in bolstering the immune system and treating cancer. Although these hopes have not been fulfilled to date, it has been effective in a few cases. It has been useful in treating a rare form of leukemia and more recently there has been success in using interferon to increase survival time in patients with malignant melanoma.

Another nonspecific defense of the body is found in complement, a complex of interrelated and interacting proteins manufactured in the liver. Complement is active in inflammation and phagocytosis and also assists the action of antibodies in the specific response if the infecting agent is not destroyed by the nonspecific defenses.

Inflammatory exudates   The increased permeability of the blood vessels allows certain fluids to escape along with the leukocytes and cellular debris. The exudate has various functions. The role of the leukocytes has already been mentioned. The fluid of the exudate also dilutes poisonous substances that may be present at the site of injury. The plasma fluid contains antibodies to microbial invasion, and fibrinogen (blood clotting factor), which can form a barrier to invaders. Fibrinogen also aids in phagocytosis by trapping microorganisms for the leukocytes.

The nature of the exudate changes according to the severity of the injury. Mild damage produces a watery exudate, which is called **serous.** More severe injury may lead to the release of more fibrin, and the exudate is then described as **fibrinous.** **Purulent** exudate, or pus, also occurs in a more severe injury, and if the lesion is deep enough to

penetrate blood vessels and allow red blood cells to escape, then the exudate is called **hemorrhagic.**

Healing

When an injury is mild, resolution occurs, with the site returning to normal. However, if there has been extensive damage, the inflammatory response does not resolve; a chronic abscess may form, pus is produced continuously, and fibrous tissue is laid down around the abscess, walling it off. If the inflammatory agent is destroyed or neutralized, healing may still occur. But if the body is unable to remove or destroy the inflammatory agent, then the result is chronic inflammation. Chronic inflammation may also occur without an acute phase as the result of certain disease processes, such as tuberculosis, syphilis, autoimmune diseases, and hypersensitivity, all of which will be discussed in later chapters.

When significant amounts of tissue have been destroyed, resolution cannot occur. Whether loss of tissue occurs from an accidental or surgical incision, physical or chemical agents, **ischemia,** or severe inflammation leading to necrosis (cell death), the tissue is replaced by **regeneration** and **repair.** The replacing of lost tissue by tissue of the same type is regeneration. This type of healing is referred to as primary healing and occurs most often when a surgical incision has been made as shown in Figure 3-5. The replacing of lost tissue by granulation tissue, which becomes a fibrous connective-tissue scar, is repair and referred to as secondary healing. Most cells in

permeability	per-me-a-BIL-i-tee
diapedesis	di-a-ped-E-sis
chemotaxis	ke-mo-TAK-sis
phagocytosis	fag-o-si-TO-sis
bradykinin	brad-e-KI-nin
prostaglandin	pros-ta-GLAN-din
leukotrienes	loo-ko-TRI-enz
fibrinous	FI-brin-us
purulent	PURE-yu-lent
hemorrhagic	hem-o-RAJ-ik
ischemia	is-KEE-me-a

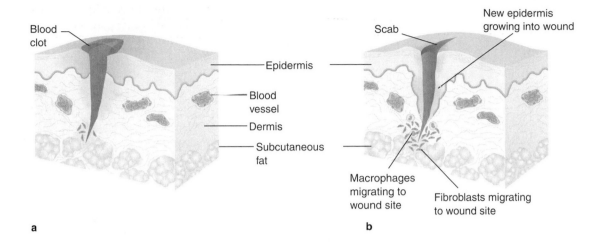

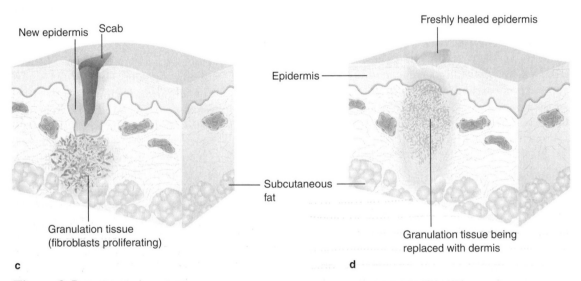

Figure 3-5

Tissue Repair. (a) Fresh wound cuts through the epithelium (epidermis) and underlying connective tissue (dermis), and a clot forms. (b) Approximately 1 week after the injury, a scab is present, and epithelium (new epidermis) is growing into the wound. (c) Approximately 2 weeks after the injury, the epithelium has grown completely into the wound, and granulation tissue has formed. (d) Approximately 1 month after the injury, the wound has completely closed, the scab has been sloughed, and the granulation tissue is being replaced with dermis.

the body have some capacity to regenerate, with the exception of central nervous system (CNS) nerve cells, skeletal cells, and cardiac muscle cells.

If neurons are destroyed in the CNS, they are permanently lost. In the peripheral nervous system (PNS), regeneration may occur if the cell body is not destroyed. Healing in any part of the body follows the same pattern, beginning with the inflammatory reaction and ending with resolution or regeneration and repair. There are local variations, depending on the type of tissue involved.

Factors Affecting Inflammation and Healing

For some individuals, in some cases, the inflammatory response and healing may be impaired. Many factors can lead to slow healing or no healing. One of the most crucial factors in an effective inflammatory response is an adequate blood supply. If the blood supply to the area of injury is impaired for any reason, the inflammatory response will be slow and healing prolonged. Nutrition is another important factor. Lack of sufficient protein, vitamin C, and zinc have been shown to delay healing, and adequate calcium and vitamin D are crucial in the healing of bones.

Although age has been thought by some to be a factor in slow healing, there is little to support this idea, and if healing in the elderly does occur more slowly, it probably is due to malnutrition or inadequate circulation. Antiinflammatory drugs such as the **glucocorticoids** inhibit inflammation and wound healing if they are present in large amounts. The presence of infection or foreign bodies will also impede healing. Diabetics have an increased susceptibility to infection, and this along with other deficiencies caused by the disease lead to inadequate healing.

Natural Specific Immunity

There are two kinds of specific immunity to disease: (1) **humoral,** or **antibody-mediated immu-**nity, and (2) **cell-mediated immunity.** Both kinds are provided by the action of lymphocytes. In humoral immunity, *B lymphocytes,* or *B cells,* produce antibodies that protect against extracellular antigens such as bacteria, toxins, parasites, and viruses outside of cells. In cell-mediated immunity, *T lymphocytes* (*T cells*) produce **lymphokines,** which provide protection against intracellular antigens such as viruses, intracellular bacteria and fungi, and tumors, and regulate humoral and cell-mediated immune responses. Three types of T cells have been identified. Helper T cells are needed for antibody production by B cells. Killer T cells are active in destroying foreign cells and in the rejection of tissue transplants. Suppressor T cells act to suppress the production of antibodies. They keep the immune response from getting out of control.

The Combined Immune Response

When a microbial invader (**antigen**) enters the body, chemical messages are sent out from the point of entry, and phagocytes, B cells, and T cells all arrive at the scene. As the phagocytes begin to attack, antigens reach the B and T cells, which begin clonal expansion. B cells form immunoglobulin (antibodies), which participates in the inflammatory response. Antibodies attach to antigen on the surface of the microbes, causing clumping and immobilization. Complement is activated in response to this action and enhances the phagocytosis of the invaders by causing destruction of the invader's cell membrane (Figure 3-6). In the meantime, more T cells have been produced, T lymphocytes have combined with microbial antigens, and other chemicals are released. If the effort is successful, B and T lymphocytes withdraw, and **macrophages** perform the cleanup.

---

glucocorticoid   gloo-ko-KORT-i-koid
lymphokines   LIM-fo-kins

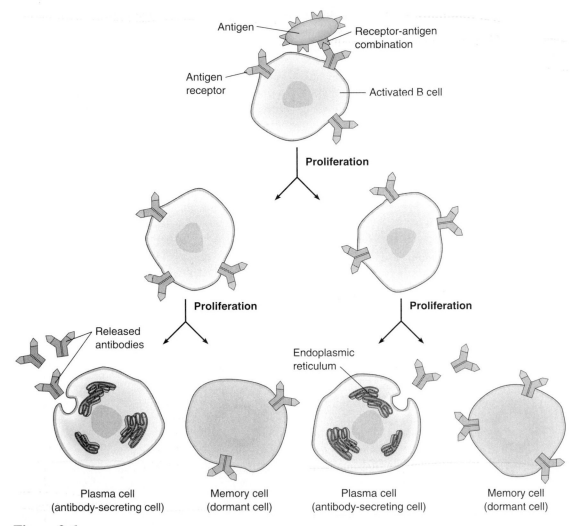

Antigen

Receptor-antigen combination

Antigen receptor

Activated B cell

Proliferation

Proliferation

Proliferation

Released antibodies

Endoplasmic reticulum

Plasma cell (antibody-secreting cell)

Memory cell (dormant cell)

Plasma cell (antibody-secreting cell)

Memory cell (dormant cell)

Figure 3-6

The immune response is a coordinated effort to destroy foreign invaders (antigens). It involves four varieties of lymphocytes: macrophages, neutrophils, B cells, and T cells. Macrophages engulf invading antigens such as bacteria and at the same time, inform other lymphocytes of the attack. B cells and helper and killer T cells swarm around the macrophages and begin to multiply. Suppressor T cells take their cue from the number of antigens as to when to suppress the response. All four varieties of lymphocytes produce active cells and memory cells. Memory cells stay in the bloodstream and are prepared in case the same antigen attacks again. The interaction and multiplication of these cells provides a strong defense against invaders.

ACQUIRED IMMUNITY

We have been discussing natural immunity to disease. Everyone is born with these defense mechanisms, but we also acquire immunity to disease.

Acquired immunity can be acquired naturally or artificially, and it can be active or passive. Thus there are four kinds of acquired immunity: active natural, active artificial, passive natural, and passive artificial.

Active Natural Immunity

Active natural immunity occurs when an individual is exposed to a disease-causing microorganism and the body learns to produce the antibodies necessary to destroy the organism. Normally the symptoms and the disease will be present with the first infection (in some cases the person may be asymptomatic yet still produce the antibodies). On subsequent exposure, the body is prepared with the specific antibodies, and the individual is immune to the disease. Most people over forty years of age were infected with the mumps virus as children. When exposed to mumps as an adult, they do not become ill. (Mumps is one childhood disease that does not always produce apparent symptoms.)

Active Artificial Immunity

Active artificial immunity occurs through vaccination with a form of the disease microorganism. It may be dead, attenuated (weakened), or altered so that it will not produce the disease but will cause the body to produce antibodies. Because the body has learned to make the antibodies, this type of vaccination is long lasting and preferable. Most

people under twenty years of age have received the measles, mumps, and rubella (MMR) vaccine and will not become sick with these diseases. Recommendations for vaccinations for children are shown in Table 3-1.

Passive Natural Immunity

Passive natural immunity results from the transfer of antibodies from a mother to her baby through the placenta. The mother has been exposed to a number of pathogenic organisms during her life, and this protection is passed on to the baby in the form of antibodies. If the mother nurses the baby, then more protection is gained by antibodies in the milk. However, in both cases, because the baby's body has not learned to make the antibodies, the protection lasts only for a few months until the antibodies are broken down.

Passive Artificial Immunity

Passive artificial immunity is acquired through inoculation with antibodies. Because it gives protection only as long as the antibodies are not used

TABLE 3-1   **Recommended Childhood Immunization Schedule, (1995)**

Vaccine	Birth	2 Months	4 Months	6 Months	12 Months	15 Months	18 Months	4–6 Years	11–12 Years	14–16 Years
Hepatitis B	HB-1	HB-2		HB-3						
Diphtheria-Tetanus-Pertussis (DTP)		DTP	DTP	DTP	DTP or DTap ≥ at 15 months			DTP or DTaP	Td	
Haemophilus influenzae type b		Hib	Hib	Hib	Hib					
Poliovirus		OPV	OPV	OPV				OPV		
Measles-Mumps-Rubella					MMR				MMR or MMR	

Source: CDC, MMWR, June 16, 1995, p. 2

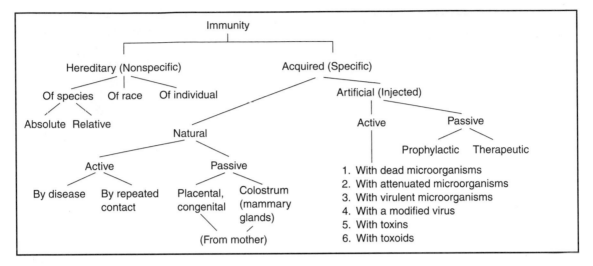

Figure 3-7
Diagram of types of immunity

or eliminated from the system, this type of therapy is generally reserved for those who have been exposed to a disease such as rabies or tetanus or are at high risk for an infection because of age or physical condition. Immune serum or serum containing antibodies, which is given to counteract one or more specific **toxin**(s), is also referred to as **antisera** or **antitoxin.** Figure 3-7 is a model of the different types of immunity.

IMMUNE DISORDERS

Because the body's response to foreign invaders is so complex, there are times when it may malfunction. Instead of protecting us from disease and discomfort as it does most of the time, the immune response may become overactive or misdirected. The conditions that then occur are referred to as hypersensitivity (allergies) and autoimmune disorders.

Hypersensitivity (Allergies)

Allergies occur because of an inappropriate reaction of the immune system. As has been discussed previously in this chapter, the function of the immune system is to recognize foreign invaders

(antigens), such as bacteria and viruses, and to form antibodies and sensitized lymphocytes that will interact with these disease agents when next encountered and destroy them. In allergies, for some unknown reason, the immune system forms antibodies against harmless substances because they are identified as potentially harmful antigens.

One out of seven people in the United States today has an allergy. The substance that causes an allergic reaction is called an allergen, and these allergens can be introduced into the body by different routes. These routes are inhalation, ingestion, injection, and direct contact. The list of possible allergens is endless, and in many cases there is an inherited tendency to develop an allergy. Some of the most common allergens are pollen, animal dander, and other particulates in the air; milk, strawberries, and almost any other food; penicillin and many other drugs; poison ivy and other plant life; synthetic materials, chemicals, and insect venom.

The symptoms are also diverse, ranging from a mild rash to life-threatening anaphylactic shock (Figure 3-8). Most allergic reactions are acute and not recurrent, because the allergen is readily identified and can be avoided. However, the most com-

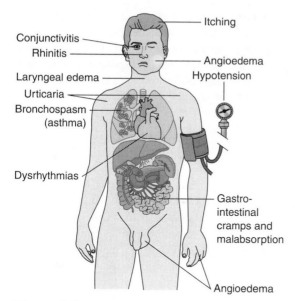

Itching
Conjunctivitis
Rhinitis
Angioedema
Hypotension
Laryngeal edema
Urticaria
Bronchospasm
(asthma)

Dysrhythmias

Gastro-
intestinal
cramps and
malabsorption

Angioedema

Figure 3-8

Hypersensitivity reactions may affect various body systems.

mon allergic reaction, allergic rhinitis, is often a chronic condition.

Allergic Rhinitis

Allergic rhinitis, generally called hay fever, is a reaction to an airborne allergen. For some individuals it may be a seasonal problem, caused by certain pollens, whereas for others it is year-round and caused by many different allergens.

Cause

A predisposition to allergic rhinitis is inherited. The major allergens that induce the reaction are pollen, mold spores, house dust, animal dander, cigarette smoke, and upholstery.

Symptoms

Histamine and other chemicals released by the body in response to an allergen are responsible for the allergic reaction. For some individuals, the symptoms may be mild, with runny nose; watery, itchy eyes; and sneezing. For others, however, these may be accompanied by malaise, fever,

headache, and sinus pain. In perennial allergic rhinitis, chronic nasal obstruction is common and often results in eustachian tube obstruction and if untreated may lead to asthma, **otitis media** (middle ear infection) with hearing loss, and other respiratory problems.

Prevention

The best method of prevention is desensitization and avoidance of allergens.

Treatment

Antihistamines will reduce symptoms. Nasal sprays may be used, but continued use can cause a **rebound effect** when the drug is suddenly discontinued, leading to a return of the allergic symptoms. Decongestants are of little value. A process called desensitization is considered to be the most effective treatment. For a person to undergo desensitization, specific allergens must be identified. The specialist will then administer repeated small doses of the allergen until the person no longer has an allergic reaction. Sometimes a change of residence is recommended to provide an environment as free of the allergen as possible.

Urticaria and Angioedema

Urticaria is a skin condition that is more commonly called hives. It is characterized by the development of itchy wheals (raised white lumps surrounded by an area of red inflammation).

Sometimes a more severe condition called angioedema (swelling in areas of skin, mucous membranes, or internal organs) occurs with urticaria, or it may occur by itself. These reactions may occur in twenty percent of the population at one time or another.

Cause

It is sometimes difficult to identify the cause, but urticaria and angioedema are often due to a reaction to a particular food, food additive, insect sting,

---

otitis media   o-TI-tis ME-dea
urticaria   ur-ti-KA-re-a

or drug. In any case, the reaction is thought to be related to the release of histamine. In some individuals, exposure to cold, heat, water, or sunlight may also cause urticaria and angioedema. There are also a number of other disorders that can cause these reactions, including Hodgkin's disease, systemic lupus **erythematosus,** and psychogenic disease.

Symptoms

The main symptom of urticaria is a rash. Itchy, raised white lumps surrounded by an area of red inflammation appear. These lesions vary in size, and large ones may merge into large patches. Angioedema produces sudden swellings in the skin, throat, and other areas.

Prevention

Avoidance of allergens, if possible, is the best means of prevention.

Treatment

Antihistamines can ease the itching and swelling for every kind of urticaria. Medicated lotions can also reduce the discomfort from itching.

Asthma

Asthma attacks can be terrifying experiences for everyone involved because of the difficulty the victim has in breathing. Spasms of the bronchial tubes, increased mucous secretion, and swelling of the mucous membranes are responsible for the airway obstruction.

Extrinsic asthma begins in childhood and is usually accompanied by other allergies, such as allergic rhinitis. In *intrinsic* asthma, which is more common in adults, no extrinsic allergen can be identified. Most of these cases are preceded by a severe respiratory infection. About one in ten children experiences asthma as does one in twenty of the general population. It can strike at any age, but half of all cases occur in children under ten years of age, and it affects twice as many boys as girls in this age group. When it occurs in the ten- to thirty-year-old age group, the incidence is equal among the sexes.

Cause

A predisposition for asthma seems to be inherited, because three-fourths of children with two asthmatic parents have the disorder, and about one-third of asthmatic children share the disease with at least one other member of the family. Extrinsic asthma attacks are brought on by exposure to allergens, whereas attacks of intrinsic asthma can be due to a number of factors, including emotional stress, fatigue, endocrine changes, temperature and humidity changes, and exposure to noxious fumes. Many asthmatics have both intrinsic and extrinsic asthma.

Symptoms

Asthma attacks may begin abruptly or insidiously. An acute attack leads to sudden difficulties in breathing, wheezing, tightness in the chest, and a cough with thick, clear or yellow sputum. The victims may be unable to speak and feel as if they are suffocating. If the attack comes on gradually, these symptoms are mild at first but may progress to become as severe as the acute attack. Without treatment, the disease can lead to respiratory failure and death.

Prevention

In extrinsic asthma, avoidance of known allergens is the best prevention. For intrinsic asthma, predisposing factors need to be avoided or removed as much as possible.

Treatment

Acute attacks may be relieved by a number of drugs. For persistent asthma, adrenocortical hormones may be required. These hormones provide dramatic relief but cannot be used on a long-term basis because of dangerous side effects. A new drug, Azamacort, can be inhaled but it does not help acute attacks. However, it can be used over a longer time without the same dangerous side effects as the corticoids. Sedatives and expectorants are sometimes used. Controlling the predisposing factors and removing allergens is considered to be the best treatment.

AUTOIMMUNITY

Rheumatoid Arthritis

Rheumatoid arthritis is a chronic systemic inflammatory disease that primarily attacks peripheral joints and surrounding muscles, tendons, liga-ments, and blood vessels. The disease generally progresses slowly but is potentially crippling, and ten percent of its victims suffer total disability.

One of the distinguishing characteristics of the disease is the tendency for the pain that occurs as a result of the inflammation to fluctuate in severity, at times even disappearing altogether for a time (spontaneous remission). This characteris-tic has resulted in many claims of miraculous cures by different methods when in fact the "cure" received credit for what was a natural decrease in pain or natural remission at an opportune time. Many unscrupulous quacks have taken advantage of this phenomenon to promote their worthless products.

The disease occurs worldwide but is found three times as often in women as in men. Although rheumatoid arthritis can occur at any age, it gener-ally appears in women between the ages of thirty and sixty. More than six and a half million people are affected in the United States.

Cause

The cause is unknown. However, the most widely held theory is that it is an autoimmune disease. The belief is that the changes in the joints are related to an antigen-antibody reaction that is poorly under-stood. Individuals who get rheumatoid arthritis are believed to have a genetic susceptibility.

Symptoms

Rheumatoid arthritis develops insidiously with non-specific symptoms. These include fatigue, malaise, anorexia, persistent low-grade fever, weight loss, lymphadenopathy, and vague joint pain. Later, more specific symptoms appear in affected joints. They may stiffen after use and become tender and painful. At first the pain occurs only upon moving the joint, but eventually it is present even at rest. As the disease progresses, joint function diminishes. Deformities are common: joints may swell and wrists and fingers assume unnatural positions (Figure 3-9). The most common overt sign is the gradual appearance of rheumatoid nodules, usually in pressure areas. Inflammation of the blood vessels

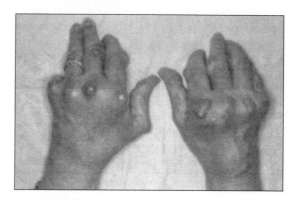

Figure 3-9
Rheumatoid arthritis

can lead to skin lesions and leg ulcers. Other com-plications of rheumatoid arthritis include osteo-porosis, myositis, cardiopulmonary lesions, **lymph-adenopathy,** and peripheral neuritis.

Prevention

No preventive measures are known at present.

Treatment   *rest*

No modern drug has proved as effective for reliev-ing the pain and inflammation of rheumatoid arthritis as aspirin. Unfortunately, many individu-als cannot tolerate aspirin and develop stomach problems. Nonsteroidal antiinflammatory drugs (NSAIDs) have been effective but may also cause stomach problems. Corticosteroids are very effec-tive but have prohibitive side effects. Gold salts and immunosuppressives are used when other therapies are not effective. Methotrexate, a drug originally used in cancer chemotherapy, has been found to be effective, in much smaller doses, for rheumatoid arthritis but is generally a second-line choice. Rest is of great importance during the acute phase, with eight to ten hours of sleep every night and frequent rest periods between daily activities. Physiotherapy helps to restore function *exercise* and prevent crippling deformities. In advanced disease, surgical repair may be necessary. *joint replacement & repair.*

erythematosus	er-i-the-ma-TOS-is
lymphadenopathy	lym-fad-en-OP-a-the

✱ Diagnosis = By Lab & X-rays

✱ exacerbations = increase in symptoms

remissions = symptoms subside temporarily mild symptoms

Lupus Erythematosus

This chronic inflammatory disorder of the connective tissues appears in two forms, cutaneous and systemic. Cutaneous lupus erythematosus is a mild form that affects only the skin, whereas the systemic kind affects the skin and a number of organ systems and can be fatal. Systemic lupus erythematosus (SLE) resembles rheumatoid arthritis in that there are times of complete remission and at different times the symptoms may be mild or severe.

The disease occurs eight times more frequently in women than in men, and this increases to fifteen times more often for women during childbearing years. The disease is found worldwide but is more prevalent among Asians and blacks. *3X more*

Cause   *500000 in US diagnosed*

Physical or mental stress, streptococcal or viral infections, exposure to sunlight or ultraviolet light, immunization, pregnancy, and abnormal estrogen metabolism may make a person more susceptible to SLE. Individuals who develop cutaneous lupus erythematosus go on to SLE in about five percent of the cases. The exact cause of these diseases is unknown, but evidence suggests an autoimmune defect.

Symptoms

There are a variety of symptoms that may occur in individuals with SLE. They may appear suddenly or slowly and, in ninety percent of patients, are similar to arthritis symptoms. Other symptoms include fever, weight loss, malaise, fatigue, and skin rashes. A butterfly rash over the nose and cheeks occurs in less than fifty percent of the patients (Figure 3-10). Skin lesions generally appear in areas exposed to light. Individuals who have the more serious form of the disease can develop myocarditis, renal involvement leading to kidney failure, convulsive disorders, and other complications that can lead to death. In cutaneous lupus erythematosus, there are raised, red, scaling

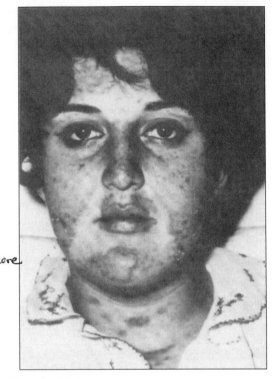

Figure 3-10
Lupus erythematosus.

plaques that, if not treated, can lead to scarring and permanent disfigurement. These lesions can appear anywhere on the body, but they usually erupt on the face, scalp, ears, neck, and arms.

Prevention

No preventive measures are known at present.

Treatment

If the disease is mild, little or no treatment is required. For the systemic form, corticosteroids are the treatment of choice. Some individuals who are particularly sensitive to light need to wear protective clothing and use a screening agent when out in the sun.

- Surgery if joints are bad
- steroids
- non steroidal anti inflam -
  ex- advil

SUMMARY

The cell is the basic structural unit of all life. Injury and death of cells caused by outside agents can lead to aging, disease, and death of the individual.

The many theories of aging can be divided into two categories, programmed theories and error theories. Two of the theories, the telomerase and free radical theories are receiving intense interest today. However, many scientists feel that the quality of life in old age must be improved before lengthening the life span is practical.

The human body is protected by *natural immunity* and *acquired immunity*. In natural immunity there are nonspecific and specific defense mechanisms. Nonspecific mechanisms are the external barriers to injury and infection, such as the skin and mucus and the inflammatory response. The body is also able to repair damage to tissue, but there are factors that influence the speed and extent of repair possible. Specific defense mechanisms are composed of antibody-mediated and cell-mediated responses.

B cells, T cells, and complement are all active in the immune response to infection.

There are four kinds of acquired immunity. Acquired active natural immunity is present after an individual has been exposed to a disease and the body has learned to produce antibodies. Acquired active artificial immunity occurs when an individual has been vaccinated with a disease agent. Acquired passive natural immunity results from the passage of antibodies from the mother to the fetus or baby. Finally, acquired passive artificial immunity is a result of inoculation with antibodies.

The immune system sometimes malfunctions, and this leads to conditions referred to as hypersensitivity and autoimmune disorders. The most common hypersensitivity disorders are allergic rhinitis, urticaria and angioedema, and asthma. Two of the most common autoimmune disorders are rheumatoid arthritis and lupus erythematosus.

QUESTIONS FOR REVIEW

1. Briefly explain the function of the major organelles in the human cell.
2. What is the telomerase theory of aging?
3. What is the theory of free radicals pertaining to aging?
4. What are the external barriers to infection in natural, nonspecific immunity?
5. How do the external barriers protect us from disease?
6. What do the "friendly" bacteria do to protect us from disease?
7. What produces the inflammatory response?
8. What are the signs of inflammation?
9. Explain what occurs during the inflammatory response.
10. What is chemotaxis?
11. What are the principal chemical mediators of the inflammatory response?
12. How does interferon work to assist the body in the inflammatory response?
13. What is complement?
14. What are inflammatory exudates, and how do they perform in the inflammatory response?
15. When does resolution occur, and when do regeneration and repair occur in the inflammatory response?

16. What factors cause a difference in the time required for healing?
17. How are humoral and cell-mediated immunity different?
18. What occurs during the combined immune response?
19. What is the difference between acquired active natural immunity and acquired active artificial immunity?
20. What is the difference between acquired passive natural immunity and acquired passive artificial immunity?
21. How are *autoimmune* and *hypersensitivity* defined?
22. What are the characteristics of allergic rhinitis, urticaria, angioedema, and asthma?
23. What are common allergens or risk factors, symptoms, prevention, and treatment for:
    a. Allergic rhinitis?
    b. Urticaria and angioedema?
    c. Asthma?
24. What are the characteristics of rheumatoid arthritis and lupus erythematosus?
25. What are the risk factors, symptoms, prevention, and treatment for:
    a. Rheumatoid arthritis?
    b. Lupus erythematosus?

FURTHER READING

Bousquet, J. 1999. Rapid symptom relief in rhinitis. *Clinical and Experimental Allergy* 29:25.

Day, J. 1999. Pros and cons of the use of antihistamines in managing allergic rhinitis. *Journal of Allergy and Clinical Immunology* 103:395.

de Bono, J., and L. Hudsmith. 1999. Occupational asthma: a community based study. *Occupational Medicine* 49:217.

De Bruin-Weller, M.S., et al. 1999. Repeated allergen challenge as a new research model for studying allergic reactions. *Clinical and Experimental Allergy* 29:159.

Eyles, Jim E. 2000. Intranasal Administration of influenza vaccines: current status. *BioDrugs* 13:35.

Gariballa, S.E., and A.J. Sinclair. 1999. Cerebrovascular disease and oxidative stress. *Reviews in Clinical Gerontology* 9:197.

Godnic-Cvar, J., et al. 1999. Respiratory and immunological findings in brewery workers. *American Journal of Industrial Medicine* 35:68.

Hanson, L.A. 1998. Breastfeeding provides passive and likely long-lasting active immunity. *Annals of Allergy, Asthma, and Immunology* 81:523.

Hesselmar, B., et al. 1999. Does early exposure to cat or dog protect against later allergy development? *Clinical and Experimental Allergy* 29:611.

Holt, S.E., et al. 1999. Resistance to apoptosis in human cells conferred by telomerase function and telomere stability. *Mol Carcinog* August, 241.

O'Connor, G.T., and D.R. Gold. 1999. Cockroach allergy and asthma in a 30-year-old man. *Environmental Health Perspectives* 107:243.

Schaefer, O.P., and J.M. Gore. 1999. Aspirin sensitivity: the role for aspirin challenge and desensitization in postmyocardial infarction patients. *Cardiology* 91:8.

Schell, H.M. 1999. The immunocompromised host and risk for cardiovascular infection. *Journal of Cardiovascular Nursing* 13:31.

Schwartz, Robert S. 1999. The new immunology—the end of immunosuppressive drug therapy? *New England Journal of Medicine* 340:1754.

Shore, S., S. Shinkai, and S. Rhind, et al. 1999. Immune responses to training: How critical is training volume? *Journal of Sports Medicine and Physical Fitness* 39:1.

Sly, R.M. 1999. Changing prevalence of allergic rhinitis and asthma. *Annals of Allergy, Asthma and Immunology* 82:233.

Strauss, Evelyn. 1999. Anti-immune trick unveiled in salmonella. *Science* 285:306.

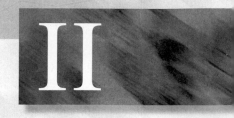

Infectious Disease

Since the relationship between disease and bacteria was discovered by Pasteur, Lister, and Koch in the nineteenth century, great strides have been made in the fight against infectious disease. Effective treatment and cures have been found for many diseases that at one time led to much suffering, scarring, crippling, and death.

More important than being able to treat and cure infectious disease, however, is the ability to prevent it from occurring. Jenner's discovery of the smallpox vaccination in the eighteenth century provided the means for preventing and eventually eradicating this disfiguring and potentially fatal disease, and today we are able to prevent infection with a number of diseases by vaccination or inoculation.

In the past three decades, doctors, scientists, and health educators have begun to focus their attention, not on what causes people to get sick, but what causes some people, exposed to the same diseases, to stay well. This change in focus has coincided with rapid development in the

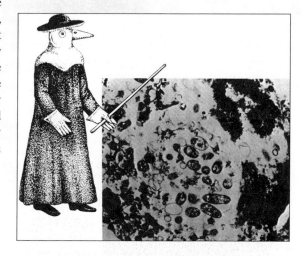

Doctor's protective wear from fourteenth-century plague epidemic.

Electron micrograph of *Legionella pneumophila (right).*

science of immunology. Increasing evidence of a mind-body link in the development of disease and disorders has led to a new discipline, psychoneuroimmunology, mentioned in Chapter 2.

All persons may be created equal in their right to "life, liberty and the pursuit of happiness" but they are not created or born equal in biochemical makeup. About ten percent of the population never have a cold. In any disease epidemic some individuals escape the disease even though they have never had an apparent infection or been vaccinated against it. Everyone reacts differently to drugs of any kind. One glass of wine may make some people relaxed and sleepy although others can consume two or three glasses with little or no observable effect. Likewise, medicinal drugs have to be adjusted in dosage for each person to gain the best therapeutic level. We are all born with an immune system that protects us from disease but even our immune systems vary in effectiveness. Regardless

of how strong an immune response we have at birth, its effectiveness can be increased (or decreased) by our lifestyle.

As indicated in the first chapter, people must take responsibility for their own health. A physician can diagnose and advise a patient, but each individual makes the decision whether to follow that advice. In many cases, it involves a change in lifestyle to reach an optimum level of health. That "best" level is different for each person but years of research have demonstrated the effectiveness of a healthy lifestyle including good nutrition, regular exercise, and stress management (mental and emotional health). Most people know that positive changes in lifestyle can provide protection against heart disease and cancer, but many do not know that these changes will increase resistance to infectious disease also. The factors involved in improving resistance to infectious (and noninfectious) disease are shown in the illustration below.

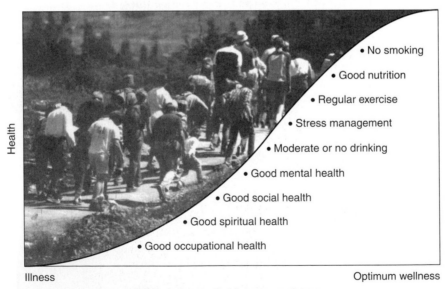

Lifestyle factors that increase resistance

Bacterial Diseases Acquired through the Respiratory Route

OBJECTIVES

1. *Explain the positive and negative effects that lifestyle can have on our susceptibility to disease.*

2. *Identify common upper respiratory infections.*

3. *Identify the two most common forms of pneumonia.*

4. *State environmental conditions conducive to Legionnaires' disease.*

5. *Discuss the connection between streptococcal sore throat, scarlet fever, and rheumatic fever.*

6. *Name and describe the stages of whooping cough.*

7. *Explain why diphtheria may still be a problem today.*

8. *Explain the processes involved in primary and secondary tuberculosis.*

9. *Apply techniques to prevent the spread of bacterial diseases acquired through the respiratory route.*

10. *Discuss characteristics, transmission, symptoms, treatment, prevention, and control for bacterial diseases acquired through the respiratory route.*

BRIEF REVIEW OF THE RESPIRATORY SYSTEM

Normal respiration requires efficient action of the diaphragm, a clear route to the lungs, healthy bronchial tubes, and effective diffusion of gases (Figure 4-1). Oxygen that is inhaled must be diffused across the alveolar-capillary membrane into the blood; at the same time, carbon dioxide is being diffused from the blood across the same membranes, into the lungs for exhalation.

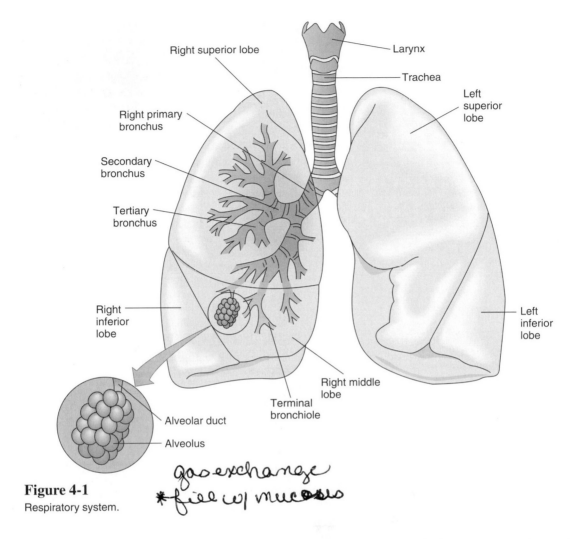

Figure 4-1
Respiratory system.

gas exchange
*fill w/ mucous

Air usually enters the body through the nose. During periods of exertion, it may enter through the mouth, but the nose is a preferable point of entry for several reasons. First, the cilia (fine hairs in the nasal cavity) protect against dust and other particles from the air. Next, particles that may slip through the cilia are caught in the thick, sticky, mucous lining of the nasal cavity, allowing only clean air to pass to the lungs. Third, air is warmed in the nasal cavity, and, finally, moisture is added.

Air passes from the nose backward and downward through the pharynx to the larynx. The larynx contains the vocal cords, through which the air passes on its way to the trachea. The trachea branches into the right and left bronchial tubes, which in turn branch into bronchioles, which ultimately end in the alveolar sacs. It is here that the cycle of oxygen diffusion into the blood and CO_2 diffusion out of the blood occurs.

UPPER RESPIRATORY INFECTIONS (URIs)

Infection of the upper respiratory tract is caused most frequently by bacteria and viruses. These infections are generally superficial and may be acute, chronic, or recurrent. Pharyngitis, laryngi-

Tylenol doesn't bring down swelling

tis, tonsillitis, and sinusitis are due to infection of the pharynx, larynx, tonsils, and sinuses, respectively (Figure 4-2). They are usually preceded by the common cold. An extension into the eustachian tube of the disease agents that cause pharyngitis may lead to **otitis media** (inflammation of the middle ear). The relationship between the pharynx, eustachian tube, and middle ear can be seen in Figures 4-2 and 4-3.

The most important agents of bacterial pharyngitis and laryngitis are streptococci and *Staphylococcus aureus.* Other disease agents may be involved in sinusitis and *otitis media.* The incu-

bation period for these URIs is short (one to two days) when person-to-person transmission is involved. It is not known how long the infections take to develop if they are endogenous. URIs are communicable as long as they are active. Natural resistance to the disease agents that cause these infections is present in individuals whose mucous membranes are not compromised. Colds and other

Staphylococcus aureus	Staph-il-o KOK-us AU-re-us

[handwritten: ear infection]

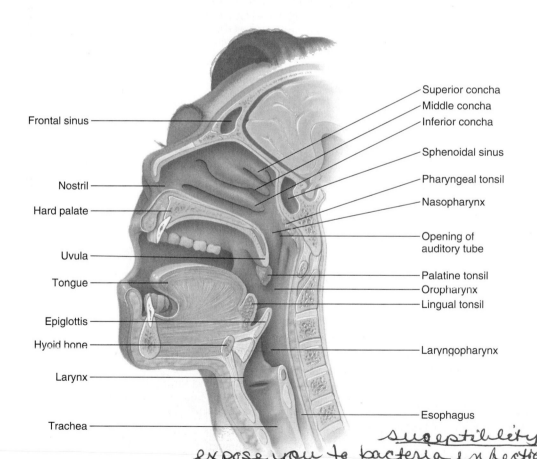

Frontal sinus

Nostril

Hard palate

Uvula

Tongue

Epiglottis

Hyoid bone

Larynx

Trachea

Superior concha

Middle concha

Inferior concha

Sphenoidal sinus

Pharyngeal tonsil

Nasopharynx

Opening of auditory tube

Palatine tonsil

Oropharynx

Lingual tonsil

Laryngopharynx

Esophagus

Figure 4-2
Upper respiratory system.

[handwritten: susceptibility expose you to bacteria infection: Stress, eating right, smoke, pollen toxic fumes (nail salon)]

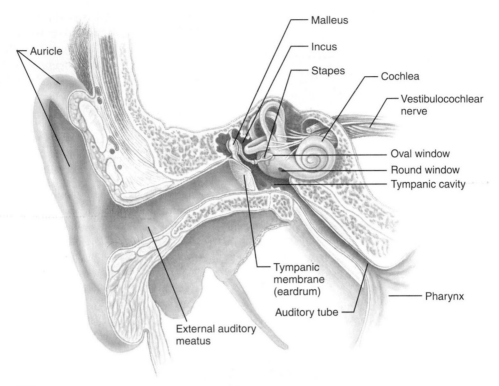

Figure 4-3
External, middle, and inner ear.

viral infections, inhalation of toxic vapors or smoke, excessive dryness, and pollen or dust allergies all may predispose an individual to bacterial infections.

Transmission

Human beings are the reservoir for the organisms that are most often responsible for URIs. If the infection is transmitted from person to person, it is generally by airborne droplets but may also be by direct or indirect contact with secretions from the nose and throat of an infected person.

Symptoms

Individuals with pharyngitis experience a sore throat and slight difficulty in swallowing. Laryngitis involves pain in the area of the larynx and hoarseness or loss of voice. In sinusitis, there is pain of the sinuses involved, and otitis media causes earache. Individuals with these infections

may also have a low fever, headache, and muscle and joint pain.

Prevention #1 defense

Washing the hands regularly, particularly after contact with people during times when these infections are known to be prevalent, is a good preventive measure along with avoidance of predisposing factors mentioned earlier.

dishwasher
Control

Those who have a URI need to practice careful personal hygiene, disposing of any contaminated tissues in closed paper or plastic bags and washing their hands frequently and carefully. Drinking or eating utensils should be thoroughly washed.

Treatment

Treatment for URIs caused by bacteria is with antibiotics.

cold — mucus sits there for a while, and it becomes a bacterial infection.

SINUSITIS

According to Rachelefsky, et al., in *Patient Care,* sinusitis is "the most frequently reported chronic disease in the U.S., with thirty-five million Americans suffering from the condition." Several disease agents, including pneumococci and ***Haemophilus influenzae*** can cause sinus infection. Infection occurs when the sinus passages are blocked, which can occur with a number of conditions. Chronic sinusitis may be the result of allergic rhinitis, nasal edema, persistent bacterial infection, or a purulent acute sinusitis.

Transmission

Pneumococci are natural inhabitants of the human body and can cause disease when resistance is lowered. *H. influenzae* is transmitted by airborne droplets or secretions from the nose and throat.

Symptoms

The symptoms of acute sinusitis include fever; congestion; sore throat; thickened, discolored nasal discharge; and a cough. Because of the proximity of the paranasal sinuses to the roots of the teeth, there can be tooth pain (Figure 4-4). Tenderness or swelling can sometimes be found over the affected sinuses. The symptoms for chronic sinusitis are not as distinct. Usually there is congestion, cough, and postnasal discharge.

Prevention

Maintaining a lifestyle that produces the optimal level of resistance for each individual is the best

---

Haemophilus influenzae   He-MOF-il-us in-flu-ENZ-i

---

if sinus passageways are small — infection is more likely.

pain

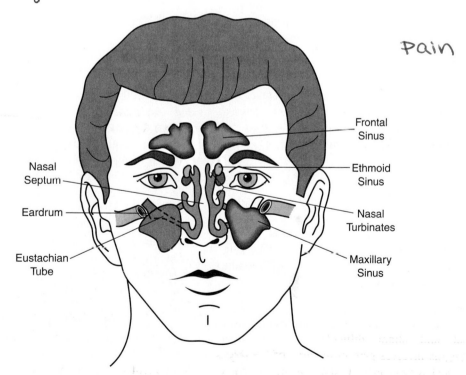

Figure 4-4
Sinuses.

Nasal Septum

Eardrum

Eustachian Tube

Frontal Sinus

Ethmoid Sinus

Nasal Turbinates

Maxillary Sinus

antihistamine = drys things up

de-congestant = keeps things running.

*Steroids - reduce swelling *sinuses can drain*

Steroids

means of prevention. Whenever a cold lasts more than a week and the nasal discharge becomes discolored, a physician should be consulted.

Control
Control is the same as for other URIs, although chronic sinusitis may no longer be infectious.

Treatment
Antibiotics may be prescribed by a physician.

STREPTOCOCCAL SORE THROAT (PHARYNGITIS)

Because sore throat caused by *Streptococcus pyogenes* can lead to more serious illness it will be dealt with in more detail, as will the possible **sequelae:** rheumatic fever, rheumatic heart disease, and glomerulonephritis (infection of the kidneys). Ninety-five percent of all bacterial sore throats are caused by *S. pyogenes.* They are most common in children six to twelve years of age and from October to April. Up to twenty percent of schoolchildren are thought to be carriers. *Otitis media* or acute sinusitis are the most frequent complications.

Transmission
Transmission is by direct or intimate contact with an individual with active pharyngitis or a carrier. Ingestion of contaminated food may lead to sudden outbreaks of streptococcal sore throat.

Symptoms
A temperature of 101 to 104°F, severe sore throat, swollen glands and tonsils, malaise and weakness, anorexia, and occasional abdominal discomfort are included in the symptoms. Up to forty percent of small children have symptoms too mild for diagnosis, and all symptoms that do occur tend to disappear in a week.

Prevention
Although strep sore throat is generally severe enough for the individual to seek medical attention, symptoms may be milder in children. Any child who has a sore throat that is constant, and is accompanied by fever and other signs of infection,

should be seen by a doctor. The public needs to be educated about the possible sequelae of strep sore throat. Information on means of transmission should be widely published. Avoidance of close contact with infected persons and proper food handling are the best means of prevention.

Control
In an outbreak of strep sore throat, the source of infection and manner of spread should be investigated, because these can often be traced to a carrier. Milk and food supplies should be checked for contamination. In special circumstances, antibiotics may be given **prophylactically.**

Treatment
Although there is an increasing problem with drug-resistant bacteria, *S. pyogenes* has not developed resistance at this writing. Penicillin and other antibiotics are still effective treatment and should be administered for ten days. If the treatment is given within the first twenty-four to forty-eight hours, the illness may be milder, and the risk of complications is diminished. Bed rest is also recommended.

RHEUMATIC FEVER *Rheumatic valve - heart*

Rheumatic fever is a disease of childhood that does not stand alone. It is always preceded by another streptococcal infection, often strep sore throat, and it may lead to heart or kidney disease. As with many other bacterial diseases, it is no longer as serious as it once was and is becoming rare since the availability and use of antibiotics. However, because not everyone gets treatment for a sore throat and because the symptoms of rheumatic fever may be mild enough to go unnoticed, it is still a potentially dangerous disease. It is possible for damage to be done to the heart that may not become apparent until much later in life.

Why infection with *S. pyogenes* sometimes leads from strep sore throat to rheumatic fever to rheumatic heart disease or to other tissue damage is not known. It is thought that altered host resistance and a hypersensitivity reaction (antibodies

malaise = weak

[handwritten note top left: Strep does permanent damage to heart valve]

manufactured to combat the streptococci attacking the heart and joints) are factors. Rheumatic fever is more prevalent in some families and in lower socioeconomic groups, perhaps because of malnutrition and crowded living conditions. It is a disease of childhood but is often recurrent, especially without adequate treatment.

Transmission
Rheumatic fever cannot be transmitted from one person to another, because it is not a bacterial infection but a hypersensitivity reaction. If the person still harbors the streptococcal organism that preceded the rheumatic fever, then transmission of that organism can occur.

Symptoms
Fever and migratory joint pain are most commonly the early symptoms of rheumatic fever. Some individuals have the infection but do not suffer joint pain. Other symptoms include abdominal pain, a rash, nodules under the skin, cardiac involvement, and up to six months later, chorea (involuntary muscular twitching of face or limbs).

Prevention
The public needs to be educated on the relationship between a streptococcal infection and rheumatic fever. The best prevention for rheumatic fever is immediate antibiotic treatment.

Control
In recurrent episodes of rheumatic fever in a family or in epidemic situations, an investigation needs to be carried out to find all carriers and administer proper treatment. Contact investigation (finding those known to have been exposed to the disease and testing each one for possible infection) should be pursued. Any unusual grouping of cases should be investigated for the possibility of contaminated milk or foods. In some circumstances, penicillin or another antibiotic may be given prophylactically.

Treatment
Immediate treatment of the primary infection with antibiotics will eradicate the organism, relieve the symptoms, and prevent development of hypersen-

sitivity-related complications. Penicillin is the drug of choice, but for those allergic to it, erythromycin and other antibiotics can be used.

SCARLET FEVER
Scarlet fever is generally preceded by streptococcal sore throat. It occurs when the pathogenic organism *S. pyogenes* produces erythrogenic *[handwritten: =redness]* toxin. Many individuals are immune to this toxin, but if they are not, then scarlet fever is the result. The incidence and severity of scarlet fever have been declining, probably as a result of the frequent use of antibiotics. Penicillin and other antibiotics are extremely effective in destroying the streptococcal organisms. Humans are the reservoir for the streptococci that are responsible for scarlet fever. The incubation period is rarely more than three days. Communicability generally ends after twenty-four to forty-eight hours of antibiotic treatment. Almost everyone is susceptible, although some individuals may have immunity, as noted above.

Transmission
[handwritten: can't spread scarlet fever we catch - strep throat - turns into scarlet fever]
Transmission is by droplet spread, direct contact, and indirect contact with temporarily contaminated environmental sources, including milk or food.

Symptoms
The infected individual has a sore throat, rash, nausea, vomiting, and fever. A distinctive symptom for scarlet fever is the strawberry tongue, which at first has red papillae showing through a furry white coat. In two or three days the tongue loses the white coat and gradually becomes red. The rash is fine, blanches on pressure, and resembles sunburn with goosebumps. It usually appears first on the upper chest, then spreads to the neck, abdomen, legs, and arms, sparing the soles and palms. The cheeks are

pyogenes	PY-o-genes
sequelae	se-KWE-li
prophylactically	pro-fi-LAK-tic-lee

flushed, with pallor (paleness) around the mouth. Desquamation (shedding of skin) that occurs during convalescence can be seen. Figure 4-5 shows how the signs and symptoms of scarlet fever develop.

Prevention

Preventive methods are the same as for the other streptococcal diseases already discussed.

Control

Isolation is not necessary if antibiotics are given immediately. Disinfection of all items contaminated with purulent discharge, and other hygienic measures, will control the infection.

Treatment

Penicillin is the drug of choice. Streptococci are also susceptible to erythromycin and clindamycin. Adequate levels of antibiotics need to be maintained for ten days.

PNEUMONIA   3 types

Pneumonia and influenza are the only communicable diseases that still hold a place among the top ten causes of death in the United States. The two are placed together on the chart because death from pneumonia is often preceded by influenza.

Pneumonia is an acute infection of the lungs and can be caused by every infectious agent except **helminths** (Table 4-1). However, bacterial pneumonia is the most common type and is the fifth leading cause of death among the elderly and debilitated.

There are three ways to classify pneumonia: (1) disease agent, (2) location, and (3) type. It may be bronchial, involving the bronchial tubes and alveoli (see Figure 4-1); lobular, involving part of a lobe; or lobar, involving the entire lobe (see Figure 4-1). Pneumonia is also referred to as primary, resulting from inhalation or aspiration of a pathogen, or secondary, involving spread of bacteria from another location. *[handwritten: usually results in death — inhaling liquid]*

Pneumococcal and mycoplasmal pneumonia will be discussed in this chapter and also a type of pneumonia that has been recognized only since 1976, Legionnaires' disease.

Pneumococcal Pneumonia

Pneumococcal pneumonia, caused by *Streptococcus pneumoniae,* is the most common type of pneumonia and is more frequent among the very young and the very old. It is also commonly a cause of death among alcoholics. Pneumococci are natural inhabitants in the upper respiratory tract of healthy per-

[handwritten: alcoholics = poor nutrition — lowered immune system]

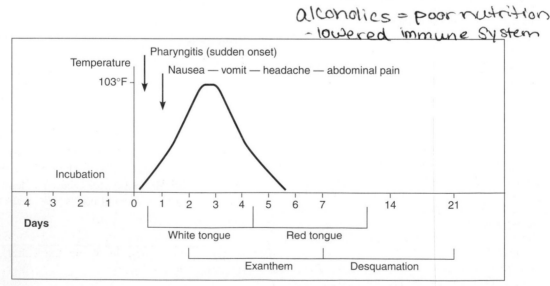

Figure 4-5
Evolution of signs and symptoms of scarlet fever.

TABLE 4-1	Examples of Pathogens that Can Cause Pneumonia
PATHOGEN	**COMMENTS**
BACTERIA	Many bacteria are capable of causing pneumonia. Some, like *Streptococcus pneumoniae* cause primary pneumonia, whereas the pneumonia caused by others is secondary (to another infection)
S. pneumoniae	Most common primary cause (seventy percent of cases)
H. influenzae	Once thought to cause influenza but other organisms found to be the cause; increasingly common in hospitals (nosocomial)
Staphylococcus aureus	Common inhabitant of human body (opportunistic) antibiotic resistant
Klebsiella pneumoniae	Secondary to another infection
Legionella pneumophila	Legionnaires' disease
Mycoplasmal pneumonia	Primary atypical pneumonia
Chlamydia pneumoniae	Most frequent in young adults but disease has occurred in all ages
Chlamydia trachomatis	Congenital; secondary to mother's genital infection with chlamydia
VIRUSES	
Respiratory syncytial	Infants and children
Adenovirus	Usually affects young adults
Influenza (A, B, C)	More in infants and elderly
FUNGI	
Aspergillus fumigatus	Opportunistic
Pneumocystis carinii	Opportunistic; AIDS patients extremely susceptible
PROTOZOA	
Toxoplasmoses gondii	Compromised immune system causes susceptibility

sons. The incubation period is uncertain but is probably one to three days. With antibiotic therapy, an infected individual will become noninfectious within twenty-four to forty-eight hours. Without treatment, the individual will be able to communicate the disease as long as discharges contain virulent pneumococci in significant numbers. Most people have good resistance to the organism, but any factor causing injury to lung tissues may lower that resistance. Viral respiratory infections, chronic lung disease, and exposure to irritants in the air are some factors responsible for lowered resistance.

Transmission

Casual contact with an individual who has pneumonia does not generally lead to infection. Transmission occurs by droplet spread, direct oral contact, or indirectly through fomites (inanimate objects that have been contaminated with respiratory discharges).

Symptoms

The onset of pneumococcal pneumonia is usually sudden, with chills, fever, chest pain, difficult breathing, and cough. The sputum may be bright red or rusty with blood. Pleurisy (inflammation of the external membrane surrounding the lung) may also be present, causing sharp pain during breathing or coughing. In some cases, particularly in the elderly, the onset of pneumonia is more insidious, with X ray examination producing the first evidence. In children under two years of age, vomiting and convulsions may be the initial signs.

Prevention

A vaccine is available and is recommended for high-risk individuals, including the elderly, the debilitated, and alcoholics.

---

helminths   hell-MINTHS

Control

Generally no measures are necessary unless an outbreak is a threat, in which case crowding should be avoided, especially in populations with low resistance, such as pediatric wards, geriatric institutions, and military hospitals.

Treatment

S. pneumoniae has become resistant to some forms of penicillin and other drugs. There are still antibiotics that can be used but the increasing resistance of microorganisms to antibiotics is a growing threat to the progress made in controlling bacterial disease.

Mycoplasmal Pneumonia   *walking pneumonia*

It is estimated that twenty percent of all pneumonias are caused by *Mycoplasmal pneumoniae.* This small, unusual bacterium is responsible for what has been called walking pneumonia. It is considered a primary atypical pneumonia, pneumonia that begins in the lower respiratory tract and does not produce the typical **exudative** (fluid-causing) response in the lungs. The disease occurs worldwide, with the greatest incidence during the fall and winter months in temperate climates. Humans are the reservoir of infection. **Mycoplasmal** pneumonia may be very mild or asymptomatic in children under five years of age and is more frequent among school-age children and young adults. The incubation period is usually about two weeks, and the disease is probably most communicable during the first week of apparent illness. Premature infants, those who have chronic debilitating diseases, and those in whom the immune system is compromised are more susceptible to mycoplasmal pneumonia.

Transmission

Infection is transferred by direct and indirect contact with respiratory secretions.

Symptoms

The onset of mycoplasmal pneumonia is insidious, with headache, malaise, and cough. The cough often occurs in sudden episodes (paroxysms), and there is usually substernal (under the chest bone) pain. The illness lasts from a few days to a month or more, and because symptoms are often mild, the infection may not be recognized as pneumonia. There generally are no complications, and fatalities are rare.

Prevention

No vaccines are available. Avoidance of crowding in living and sleeping quarters, especially in institutions, barracks, and on shipboard can decrease the risk.

Control

Investigation of contacts may identify cases of treatable disease. Proper sanitary measures including disposal of articles contaminated with respiratory secretions will help to control the spread of the infection.

Treatment

The mycoplasmal bacteria are resistant to penicillin, but erythromycin or tetracycline is effective in treating the disease.

Legionnaires' Disease   *classified as a pneumonia*

The epidemic of respiratory illness that swept through a group of people attending a state convention of American Legionnaires in Philadelphia during the summer of 1976 has already been mentioned as one of the emerging diseases since the early 1970s. Before the epidemic ended, it took 29 lives and hospitalized 182 people of the 5000 or more who had gathered for the convention. Epidemiologists worked around the clock in a search for the cause of the illness and death. Finally, bacteria were discovered in the cooling towers of the hotel headquarters for the convention and were identified as ***Legionella pneumophila.***

Although the organism had not been named before this time, it had been described as early as 1947 and probably had been the unrecognized cause of some cases of pneumonia for many years. The rise in reported cases shown in Figure 4-6 is partially due to increased recognition and reporting of the disease after the Legionnaires' convention.

Other types of *L. pneumophila* have been responsible for milder forms of respiratory illness.

CASE STUDY

Legionellosis

On October 15, 1996, a district health department in southwestern Virginia received a report from a hospital (hospital A) that fifteen patients had been admitted during October 12–13 with unexplained pneumonia. On October 21, another hospital (hospital B), located approximately fifteen miles from hospital A, reported its pneumonia census to be higher than expected for the first two weeks of October. On October 23, the district health department was informed about three area residents with legionellosis. Based on a review of the records, twenty-three cases eventually were identified. Twenty-two were hospitalized, and two died. The mean age of the patients was sixty-five years with a range of forty-two to eighty-six years and most (seventeen) were male.

The patients were asked about their activities during the two weeks before onset of illness. A history of having visited a large home improvement center during the two weeks before onset of illness was reported by fourteen (93%) of the fifteen cases compared with twelve (27%) of forty-five controls. Samples were collected and cultured for the presence of *Legionella* from water sources in the home improvement center, including a whirlpool spa, spa filters, a greenhouse sprinkler system, a decorative fish pond and fountain, potable water fountains, urinals, and hot and cold water taps in the store's restrooms.

The bacteria responsible for Legionnaires' disease were isolated from one of the filters of one of the whirlpool spas. All of the other possible sources tested negative. The people infected did not enter the water, but all most likely contracted the disease by spending time in the area or just walking by.

Source: Adapted from *Morbidity and Mortality Weekly Report* 46:83, 1997.

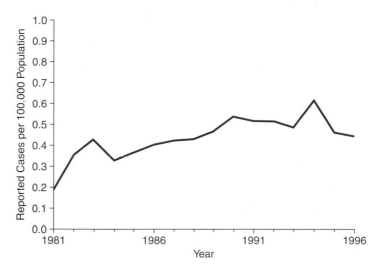

Figure 4-6
Legionellosis by year, United States, 1981–1996.

exudative EKS-u-da-tiv
mycoplasmal MI-ko-plas-mal
Legionella pneumophila Le-gin-EL-la nu-mo-FIL-a

The organism thrives in warm, moist conditions, and its reservoir is in soil and water. The disease has been diagnosed in most states in the United States and in some foreign countries. Outbreaks are recognized more often in the summer and autumn. The incubation period is two to ten days, most often, five to six days. Susceptibility to the organism is general, but the disease is uncommon in those under twenty years of age. Mortality rates in Legionnaires' disease have run as high as fifteen percent in hospitalized patients. Generally fatalities occur among those whose immunity is compromised.

Transmission

Outbreaks of this disease have revolved around faulty air cooling systems, cooling towers, or excavation sites. In these conditions, the organism is transmitted by air from the soil or water where it resides. Humans become infected through inhalation of the bacteria that have become airborne. There is no evidence of person-to-person transmission.

Symptoms

Onset of the disease may be gradual or sudden. Nonspecific symptoms appear first, including diarrhea, anorexia, malaise, **myalgias,** and generalized weakness, headache, recurrent chills, and an unremitting fever that may reach 105°F within twelve to forty-eight hours. After this, a nonproductive cough develops that may eventually produce grayish, blood-streaked sputum. Other characteristic symptoms include nausea, vomiting, disorientation, pleuritic chest pain, and, in fifty percent of patients, **bradycardia** (slow heartbeat). Complications include congestive heart failure, acute respiratory failure, renal failure, and shock, any of which can be fatal.

Prevention

No immunization is available. Cooling towers and water supplies that have been implicated need to be disinfected.

Control

The source of infection needs to be identified when there is a cluster of cases. Because there is no evidence of person-to-person transmission, isolation of individuals with the disease is not considered necessary.

Treatment

Penicillin is not effective against *L. pneumophila.* Erythromycin and tetracycline are the drugs of choice, and if they are not effective alone, **rifampin** can be added.

WHOOPING COUGH (PERTUSSIS) 3 Stages

Since the 1940s there has been a decrease in incidence and deaths from the disease because of immunization and aggressive diagnosis and treatment. However, the incidence has increased in recent years (Figure 4-7) because of fear of vaccine-associated complications that are rare, but were given headlines in newspapers. Lately there have been reports of vaccinated older adults contracting the disease. Although the disease is not often dangerous for adults, they can transmit it to infants and children. Researchers have reported that as high as "thirty-one percent of adults with a chronic cough have an undiagnosed infection" of the bacterium that causes whooping cough.* Epidemic cycles of pertussis tend to run every three to four years, and the epidemic incidence is highest in the winter and early spring. WHO estimates that half a million people die of pertussis each year.

Bordetella pertussis, a bacillus, causes the disease. The mortality from pertussis is usually a result of secondary pneumonia in children under one year of age, but it can also be dangerous to the elderly. Humans are the only reservoir for the organism. Whooping cough is highly communicable during late incubation and in the **catarrhal** stage (when mucous membranes of the head and throat are inflamed). Once the cough is present, communicability declines until in about three weeks there is little danger to contacts even though the cough persists. If treated with antibiotics, the communicable stage lasts only five to seven days. One attack generally confers prolonged immunity.

Transmission

Transmission is primarily by direct contact with airborne droplets from respiratory discharges of

*Kathleen Flackelmann, "100-day cough," *Science News* 150:46.

myalgia - muscle pain

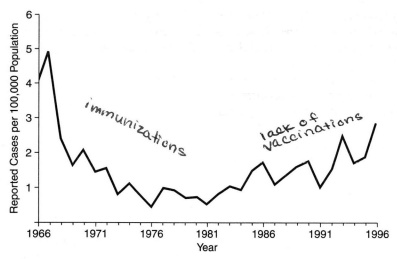

Figure 4-7

Pertussis (whooping cough) by year, United States, 1966–1996.
Source: *Morbidity and Mortality Weekly Report.* 1997. Summary of Notifiable Diseases.

infected persons. It may also be indirect from contact with contaminated objects.

Symptoms 3 Stages

There are three stages of whooping cough: the catarrhal (mentioned earlier), **paroxysmal,** and convalescent. The *catarrhal stage* has an insidious (cunning or sneaky) onset, and the symptoms resemble a cold. They may include an irritating cough, particularly at night; this may be accompanied by anorexia, sneezing, listlessness, infected conjunctiva, and sometimes a low-grade fever. The cough becomes progressively more irritating and violent and eventually paroxysmal (sudden and periodic).

This second or *paroxysmal stage* produces spasmodic and recurrent coughing that may expel tenacious mucus. The characteristic cough ends in a loud, high-pitched inspiratory whoop, and vomiting can occur because of choking on mucus. The coughing can be violent enough to cause complications such as nosebleed, detached retina, and hernias. During this stage, the individual is highly susceptible to secondary infections such as *otitis media* (middle ear infection), **encephalopathy** (brain damage), or pneumonia.

The second stage lasts about three weeks or until the paroxysmal coughing becomes less violent and less frequent.

The third stage is the *convalescent stage.* The cough may last one to two months, and even a mild upper respiratory infection may trigger it again. A summary of characteristics of the three stages is found in Table 4-2. Adults rarely experience more than a persistent cough that generally stops on its own. This is the reason for a misdiagnosis.

Prevention

Active immunization is available and should be administered at two to three months of age. A schedule is recommended for booster shots of the vaccine and should be followed to provide the best immunity. The vaccine for pertussis is generally

myalgia   my-AL-ge-a
bradycardia   brad-e-KAR-de-a
rifampin   RIF-am-pin
Bordetella   Bor-de-TEL-la
catarrhal   ka-TARR-hal
paroxysmal   par-ok-SIZ-mal
encephalopathy   en-SEF-a-lop-a-thee

TABLE 4-2	Duration and Symptoms for the Stages of Whooping Cough			
Stage	Incubation	Catarrhal	Paroxysmal	Convalescent
DURATION	7–10 days	1–2 weeks	2–4 weeks	3–4 weeks (or longer)
SYMPTOMS	None	Rhinorrhea, malaise, fever, sneezing, anorexia	Repetitive cough with whoops, vomiting, leukocytosis	Diminished paroxysmal cough, development of secondary complications (pneumonia, seizures, encephalopathy)

given in combination with that for diphtheria and tetanus and is referred to as DTP.

Control

Suspected cases should be isolated, particularly from young children and infants, until antibiotic therapy has been administered for at least five days. Close contacts who have not received the four DTP doses or have not received a DTP dose in the past three years, and are under seven years of age, should be given a dose as soon after exposure as possible. Prophylactic administration of gamma globulin may be indicated for susceptible children and adults who are exposed to whooping cough. Investigation of contacts should be performed to identify undiagnosed cases for proper treatment.

Treatment

Treatment of whooping cough is now vigorous and thorough. Infants are hospitalized, often in the intensive care unit (ICU), and fluid and electrolytes are administered. Nutritional supplements where needed, codeine and mild sedation to decrease coughing, oxygen therapy, and antibiotics may be used, depending on the case. Antibiotics are not very effective in relieving symptoms but do shorten the period of communicability.

DIPHTHERIA

At one time diphtheria was one of the leading causes of death in all parts of the world. Since the 1920s, when large-scale immunization of children began in the United States, the death rate has dropped dramatically, and the disease *was* uncommon in developed nations. However, since 1990 diphtheria has expanded to epidemic proportions in the former Soviet Union because of social upheaval and lack of health services. The WHO has declared the epidemic an international health emergency but the availability of funds has been slow. In addition, diphtheria is still an important cause of disease and death in developing nations, particularly among children. In 1995, 52,000 cases were reported worldwide and up to twenty-five percent of those infected have died.

Corynebacterium diphtheriae is the organism responsible for diphtheria. Unlike many of the other pathogenic organisms, this one does not invade other areas or tissues of the body but stays in the upper respiratory region. Here it produces a deadly exotoxin that irritates the tissue, producing a pseudomembrane (false membrane) which, along with swelling, may occlude the air passages, leading to death by suffocation. The toxin also spreads through the body, causing other serious symptoms, and often death, from its effects on the heart, nerves, and kidneys.

The reservoir of infection for the diphtheria organism is humans. The incubation period is generally two to five days, occasionally longer. The communicable period is variable, lasting up to four weeks, but the carrier state may persist for a lifetime. Infants born of immune mothers usually have passive resistance for up to six months.

An attack of diphtheria does not always confer immunity.

Transmission

Means of transmission are by direct contact, droplet spread, and indirect contact with articles soiled with discharges from infected persons. Milk that has been contaminated after pasteurization or raw milk may serve as a vehicle also.

Symptoms

The characteristic symptom of diphtheria is the thick, patchy, grayish green membrane that forms over the mucous membranes of the pharynx, larynx, tonsils, soft palate, and nose. Other symptoms include fever, sore throat, a rasping cough, hoarseness, and other symptoms similar to croup. If the pseudomembrane causes airway obstruction, then there is difficulty in breathing and possible suffocation if the disease is untreated. Complications include myocarditis, neurologic involvement, and kidney involvement.

Prevention

The only effective means of prevention is by a community program of active immunization with diphtheria toxoid. Generally it is combined with tetanus toxoid and pertussis vaccine (DTP). Children should be fully immunized before entering school. The exact schedule is up to the physician, but the first injection is generally given two to three months after birth, with one to four more being given at intervals. Special efforts should be made to see that persons who are at higher risk, such as health workers, are fully immunized and receive a booster dose every ten years.

Control

There should be strict isolation for anyone ill with pharyngeal diphtheria. All articles that come in contact with the individual who is sick should be disinfected. Any adult contacts who are food handlers should be screened to be sure they are not carriers. Antibiotics should be given prophylactically to nonimmunized contacts of the individual. Future control of diphtheria depends on continuing the education of people everywhere as to the necessity of adequate artificial active immunization.

Treatment

For treatment, diphtheria antitoxin is administered, antibiotics are used to destroy the organism, and measures taken to prevent complications.

TUBERCULOSIS (TB)

Tuberculosis is an ancient, worldwide disease, sometimes acute, more often chronic, caused by *Mycobacterium tuberculosis,* or tubercle bacillus. This bacillus has been found in Egyptian mummies from 4000 B.C. In the year 1900, two of every 1000 Americans died of tuberculosis, and twenty were ill with the disease. Great strides have been made in the prevention and control of this disease, but today, even in the United States, there are still some 30,000 cases of TB reported annually. That figure is down for the third year in a row after an eight-year surge (Figure 4-8). Although the overall decrease in the United States is good, according to the Centers for Disease Control and Prevention (CDCP) there were twenty states that reported no decrease or an increase in TB cases in 1998. Those with an increase included Arizona (28%), Minnesota (11%), Iowa (9%), Louisiana (9%), Pennsylvania (9%), and Wisconsin (7%). A comparison of rates in different states can be seen in Figure 4-9.

In 1993, WHO declared tuberculosis its first ever "global emergency." It has been estimated that twenty-two million people are infected with the tubercle bacillus worldwide. Nancy Dreher in *Current Health* states a number of factors that are involved in the reemergence of tuberculosis. (1) The compromised immune systems of those with HIV/AIDS. Tuberculosis was the leading killer of HIV-positive people in 1996. (2) Increased numbers of immigrants from countries where there are many cases and who have little or no access to health care. (3) Increased poverty, alcoholism and drug abuse, and homelessness, which make people more susceptible to TB. (4) The emergence of

---

Corynebacterium diphtheriae   Ko-rine-bak-TE-re-um dip-THE-ree-i

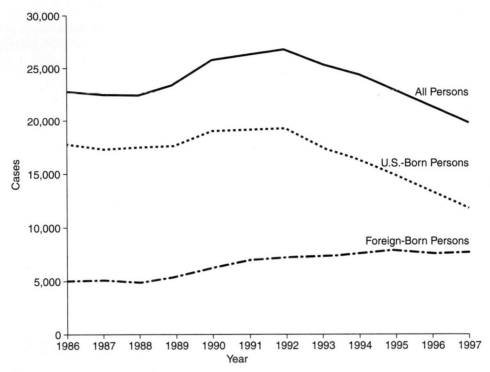

Figure 4-8

Number of persons with reported cases of tuberculosis by country of birth, United States, 1986–1997.

strains of TB that are resistant to the antibiotics used to treat the disease, leading to a fifty to sixty percent fatality rate even with treatment.

Compounding these factors is the difficulty that doctors have keeping TB-positive patients taking their medication for the full course (six months). After two to four weeks some people feel better and stop taking the prescribed drugs before they have taken enough to destroy all of the bacteria. The remaining bacteria can become drug resistant. Although the victims seem free of symptoms, they are still able to infect others.

TB is primarily a disease of the lungs, but if the organism invades the bloodstream, the liver, brain, urogenital tract, and bone can become infected. Illness and death rates increase with age and, in older persons, are higher in males than in females. There are much higher rates of the disease among the poor and among nonwhite races, and rates in cities are usually higher than in rural areas.

The primary reservoir is in humans, but in some areas the bacillus is also present in infected cattle. The incubation of four to twelve weeks is longer than for most infectious diseases. TB is communicable as long as the individual has tubercle bacilli in their sputum. The degree of communicability depends upon the intensity of infectious droplet contamination of the air. Susceptibility is general but is influenced by age, sex, race, nutrition, and general health.

Transmission

Transmission of TB may occur by direct or indirect contact with persons who have active pulmonary lesions, but the usual route is by inhalation of airborne droplets containing the bacilli. Although TB is not as easy to catch as many communicable diseases, prolonged exposure to an unrecognized active case may lead to infection. If there is an active case in a family situation, an

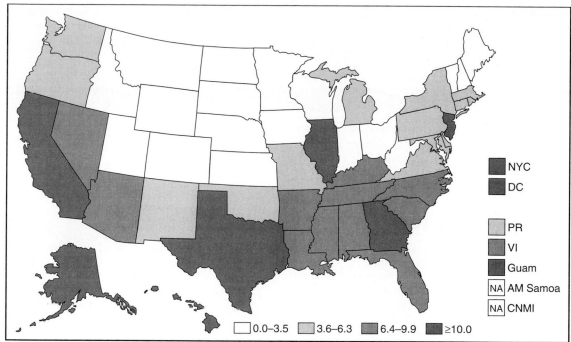

In 1995, a total of 19 states had tuberculosis rates of ≤3.5 cases per 100,000, which is the interim (e.g., year 2000) target for the elimination of tuberculosis by the year 2010.

Figure 4-9

Tuberculosis, reported cases per 100,000 population, United States and territories, 1996.

army barracks, a college dormitory, or other institutional living arrangement, prolonged exposure may lead to infection of contacts.

Symptoms

In primary TB, there are usually no symptoms. If symptoms do occur, they include fatigue, weakness, anorexia, weight loss, night sweats, and low-grade fever. The initial infection is generally controlled by the body defense mechanism, and the *M. tuberculosis* organisms are encapsulated or "walled up" in the lungs, where they cause no further damage unless something occurs to reduce the host's resistance. Secondary TB or reactivation TB usually occurs late in life or at a time when the adult victim's immune system is compromised. Symptoms of reactivation TB include a cough that produces sputum containing mucus and pus, chest pains, and, occasionally, bloody sputum.

Prevention

Vaccination with BCG (bacillus Calmette-Guérin) vaccine is not used routinely in the United States, because its use prevents the Public Health Service tracing of TB outbreaks by skin tests. Improving social conditions that increase the risk of infection with TB and education of the public are the main means of prevention in the United States.

Control

Control of TB in the United States has evolved by a number of measures. These include finding and treating TB as soon as possible; investigation of source and contacts and application of appropriate chemotherapeutic methods; frequent community surveys by skin testing and X ray examination; and continuing public education concerning the importance, origin, and control of TB.

HIV or Aids — Incidence of TB is high b/c of lack of immune symptom

Disease of lungs- can infect blood stream

Treatment

Most primary infections heal without recognition or treatment. Individuals with diagnosed TB are given **isoniazid** combined with rifampin or other antitubercular drugs. Nine months of therapy usually resolves an active case of TB.

SUMMARY

Table 4-3 summarizes the most important facts concerning the leading infectious diseases that are acquired by way of the respiratory system.

TABLE 4-3	**Bacterial Diseases Acquired through the Respiratory Route**			
Disease	**Special Characteristics**	**Transmission**	**Most Common Symptoms**	**Prevention/ Control**
UPPER RESPIRATORY INFECTIONS	Pharyngitis, laryngitis, tonsillitis, sinusitis, otitis media (complication)	Person to person or autoinfection, by direct or indirect contact	Sore throat, hoarseness, loss of voice, sinus pain, earache	Frequent hand washing
Sinusitis	URI that can become chronic from allergies, persistent infections	Airborne droplets or autoinfection	Fever, congestion, sore throat, thickened discolored nasal discharge	Healthy lifestyle
Streptococcal sore throat (pharyngitis)	Sequelae include rheumatic fever, glomerulonephritis, rheumatic heart disease, and scarlet fever	Direct contact and ingestion of contaminated food	Temperature, severe sore throat, swollen glands and tonsils, malaise, weakness, and anorexia	Avoidance of close contact with infected persons and proper food handling
Rheumatic fever	Childhood disease always preceded by another strep infection. May lead to heart or kidney disease	No person-to-person transmission but possible transmission of strep organism if victim is a carrier	Fever and migratory joint pain	Immediate antibiotic treatment for any streptococcal infection; contact investigation and treatment of sources (individuals or food)

TABLE 4-3	*Continued*			
Disease	**Special Characteristics**	**Transmission**	**Most Common Symptoms**	**Prevention/ Control**
Scarlet fever	Generally preceded by strep sore throat; *Streptococcus pyogenes* is the disease agent	Direct and indirect contact with respiratory discharges or in contaminated milk or food	Sore throat, fine rash that blanches on pressure, nausea, vomiting, fever, strawberry tongue	Same as streptococcal sore throat
PNEUMONIA	With influenza one of top ten causes of death in United States; caused by many disease agents	See specific type	See specific type	See specific type
Pneumococcal pneumonia	Most common type of pneumonia; more common among very young and very old; common cause of death among alcoholics; incubation 1–3 days or longer	Direct or indirect contact with respiratory discharges	Sudden onset of chills, fever, chest pain, difficult breathing and cough; red or rusty sputum; pleurisy often present; older people may be asymptomatic	Vaccine for high risk individuals; in an outbreak avoid crowds
Mycoplasmal pneumonia	"Walking pneumonia"; may last a month or more; incubation 6–32 days	Direct or indirect contact with respiratory discharges	Insidious onset with headache, malaise, cough—often paroxysmal, and chest pain	Avoidance of crowding
Legionnaires' disease	Pneumonia-like illness; outbreaks from faulty cooling systems, or at excavation sites. Described in	Organism exists in soil and water. Inhalation of airborne particles results in infection. No evidence of person-to-person	Sudden or gradual onset; diarrhea, anorexia, malaise, myalgia, weakness, headache, high fever, chills, followed by	Disinfection of source if a cooling system; control of dust if source is an excavation

isoniazid   i-so-NI-a-zid

TABLE 4-3	*Continued*			
Disease	**Special Characteristics**	**Transmission**	**Most Common Symptoms**	**Prevention/ Control**
Legionnaires' discase— Cont'd	1947. An unrecognized cause of pneumonia for many years; has been diagnosed in most states and in some foreign countries; incubation 2–10 days	transmission	nonproductive cough that may eventually produce grayish, blood-streaked sputum	
Whooping Cough	Highly communicable during late incubation and prodrome; increased incidence in recent years; incubation 6–20 days	Direct and indirect by contact with respiratory discharges	Three stages: Catarrhal resembles a cold. Paroxysmal produces spasmodic and recurrent coughing, sometimes expelling tenacious mucus. Cough ends in high whoop. Convalescent stage lasts 1–2 months with intermittent coughing.	Vaccination with booster shots; isolation of suspected cases; prophylactic use of IG in at-risk cases; investigation of contacts and administration of vaccine or treatment when necessary
Diphtheria	At one time, one of leading killers in all parts of world; still an important cause of disease and death in developing nations; incubation usually 2–5 days	Direct or indirect contact from infected persons; milk can also serve as a vehicle	Thick, patchy, grayish green mucous membranes of pharynx, larynx, tonsils, soft palate, and nose	Vaccination and booster shots as necessary; isolation of infected individuals; antiseptic measures, screening of contacts who are food handlers; antibiotic prophylactically to contacts

TABLE 4-3 *Continued*				
Disease	**Special Characteristics**	**Transmission**	**Most Common Symptoms**	**Prevention/ Control**
Tuberculosis	Still 30,000 cases reported annually; rates much higher among poor, nonwhite, and in urban areas. Incidence in U.S. in 1989 was 9.5 per 100,000. People with AIDS very susceptible. Antibiotic resistant strain (at least one); illness and death increase with age; incubation about 4–12 weeks	Usual route by airborne droplets; prolonged exposure to an active case necessary for infection	Usually no symptoms in primary TB. In secondary TB: productive cough, chest pains, sometimes bloody sputum	No vaccination in U.S.*; improvement of social conditions and education of the public; frequent screening by skin testing and chest X rays

Treatment of bacterial disease is generally by antibiotics.

*BCG used in some countries but detection of TB by skin test is not possible after it is used.

✳Know✳ these Ques for Test ✳

QUESTIONS FOR REVIEW

1. What means of prevention increases resistance to all infectious disease?

2. What conditions predispose people to URIs?

3. What are the sequelae of strep sore throat?

4. In what way does a strep infection lead to scarlet fever?

5. Why is it said that rheumatic fever is a disease that does not stand alone?

6. What is pleurisy?

7. What is "walking pneumonia"?

8. When was Legionnaires' disease first described?

9. What conditions are conducive to Legionnaires' disease?

10. What complications may occur from Legionnaires' disease?

11. What occurs during the three stages of whooping cough?

12. When is whooping cough most contagious?

13. What has caused the periodic rise in diphtheria in the United States?

14. What complications may occur with diphtheria?

15. What factors have led to an increase in TB in the 1980s and 90s?

16. What are the characteristics, means of transmission, symptoms, treatment, prevention, and control for the diseases covered in this chapter?

FURTHER READING

A new weapon found against Legionella: Water treatment may prevent outbreaks. *Hospital Infection Control* 26:34–5, 1999.

Acute sinusitis and the common cold. *Journal of Family Practice* 48:7, 1999.

Ahuha, G.S., and J. Thompson. 1998. What role for antibiotics in otitis media and sinusitis: symposium: fourth of four articles on common ENT problems. *Postgrad Medicine* 104:103–4.

Brandt, E.R., and M.F. Good. 1999. Vaccine strategies to prevent rheumatic fever. *Immunologic Research* 19:89.

Brown, Patricia D., and Stephen A. Lerner. 1998. Community acquired pneumonia. *The Lancet* 352:1295.

Bryan, Charles S. 1999. Treatment of pneumonococcal pneumonia: the case for penicillin G. *American Journal of Medicine* 107:63s.

DeReimer, Kathryn, et al. 1999. Preventing tuberculosis among HIV-infected persons: a survey of physicians; knowledge and practices. *Preventive Medicine: An International Devoted to Practice and Theory* 28:437.

Dowell, S.F., et al. 1998. Appropriate use of antibiotics for URIs in children: part I otitis media and acute sinusitis. *American Family Physician* 58:1113–8.

Dye, Christopher, et al. 1999. Global burden of tuberculosis: estimated incidence, prevalence and mortality by country. *Journal of the American Medical Association* 282:677–686.

Essery, S.D., et al. 1999. The protective effect of immunization against diphtheria, pertussis and tetanus in relation to sudden infant death syndrome. *FEMS Immunology and Medical Microbiology* 25:183.

Gasner, Rose M., et al. 1999. The use of legal action in New York City to ensure treatment of tuberculosis. *New England Journal of Medicine* 340:359–366.

Goldberg, M. 1999. The diagnostic challenge . . . legionellosis. *Emergency Medicine* 31:99–100.

Gregory, T. 1998. Scarlet fever. *Patient Care* 32:109.

Irwin, Richard S. 1999. Silencing chronic cough. *Hospital Practice* 34:53.

Jaramillo, Ernesto. 1999. Tuberculosis and stigma: predictors of prejudice against people with tuberculosis. *Social Science and Medicine* 48:163–172.

Kaiser, Harold B., and Michael A. Kaliner. 1999. Asthma, rhinitis, sinusitis, urticaria. *Patient Care* 33:115.

Kooll, J.L., et al. 1999. Effect of monochloramine disinfection of municipal drinking water on risk of nosocomial legionnaires' disease. *The Lancet* 353:272.

Leggiadro, Robert J., et al. Nosocomial pneumonococcal infection: an outbreak. *Hospital Practice* 34:77.

Lepine, L.A., et al. 1998. A recurrent outbreak of nosocomial legionnaires'; disease detected by urinary antigen testing: evidence for long-term colonization of a hospital plumbing system. *Infection Control Hospital Epidemiology* 19:905–10.

Levine, Orin S., et al. 1999. Risk factors for invasive pneumococcal disease in children: a population based case control study in North America. *Pediatrics* 103:656.

McCance, Kathryn L., and Sue E. Huether. *Pathophysiology: The Biologic Basis for Disease in Adults and Children. 3rd Ed.* St. Louis: Mosby, 1998.

Miller, Jon, et al. 1999. An update on selected pediatric respiratory infections. *Modern Medicine* 67:57.

Mufson, Maurice A. 1999. Bacteremic pneumococcal pneumonia in one American city. *American Journal of Medicine* 107:34s.

O'Connor, D.L. 1998. Common infections in child care. *Patient Care* 32:60–2.

O'Dowd, A. 1998. In the dock . . . a cruise ship . . . the source of an outbreak of Legionnaires' disease. *Nursing Times* 94:16.

Ostroff, Stephen M. 1999. Continuing challenge of pneumococcal disease. *The Lancet* 353:1201.

Rubins, J.B., and A.K. Puri. 1998. Pneumococcal vaccine is not always effective in the elderly. *Consultant* 38:2709.

Vitek, C.R., et al. 1999. Epidemiology of epidemic diphtheria in three regions, Russian 1994–1996. *European Journal of Epidemiology* 15:75.

Walling, Anne D. 1999. Acute sinusitis: are expensive antibiotics more efficacious? *American Family Physician* 59:999.

Woods, William A., et al. 1999. Group A streptococcal pharyngitis in adults 30–65 years of age. *Southern Medical Journal* 92:491.

BACTERIAL DISEASES ACQUIRED THROUGH THE ALIMENTARY ROUTE

OBJECTIVES

1. *Distinguish between food poisoning and foodborne illness.*

2. *State means of prevention for infections that are transmitted by food or water.*

3. *Recognize symptoms that might indicate foodborne illness.*

4. *State the ways that food and water can become contaminated with salmonella and other pathogenic bacteria.*

5. *Discuss characteristics, transmission, treatment, and control of the following:*

   Staphylococcus aureus *(intoxication)*

   Clostridium perfringens *(intoxication)*

   Botulism *(intoxication)*

   Escherichia coli *(infection)*

   Shigellosis *(infection)*

   Salmonellosis *(infection)*

   Campylobacter *enteritis (infection)*

   Cholera *(infection)*

   Typhoid fever *(infection)*

6. *Identify the following foodborne infections:* **Bacillus cereus, Vibrio parahaemolyticus, Listeria monocytogens,** *and* **Yersini enterocolitica** *as other bacteria that may be involved in foodborne disease.*

INTRODUCTION

There are a number of different terms for disease acquired through ingestion, and one that is commonly and incorrectly used is "food poisoning." It is important to understand that in foodborne illness the poison or toxin comes from bacteria and is not inherent in the food. In some cases, it is the ingestion of **preformed toxins** (poisons) from pathogenic organisms that cause the illness; at other times it is **ingestion of the organisms themselves that then produce toxins in the bowel.** There is also **food infection,** which is caused by ingesting living organisms that then colonize the intestinal tract. True food poisoning occurs when a food, such as some species of mushroom or shellfish, is ingested and illness occurs because of toxins (poisons) inherent in the mushrooms or shellfish.

There are some bacteria acquired through the alimentary route that cause only gastroenteritis (inflammation of the stomach and intestine) or only enteritis, and there are others that cause a systemic illness. Most of these are acquired from contaminated food and water. They become lethal when the individual becomes dehydrated as a result of diarrhea and/or vomiting. In developing countries, many do not have immediate access to medical facilities and children and older people are likely to die from the dehydration before they can get help.

Some of the most common bacterial diseases acquired through the alimentary route will be discussed in this chapter along with a few others that are becoming more common and are particularly dangerous. Some of the bacteria that are found in food are identified in Table 5-1.

WHO has developed "Ten Golden Rules for Food Preparation." They are listed here and are part of the preventive measures against all infections from contaminated food and water:

1. Choose food processed for safety.
2. Cook food thoroughly.
3. Eat cooked food immediately.
4. Store cooked food carefully.
5. Reheat cooked foods thoroughly.
6. Avoid contact between raw foods and cooked foods.
7. Wash hands repeatedly.
8. Keep all kitchen surfaces meticulously clean.
9. Protect foods from insects, rodents, and other animals.
10. Use pure water.

When people are camping, hiking, hunting, fishing, or otherwise spending time outdoors, for any reason, they need to be sure that any water supply is safe; if there is any doubt, all water should be boiled before drinking or use in food preparation. Streams, lakes, and ponds can easily be contaminated from various sources and are a ready source of organisms that cause foodborne illness.

STAPHYLOCOCCUS AUREUS FOOD INTOXICATION

Staphylococcus aureus is one of the most common causes of foodborne illness in the United States and the world. The illness is caused by ingesting food in which staphylococci have been multiplying and producing toxin. *S. aureus* is a natural inhabitant of the human body and is also responsible for boils and other infections. Occasionally the reservoir also may be in cows with infected udders. The interval between eating the food and the onset of symptoms may be as little as thirty minutes or as long as seven hours. Usually the incubation period is two to four hours. Most persons are susceptible to this kind of foodborne illness. The illness is short lasting and rarely fatal. Victims recover within a day or two, but the intensity of symptoms may require hospitalization. Figure 5-1 shows the pattern of outbreaks; although the disease occurs year-round, it peaks during the summer and the holiday season (November and December).

Transmission

Staphylococci grow in many foods, especially precooked hams, milk, custards, cream fillings, and salad dressing. Some of the most likely sources of this food intoxication are shown in Figure 5-2. The

TABLE 5-1	Foodborne Bacteria	
Identification	**Characteristics and Symptoms**	**Prevention/Control**
Bacillus cereus food poisoning: Associated with a wide variety of foods including meats, milk, vegetables, and fish that have been improperly stored. Few outbreaks reported—most not diagnosed because symptoms are similar to other foodborne disease	Onset of watery diarrhea, abdominal cramps, and pain 6–15 hours after eating contaminated food. May have nausea but rarely vomiting. Symptoms last about 24 hours, rarely fatal. Outbreaks common in other countries but rare in U.S.	Leftovers must be refrigerated soon after fixing—organism is not destroyed by boiling. Food needs to be reheated thoroughly and rapidly. Control is the same as for *S. aureus*
Vibrio parahaemolyticus associated gastroenteritis: Caused by ingestion of the vibrio in raw, improperly cooked, or cooked, recontaminated fish and shellfish	Symptoms include diarrhea, abdominal cramps, nausea, vomiting, headache, fever, and chills. Usually mild or moderate—duration, 2.5 days, incubation 4–96 hrs. after ingestion with mean of 15 hrs. Major outbreaks in U.S. during summer months, rarely fatal. Very common in Japan	Educate consumers on dangers of eating raw or undercooked fish. Educate food handlers and processors on preparing and storing fish. Avoid use of seawater in cooking—organism found in seawater as well as marine life
Listeriosis—*Listeria monocytogenes:* Found in a large variety of foods including raw milk, supposedly pasteurized milk, cheeses, ice cream, raw vegetables, raw and cooked poultry, all types of raw meats, and raw and smoked fish	Influenza-like symptoms are mild and disease usually not diagnosed until victim has septicemia, meningitis, encephalitis, intrauterine or cervical infections that can lead to spontaneous abortion or stillbirth. Laboratory blood analysis needed for diagnosis. CDC estimated 1600 cases/414 deaths per year in 1987	Special care needs to be taken with all animal products and raw vegetables. Pregnant women need to avoid contact with any meat, poultry, or vegetables that have not been cleaned. Thorough washing of any food that may have been fertilized with manure is necessary. Contact investigation should be carried out
Yersiniosis—*Yersinia enterocolitica:* Found in meats, oysters, fish, and raw milk. Organism is prevalent in the soil, water, and animals such as beavers, pigs, and squirrels. Has also been transmitted by blood transfusions	Gastroenteritis with diarrhea and/or vomiting; fever and abdominal pain are the most reliable symptoms. May mimic appendicitis and may also cause infections of other sites such as wounds, joints, and urinary tract. Onset usually 24–48 hours after ingestion of food or drink. CDC estimates 17,000 cases in U.S. annually. It is far more common in Japan, Northern Europe, and Scandinavia. Fatalities are rare	Use sanitary preparation of meat and other foods. Wash hands before food handling and eating, and after handling raw pork or animal contact. Protect water supplies from animal and human feces. Dispose of cat and dog feces in a sanitary manner. Remove anyone who has diarrhea from food preparation or care of young children or patients

Staphylococcus aureus	Staf-ill-oh-KOK-us AW-ree-us

[handwritten note: ↑ rate / Picnics - Holidays]

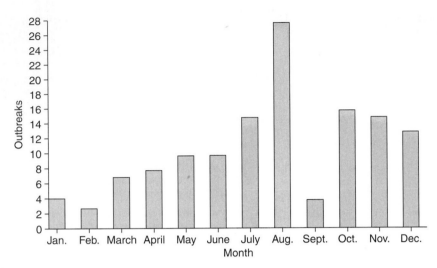

Figure 5-1

Staphylococcal food poisoning can be seen year-round but is most common during the summer and November/December holidays.

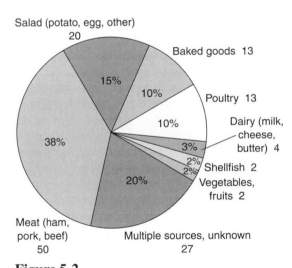

Figure 5-2

Foods implicated in staphylococcal outbreaks reported to CDC during a 5-year period.

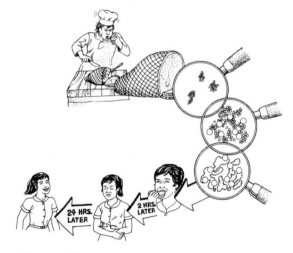

Figure 5-3

One possible means of transmission for *S. aureus* food poisoning.

source of food contamination is usually a person with an infected lesion on the hands, arms, or face. Milk from an infected cow may also be toxic. Figure 5-3 shows a possible sequence of transmission of *S. aureus*. This same progression could happen with some of the other organisms that will be discussed.

Symptoms

Staphylococcal food intoxication has an abrupt and sometimes violent onset, which helps to distinguish it from other types of foodborne illness. Nausea, vomiting, cramps, and diarrhea are the typical symptoms. The loss of fluid and violent

---

Safety Tips for Cooling and Storing Food

One way to avoid contamination of cooked foods is to refrigerate them as soon as possible. In any case they should not be allowed to sit out more than two hours. The U.S. Food Safety and Inspection Service also recommends that food cooked in large quantities should be divided into smaller containers to cool more quickly. Warm food is an ideal place for some microorganisms to multiply to an infectious dose. Many outbreaks of foodborne illness have been traced to food in large containers that was not cooled or stored correctly. Shallow containers, no more than three inches deep, are best. And if food has to be left out of the refrigerator for cooling, even for a short time, it should be covered.

---

vomiting may lead to prostration, low-grade fever, and lowered blood pressure.

Treatment

Treatment is not necessary unless the individual becomes dehydrated, in which case oral rehydration or, in extreme cases, intravenous (IV) therapy may be used to replace fluids.

Prevention

The time from the preparation of food to serving needs to be as short as possible. Proper heating or cooling procedures need to be followed, as well as using the right procedures for perishable foods. Any individual with boils, abscesses, or other infected lesions of the hands, face, or nose should be prohibited from food handling. Food handlers and others should be educated about food hygiene, sanitation and cleanliness of kitchens, proper temperature control, and personal hygiene (hand washing, cleaning fingernails, etc.). (See the preceding "Ten Golden Rules for Food Preparation.")

Control

Single cases of food intoxication are generally so mild that they are not reported. Individuals who say they have had "stomach flu" or "twenty-four hour flu" may simply be using incorrect terms for vomiting and diarrhea. Control is only necessary when there is an outbreak, and then the source of infection needs to be identified and eliminated.

CLOSTRIDIUM PERFRINGENS FOOD INTOXICATION

Food infection from **Clostridium perfringens** is generally a mild disease of short duration. It occurs worldwide wherever conditions favor increased multiplication of the organism. The incubation period is six to twenty-four hours, although the victims usually become ill in ten to twelve hours. Improper cooking and handling methods for food provide the necessary condition for the intoxication to occur. At least ten to twenty outbreaks have been reported in the United States each year for the past twenty years. Dozens or even hundreds of people are affected because institutions are a common site for the outbreaks. Figure 5-4 shows confirmed outbreaks of *C. perfringens* for a one-year period.

Transmission

Food contaminated by soil or feces and then held under conditions that allow the organism to multiply provides the means of transmission. Most outbreaks are associated with inadequately heated meats and gravies. The outbreaks are usually traced to restaurants or other businesses that prepare food but do not have adequate cooking or refrigeration facilities.

Clostridium perfringens   Kloss-TRID-ee-um
per-FRIN-gens

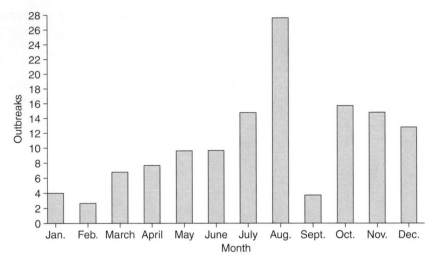

Figure 5-4

C. perfringens outbreaks.

Symptoms

Infection with *C. perfringens* generally produces much milder symptoms than those from most other food infections or intoxications. Cramps followed by diarrhea appear suddenly, and there is often nausea, but vomiting and fever seldom occur. The symptoms are present for a day or less and fatalities are rare.

Treatment

Treatment is unnecessary unless the victim becomes dehydrated.

Prevention

Outbreaks usually can be traced to places such as schools and restaurants where foods are prepared in large batches. Meat dishes are a common source. Food handlers should be educated concerning the dangers in large-scale cooking. Hot dishes should be served while still hot from original preparation. If stored, they must be cooled rapidly, and reheating must be thorough and rapid to prevent the organism from multiplying.

Control

Control is only necessary when there is an outbreak, and then the source of the intoxication needs to be identified and eliminated.

BOTULISM   *(canning)*   *Systemic Illness*

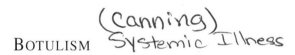

This severe intoxication from the exotoxin produced by ***Clostridium botulinum*** results in a life-threatening paralytic illness. Unlike other forms of bacterial food intoxication or infection, botulism is a systemic illness. The powerful toxin, when ingested in contaminated food, is absorbed from the intestine into the system, resulting in the paralysis of cranial and peripheral nerves. Intoxication with *C. botulinum* organisms also occurs in infants, in whom the toxin is produced by the organism in the intestines, and in wound botulism, when the organism enters a wound and anaerobic conditions are present. Infant botulism has been recognized only since 1976; wound botulism is rarely seen.

There were more outbreaks of botulism when home canning and preserving were common, but family outbreaks can still occur. There have also been some cases identified recently that were traced to commercially canned products. Incubation is usually twelve to thirty-six hours but can be longer. In shorter incubation periods, the illness is generally more severe. Everyone is susceptible to botulism if the toxin is ingested. Figure 5-5 shows reported cases by year and some

can result in paralysis

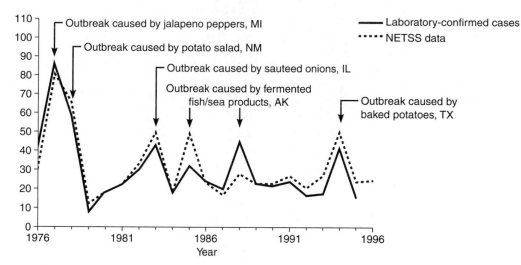

Figure 5-5

Botulism (food borne), by year, United States, 1976–1996.

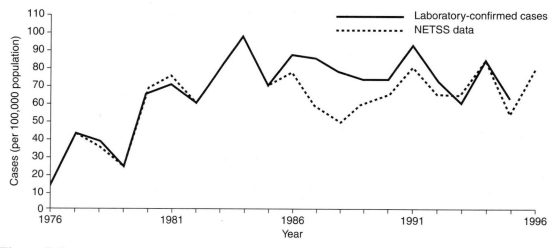

Figure 5-6

Botulism (infant), by year, United States, 1976–1996.

of the foods involved in outbreaks in the United States. Reported cases of infant botulism are shown in Figure 5-6. The case fatality rate has been under fifteen percent during the last ten years for patients who receive adequate treatment. Without treatment, about one-third of the patients may die within three to seven days after onset. Recovery may be slow and take months or even years.

Transmission

Botulism generally is the result of eating foods that have been inadequately cooked, allowing the toxin to form. The foods that have been involved

Clostridium botulinum   Kloss-TRID-ee-um bot-you-LINE-um

most often in the United States are home canned fruit and vegetables; in Europe, smoked or preserved meat and sausages; and in Japan, smoked or preserved fish. In the last ten years, two separate outbreaks of botulism have occurred in the United States involving commercially canned salmon. The largest outbreak of botulism in the United States since 1978 occurred in El Paso, Texas in April 1994. The toxin had formed in aluminum foil–wrapped baked potatoes held at room temperature for several days before they were used in a potato-based dip at a restaurant. Thirty people were affected and four required mechanical ventilation.

Symptoms

The first signs of botulism generally relate to the effects of the toxin on the nervous system. The person may experience dizziness, difficulty in swallowing, and double vision. Nausea, vomiting, and diarrhea may occur earlier, at the same time, or later. There is descending paralysis, and death usually occurs from respiratory paralysis.

Treatment

Treatment consists of intramuscular (IM) or IV administration of botulinum antitoxin.

Prevention

The best means of prevention is through effective control of processing and preparation of commercially canned and preserved foods and education of everybody who prepares and serves food. Education must also extend to those concerned with home canning and other food preservation and must include instruction in proper techniques regarding time, pressure, temperature, storage, and cooking. Any bulging cans or jars that do not seem sealed should not be opened or used.

Control

Early detection and identification of the source of botulism can save lives. Contaminated food should be boiled before discarding and buried deeply to keep animals from eating it. Contaminated utensils also need to be sterilized.

HEMORRHAGIC COLITIS (*ESCHERICHIA COLI* 0157:H7)

The organism responsible for hemorrhagic colitis is ***Escherichia coli*** 0157:H7. *E. coli* is a normal inhabitant of the intestines of all animals, including humans. Because it is the dominant species found in feces, its presence has been used as a guideline in testing water, particularly in swimming pools, to determine if the water is pure enough for swimmers. It also has a useful function in the body because it suppresses the growth of harmful bacterial species and helps in the synthesis of vitamins. There are six major categories of strains for the *E. coli* that cause diarrhea. Most of them cause a mild illness but, in 1982, a new strain appeared, *E. coli* 0157:H7 that, unlike the known strains, produced large quantities of potent toxins that cause severe damage to the lining of the intestine. The initial outbreaks were associated with two outlets of the same fast-food chain and were linked to undercooked hamburgers. In 1983 more outbreaks occurred and a new danger, hemolytic uremic syndrome (HUS) was found to occur in five percent to ten percent of the reported cases of *E. coli* 0157:H7. Children younger than five years of age are most likely to develop HUS. Much remains to be learned about this dangerous emerging disease. The incubation period is relatively long for this foodborne disease, ranging from three to eight days with a median of three to four. As long as the organism is being excreted, it is communicable. Little is known about differences in susceptibility and immunity. Reported cases of *E. coli* 0157:H7 in the United States and territories for 1996 are shown in Figure 5-7.

Transmission

Transmission of *E. coli* 0157:H7 is by ingestion of contaminated food or water and also person to person. In addition to hamburger and other meats, the organism has also been found in increasingly different sources including apple juice, cole slaw, cheese curds, jerky made from deer meat, and alfalfa sprouts. All of these have been implicated in outbreaks.

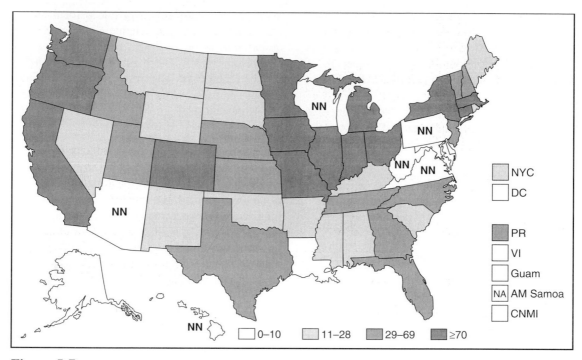

Figure 5-7

Escherichia coli 0157:H7, reported cases, United States and territories, 1996

Symptoms

Severe cramping and diarrhea are the first symptoms. At first the diarrhea is watery but, in most victims, becomes bloody. Occasionally there is vomiting but only a low-grade or no fever. The illness lasts an average of eight days. If hemolytic uremic syndrome occurs, mostly in the very young, it can lead to permanent loss of kidney function. In the elderly, HUS plus fever and neurologic symptoms can have a mortality rate as high as fifty percent.

Treatment

Most cases require no therapy, but fluid replacement may be necessary. There is some evidence that antibiotic treatment can increase the risk of complications. This is one of the areas that still needs to be investigated as far as hemorrhagic colitis is concerned.

Prevention

See the aforementioned "Ten Golden Rules for Food Preparation." The families of the people who are ill need to be educated about possible person-to-person transmission.

Control

Identify and eliminate or avoid the source when an outbreak is reported. Contact investigation and education are also important. Contacts who have diarrhea should not be allowed to work where they are involved in preparing food or working with children.

SHIGELLOSIS (BACILLARY DYSENTERY)

Shigellosis, or **bacillary dysentery,** is an acute intestinal disease caused by the bacterium

---

Escherichia coli   Esh-er-EE-she-ah KOH-lee
shigellosis   shig-e-LO-sis
bacillary dysentery   BAS-i-la-ree DIS-en-ter-e

Shigella. *Dysentery* means diarrhea with abdominal cramping and **tenesmus** (straining at stools) from any cause. The term *bacillary dysentery* is reserved for infection by the four species of *Shigella: S.* **dysenteriae,** *S.* **flexneri,** *S.* **boydii,** and *S.* **sonnei.**

Shigellosis is endemic in North America, Europe, and the tropics. Figure 5-8 shows the number of confirmed cases in the United States from 1966 to 1996. The infection is more common in children ages one to four years and in the elderly, debilitated, and malnourished. Two-thirds of the cases and most of the deaths are in children under ten years of age. It is unusual in children under six months of age. Worldwide, it is estimated that 600,000 die every year from shigellosis.

The only reservoir for *Shigella* organisms is the human intestinal tract, and infected feces are always the source of the infection. The incubation period is usually one to three days; the disease is communicable during acute infection and until the infectious agent is no longer present in feces, which is usually within four weeks after the illness. Everyone is susceptible to infection with *Shigella* organisms; drinking or ingestion of as few as ten of the organisms can lead to shigellosis.

With prompt treatment, only one percent of the cases are fatal, although in epidemics caused by *S. dysenteriae,* as high as eight percent of the cases may result in death. The graph in Figure 5-9 shows the percentage of positive specimens by age groups comparing shigellosis with campylobacter and salmonellosis.

Transmission

Transmission of shigellosis is directly by fecal-oral transmission or indirectly through contact with contaminated objects. The widest distribution of the organism is through contaminated water or food. Transmission occurs primarily through individuals who fail to wash their hands or clean their fingernails thoroughly after defecation. They can then spread the infection to others by physical contact with them or by contaminating food or water. Food can also be contaminated by flies that carry enough of the organism for it to multiply to an infectious dose in the food. When dogs ingest human feces, the infection can be passed by them to children or other susceptible persons.

Symptoms

Shigellae invade the intestinal mucosa and cause inflammation. In children, shigellosis usually produces diarrhea with tenesmus, high fever, nausea,

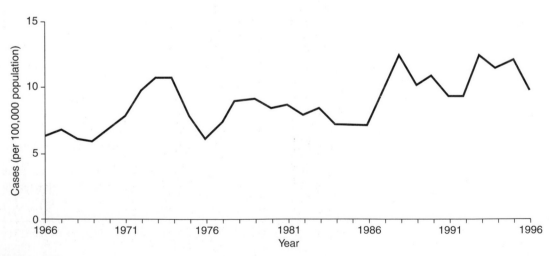

Figure 5-8

Shigellosis, by year, United States, 1966–1996.

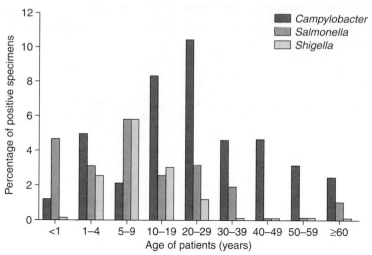

Figure 5-9

Age distribution for diarrheal diseases caused by campylobacter, salmonella, and shigella organisms.

vomiting, abdominal pain with distention, irritability, and drowsiness. Pus, mucus, and blood may appear in the stools as a result of the intestinal ulceration typical of this infection. Convulsions can be a complication in children. Shigellosis in adults produces many of the same symptoms except that adults generally do not have fever. Complications such as electrolyte imbalance and shock are rare but may be fatal in children and debilitated patients.

Treatment

Many strains of *Shigella* are resistant to antibiotics. If an effective one can be found, then the shigellae can be eliminated quickly. Antidiarrheal drugs are contraindicated, because they prolong the excretion of shigellae, fever, and diarrhea. The most important treatment is control of dehydration, with fluid and electrolyte replacement. If the illness is severe or contacts need to be protected, antibiotics may be ordered.

Prevention

There is no vaccine at present. Prevention is based on control of the human reservoir and sanitary control of environmental sources through adequate treatment of water and sewage, fly control,

and protection of food, water, and milk from human or mechanical vectors.

Control

Control measures are the same as for other diseases acquired through the alimentary route.

SALMONELLOSIS

Salmonellosis is a medical term for infection with any species of *Salmonella.* Although about 2000 species of *Salmonella* have been recognized, only ten commonly cause salmonellosis in the United States. Infection with *Salmonella* organisms can range from a symptomless carrier state to potentially fatal infections. The most frequent form of salmonellosis today is gastroenteritis. Salmonellae were not named after fish but after an American

Shigella	Shi-GEL-ah
tenesmus	te-NEZ-mus
S. dysenteriae	diss-en-TAIR-ee-i
S. flexneri	flex-NE-ri
S. boydii	BOY-dii
S. sonnei	SON-nei

CASE STUDY

Salmonellosis

During April and May 1998, a total of eleven states reported an increase in *Salmonella* infections. By June 8, a total of 209 cases were reported and at least 47 persons were hospitalized, representing an eightfold increase over the median number of cases reported in those states during 1993–1997. The states reporting increases were Illinois (49 cases), Indiana (30), Ohio (29), New York (24), Missouri (22), Pennsylvania (20), Michigan (15), Iowa (8), Wisconsin (6), Kansas (4), and West Virginia (2).

An investigation, including a case/control study, identified plain Toasted Oats cereal sold in Aldi supermarkets as the source of the salmonella. Cases were reported in more states and CDC recommended that consumers not eat plain Toasted Oats cereal produced by Malt-O-Meal until the source of the salmonella that got into the cereal could be determined.

From *Morbidity and Mortality Weekly Report* 47:462, 1998.

---

veterinarian, Daniel Salmon, who first isolated the organism from animals. An estimated five million cases occur in the United States annually. In addition to typhoid fever and gastroenteritis, salmonellosis also occurs as bacteremia, localized infection, and paratyphoid.

Foodborne Salmonellosis

Infection with salmonella from ingesting food is caused most often by *Salmonella **enteritidis.*** It has been the most common foodborne infection in the United States but is now being challenged by shigellosis and ***Campylobacter* enteritis** (see Figure 5-9). The largest single epidemic in the United States affected 285,000 persons who were infected by improperly pasteurized milk.

The rate of infection is highest for babies and young children. It is estimated that there are five million salmonella infections in the United States each year. The incubation period varies but is usually about twelve to thirty-six hours. Communicability lasts for the duration of the infection, which can be several days to several weeks. A small percentage of infected adults and children over five years of age excrete the organism for over one year. Everyone is susceptible to salmo-

nella infection from food. Figure 5-10 indicates the reported cases in the United States from 1966 to 1996.

Transmission

Salmonella infections leading to gastroenteritis are generally transmitted by ingestion of (1) food derived from an infected animal, (2) food contaminated during storage by the feces of infected animals, especially rodents, or (3) food contaminated by an infected person during its processing or preparation. Foods that are often found to be the source of salmonella infection include commercially processed meat products, inadequately cooked poultry or poultry products, raw sausages, lightly cooked foods containing eggs or egg products, and unpasteurized milk or dairy products, including dried milk. Turtles also carry salmonella and have been banned as pets because of the potential for infection.

Symptoms

When individuals become infected from eating contaminated food, there is generally a sudden onset of nausea, vomiting, abdominal pain, and diarrhea, often accompanied by fever and chills. Arthritic symptoms may follow three to four weeks after onset of acute symptoms.

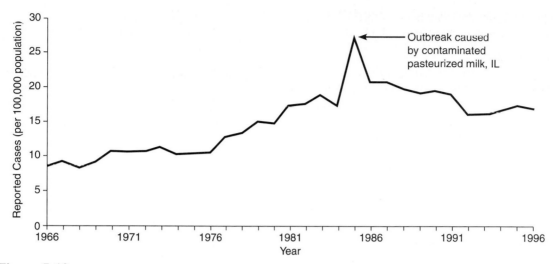

Figure 5-10
Salmonellosis (excluding typhoid fever), by year, United States 1966–1996.

Treatment

There is no specific treatment indicated for salmonella gastroenteritis unless dehydration occurs. Rehydration and electrolyte replacement may be necessary in extreme cases. Because the use of antibiotics may prolong the carrier state and lead to resistant organisms, they are only given in high-risk cases such as infants under two months of age, the elderly, the debilitated, and those with continued high fever or with indications that the infection has spread beyond the intestines.

Prevention

Meats, eggs, and milk must be protected by sanitary processing. Stored foods should be safeguarded from possible contamination by rodent feces. Food handlers and methods for preparing foods in public places should be under the continuing supervision of local health departments. Carriers must be restricted from food handling. Food handlers and the public should be continuously educated as to the sources and transmission of salmonella infection. Infection in domestic animals, fowl, and pets must be controlled.

Control

Individuals with salmonella infection need to be instructed in using proper hand-washing tech-niques. Symptomatic individuals should be excluded from food handling. They should not be allowed to return to work until stool cultures are negative. Those who come into direct contact with individuals with salmonellosis should be checked for infection. It is required that salmonella gastroenteritis be reported to local health authorities.

CAMPYLOBACTER ENTERITIS

This disease is caused by **Campylobacter jejuni** and is responsible for five percent to eleven percent of all cases of diarrhea and dysentery in the United States. The organism was recognized recently as an important cause of foodborne infection and is thought to cause more illness than salmonellae. Duration of the symptoms is generally two to five days but may last as long as ten days or more, especially in adults, and there may also be relapses. *C. jejuni* is harbored in animals, poultry, and humans; dogs are frequent carriers. The disease is communicable from several days to several weeks,

---

enteritidis   en-ter-IT-id-is
Campylobacter jejuni   KAM-peh-low-back-ter je-JUNE-ee

depending on the length of infection. Lasting immunity develops after an initial infection.

Transmission

Campylobacter bacteria are transmitted in food or water and may also be contracted by contact with infected pets, wild animals, or infected children. One means of transmission has been identified as youth activities (often field trips to dairy farms) during which children drink raw milk (Figure 5-11).

Symptoms

Symptoms include diarrhea, abdominal pain, malaise, fever, nausea and vomiting, and blood in the stools. The victim can be asymptomatic or very sick. Sometimes there are symptoms resembling typhoid and, rarely, meningitis can occur.

Treatment

Generally no treatment is needed unless it is rehydration and electrolyte replacement. In special cases, antibiotics may be used.

Prevention

All food derived from animal sources and poultry should be thoroughly cooked, milk pasteurized, and water supplies purified. Recognition and control of infection in domestic pets is also necessary.

Hand washing after animal contact and contact with chickens will also aid in prevention.

Control

Individuals with the infection should be excluded from any food preparation. In case of an outbreak, the source of infection needs to be identified and eliminated or isolated.

CHOLERA

Cholera is an acute gastrointestinal infection caused by ***Vibrio cholerae.*** The disease is caused by an exotoxin produced by the organism. Severe, untreated cases of cholera may be fatal in as many as fifty percent of its victims. With treatment, it is fatal in fewer than one percent. There was no known indigenous cholera in the Western Hemisphere between 1911 and 1973. Beginning with one case in Texas in 1973 that had no known source, sporadic cholera infections have continued to occur in the United States. A disease that had been limited to Asia and the Eastern Hemisphere spread west until in 1994 a total of more than 950,000 cases were reported in twenty-one countries in the Western Hemisphere. Only thirty-one

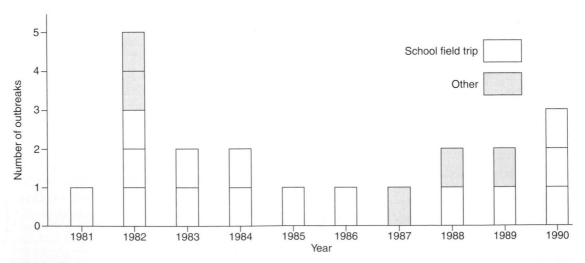

Figure 5-11

One means of campylobacter transmission is identified as youth activities such as field trips.

of these were reported in the United States, but with immigrant and returning travelers, that number could easily increase. Cholera occurs more frequently among lower socioeconomic groups and more often during the warmer months. Humans are the only known reservoir, although there is a possibility of environmental reservoirs.

The incubation period is generally two to three days; communicability lasts as long as stools are positive, usually only a few days after recovery. A carrier state may last for months. Susceptibility to cholera varies. Attack rates, even in severe epidemics, rarely exceed two percent. In endemic areas, cholera is predominantly a disease of children. In these areas, most persons acquire antibodies by early adulthood. However, when cholera spreads to areas where it has not been endemic, adults are at least as susceptible as children. Reported cases of cholera in the United States and territories are shown in Figure 5-12. Figure 5-13 shows the areas in the world reporting cholera cases in 1997.

Transmission

Cholera is transmitted through feces or vomitus of carriers or persons with active infections. Epidemic spread usually results from contaminated water supplies. Food is involved more often in sporadic cases in endemic areas. Hands, utensils, clothing, and flies may contaminate food or carry the infection directly to the mouth.

Symptoms

The symptoms of cholera are acute, painless, and profuse watery diarrhea and effortless vomiting. White flecks appear in the stools as they increase ("rice water stools"). Because of the massive loss of fluid, many symptoms occur, including thirst, weakness, wrinkled skin, sunken eyes, pinched facial expression, muscle cramps, and cardiovascular problems. Collapse, shock, and death may

Vibrio cholerae VIB-ree-oh KAHL-er-ee

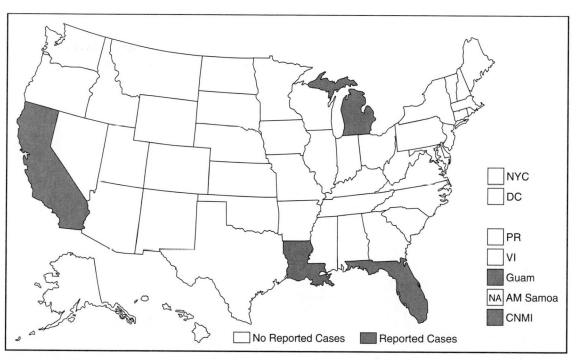

Figure 5-12
Cholera, reported cases, United States and territories, 1996.

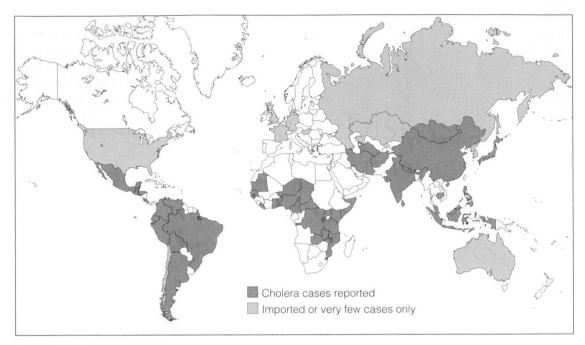

Figure 5-13

Countries and areas reporting cholera in 1997.

follow if the patient is not continuously rehydrated until the infection subsides.

Treatment

An electrolyte solution must be given immediately and continuously to replace lost fluids. In mild cases, oral fluid replacement is adequate. Tetracycline and other antibiotics are used if symptoms persist and are effective in reducing the duration and volume of diarrhea as well as speeding the elimination of the bacteria from the feces.

Prevention

Proper sanitation and vaccine are the best methods of prevention. The routine use of cholera vaccine is not recommended. However, people traveling to epidemic areas in other countries may be required to have a vaccination.

Control

Control methods are the same as they are for other diseases acquired through the alimentary route.

TYPHOID FEVER   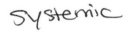 *Systemic*

In the last decade of the nineteenth century, it was recognized gradually that well persons who were carriers of pathogenic organisms were responsible for a significant number of new cases of disease. In 1906, the identification of an Irish cook, Mary Mallon, who had been the cause of seven epidemics of typhoid fever in six years, highlighted the importance of the *chronic carrier.* "Typhoid Mary" became the symbol around the world for a carrier of disease.

Salmonella typhi, the organism that causes typhoid fever, is the only species of *Salmonella* whose reservoir is only in humans. The disease has become comparatively rare in the United States since the advent of sanitation and immunization procedures. The majority of cases occur in individuals exposed to *S. typhi* during international travel. The yearly incidence of typhoid fever worldwide is an estimated seventeen million cases with 600,000 deaths. The fatality rate for untreated individuals is ten percent and for those who get treatment, three percent. Typhoid results most frequently from drinking water that has been contaminated with body discharges from a carrier. The incubation period is usually one to three weeks; communicability usually lasts from the first week through the end of convalescence but can last longer. In about ten percent of patients, the typhoid bacilli are discharged for three months after the onset of symptoms, and two percent to five percent become carriers. Susceptibility is general but usually declines with age. The number of reported cases in the United States from 1966 to 1996 is shown in Figure 5-14.

Transmission

Typhoid bacilli are transmitted by food or water that has been contaminated with the fecal matter or, less commonly, urine, of an infected person or carrier. Among some of the common foods responsible for transmission of typhoid are shellfish from contaminated beds, raw fruits, vegetables, milk, and milk products contaminated by food handlers who are carriers or unidentified cases. Flies have also been known to be carriers when they infect foods in which the organisms can multiply sufficiently to cause the disease.

Symptoms

Unlike most other *Salmonella* infections that generally produce only acute gastroenteritis, typhoid is a systemic disease. If individuals ingest *S. typhi,* they may soon have gastric and intestinal symptoms, but these usually subside before the classic symptoms of typhoid fever begin. Within the first week, these symptoms include anorexia, myalgia, malaise, headache, and fever.

During the second week the fever rises to 104 or 105°F, usually in the evening, and it is accompanied by chills, sweating, weakness, delirium, increasing abdominal pain and distention, diarrhea or constipation, cough, moist rales (chest sounds on breathing), enlarged spleen, and rose spots, especially on the abdomen. During the third week there is persistent fever, increasing fatigue, and weakness, as the symptoms gradually subside. Complications include intestinal perforation or hemorrhage, abscesses, blood clots in the legs and head, pneumonia, **osteomyelitis, myocarditis,** and acute circulatory failure.

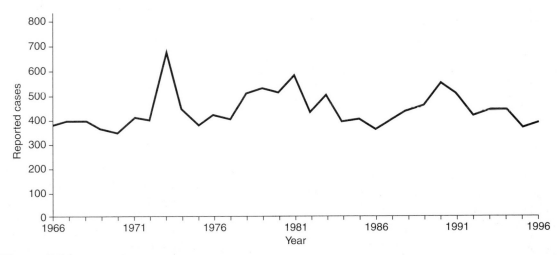

Figure 5-14
Typhoid fever, by year, United States, 1966–1996.

Treatment

A number of different antibiotics can be used to treat typhoid fever. Selection is based on the sensitivity of the strain of *S. typhi* involved. Symptomatic treatment includes bed rest and replacement of fluids and electrolytes. Various medications may also be used to relieve diarrhea and control cramps. Further treatment depends on the symptoms and kinds of complications that may occur.

Prevention

Immunization is not routinely recommended in the United States or for travel to developed areas. Individuals at high risk because of occupation, travel to endemic areas, or living conditions where typhoid could be introduced should be given the vaccine. Prevention of typhoid depends on adequate protection of water supplies; sanitary disposal of human excreta; pasteurization of milk and dairy products; fly control; scrupulous cleanliness in preparing food at home and in public eating places; careful controls on shellfish sources and cooking; and identification and supervision of typhoid carriers. Even city water must be boiled in the wake of a flood, tornado, or hurricane if there is any chance of ruptured water lines.

Control

Hospital care with proper sanitary precautions is recommended, particularly if the patient cannot be given adequate nursing and the necessary sanitary conditions cannot be maintained at home. An investigation should be conducted to determine the actual or probable source of infection for every case. Necessary measures should be taken to control any carriers who may be identified.

SUMMARY

Table 5-1 summarizes principal data regarding the most important diseases contracted through the alimentary route.

TABLE 5-1	Diseases Acquired through the Alimentary Route			
Disease	Special Characteristics	Transmission	Major Symptoms	Prevention/ Control
S. aureus food intoxication	Short incubation, 2–4 hrs; short duration; rarely fatal	Ingestion of food containing toxin	Abrupt, violent onset, nausea, vomiting, diarrhea	Safe food preparation
C. perfringens food intoxication	Mild, short duration; incubation 6–24 hrs	Ingestion of food containing organism	Mild cramps, diarrhea	Same as *S. aureus*
Botulism	Life-threatening illness; affects the nervous system; fatality rate under 15% with treatment, around 33% without treatment; incubation 12–36 hrs	Ingestion of food containing toxin	Dizziness, difficulty in swallowing, double vision, nausea, vomiting, diarrhea, descending paralysis. Shorter incubation equals more severe disease	Same as *S. aureus*

Disease	**Special Characteristics**	**Transmission**	**Major Symptoms**	**Prevention/ Control**
E. coli 0157:H7 Hemorrhagic	Most dangerous strain of *E. coli;* may lead to hemolytic uremic syndrome (HUS); incubation usually 12–72 hrs	Ingestion of food or water contaminated with the organism (rarely by direct fecal contact)	Diarrhea; stools may contain blood and pus	Protection of water supplies; sanitary disposal of human excreta; pasteurization; safe food preparation; controls on shellfish; identification and supervision of carriers; education of everyone on importance of hand washing
Shigellosis	Also called bacillary dysentery; more common in children, elderly, debilitated, malnourished; infected human feces only source; incubation usually 1–3 days	Ingestion of food or water contaminated with the organism; fecal-oral route	Diarrhea, tenesmus, nausea, high fever, vomiting, irritability, abdominal pain and distention, drowsiness, blood and pus in stools	Same as *E. coli*
Foodborne Salmonellosis	Common foodborne infection; incubation usually 12–36 hrs	Ingestion of food or water contaminated by the organism	Sudden onset headache, abdominal pain, nausea, and sometimes vomiting	Safe preparation of food; eggs, meat, and milk must be protected by sanitary processing; do not allow carriers or individuals with diarrhea to handle food; control infections in domestic animals and pets

TABLE 5-1 *Continued*

TABLE 5-1	*Continued*			
Disease	**Special Characteristics**	**Transmission**	**Major Symptoms**	**Prevention/Control**
Campylobacter Enteritis	Recognized recently; rivals *Salmonella* as most common foodborne infection; incubation usually 2–5 days	Ingestion of food or water contaminated with the organism	Diarrhea, fever, abdominal pain, malaise, nausea, vomiting; stools may be watery and contain blood and pus	Thorough cooking of food from animal sources; pasteurization of milk; control of infection in pets; hand washing after contact with animals and chickens
Cholera	Fatal in up to 50% if untreated; incubation usually 2–3 days	Ingestion of food or water contaminated with the organism	Acute, painless, profuse, watery diarrhea and effortless vomiting	Same as *E. coli*
Typhoid fever	"Typhoid Mary" carrier state; rare in U.S. today; incubation usually 1–3 weeks depending on dosage	Ingestion of food or water contaminated with the organism	Systemic disease: fever, anorexia, malaise, headache, myalgia, rose spots on abdomen, constipation or diarrhea	Same as *E. coli*

Treatment for bacterial diseases is generally antibiotics. However, many of the foodborne diseases are so mild that antibiotic treatment is not necessary. When diarrhea and vomiting are severe and prolonged, fluid and electrolytes may need to be replaced. In the case of botulism, an antitoxin is administered to counteract the poison.

QUESTIONS FOR REVIEW

1. In what three ways can people be "poisoned" by food?
2. What foods are the most likely to become the source of staphylococcal food poisoning?
3. What procedures should be followed in food preparation to prevent foodborne diseases?
4. Why is there sometimes a problem in the reporting and control of foodborne disease?
5. What conditions may lead to the transmission of *C. perfringens* in food?
6. Where do outbreaks of *C. perfringens* commonly occur?
7. In what way is botulism a dangerous form of foodborne illness?
8. Why have the cases of botulism decreased in this century?
9. What are the symptoms and prevention for botulism?
10. What measures are taken to prevent *E. coli* infection?
11. What population groups are more susceptible to shigellosis? Why?
12. What is dysentery?

13. What are the symptoms of shigellosis in children?

14. What are the sources and means of transmission for *Salmonella* infection?

15. What pets have been found to harbor salmonellae?

16. What measures will aid in the prevention of *C. jejuni?*

17. What is the fatality rate for cholera when it is untreated? Treated?

18. Where and when is cholera most likely to occur?

19. What is a distinctive symptom of cholera?

20. What is the main cause of death from cholera?

21. How is cholera prevented?

22. What is the story about Typhoid Mary and why is it important?

23. How does typhoid differ from other *Salmonella* infections?

24. What are the symptoms, complications and prevention for typhoid fever?

FURTHER READING

Abelluck, Pam, and Christopher Drew. 1998. From a farm in California to outbreak of food poisoning in the east. *The New York Times,* January 5.

Ahmed, F., D.J. Clemens, and M.R. Rao, et al. 1997. Epidemiology of shigellosis among children exposed to cases of *Shigella* dysentery: a multivariate assessment. *American Journal of Tropical Medicine and Hygiene* 56:258.

Angulo, F.J., Taylor J. Getz, and K.A. Hendricks, et al. 1998. A large outbreak of botulism: The hazardous baked potato. *Journal of Infectious Diseases.* 178:172.

Are we gaining ground on food-borne pathogens? *Consultant.* 39:1475, 1999.

Bad Bug Book. "Foodborne pathogenic microorganisms and natural toxins handbook," U.S. Food and Drug Administration, Center for Food Safety & Applied Nutrition, [http://vm.cfsan.fda.gov/~mow /intro. html], last update, April 6, 1998.

Charatan, Fred. 1999. New York outbreak of e-coli poisoning affects 1000 and kills two. *British Medical Journal* 319:873.

Chlamydia pneumoniae and cardiovascular disease. 4:4. www.cdc.gov/ncidod/eid/vol4no4/campbell.htm.

Cholera outbreak among Rwandan refugees— Democratic Republic of Congo, April, 1997. *Morbidity and Mortality Weekly Report* 47:389, 1998.

Collins, Janet T. 1997. Impact of changing consumer lifestyles on the emergence/reemergence of foodborne pathogens. *Emerging Infectious Disease* 3:471.

Cote, Timothy R., Helen Convery, Donald Robinson, and Alan Ries, et al. 1995. Typhoid fever in the park: epidemiology of an outbreak at a cultural interface. *Journal of Community Health* 20:451.

Fang, T.J., et al. 1999. Microbiological quality and incidence of staphylococcus aureus and bacillus cereus in vegetarian food products. *Food Microbiology* 16:385.

Food-borne antibiotics-resistant campylobacter infections. *Nutrition Reviews.* 57:224, 1999.

Friedman, C.R., C. Torigian, and P.J. Shillam, et al. 1998. An outbreak of salmonellosis among children attending a reptile exhibit at a zoo. *Journal of Pediatrics* 132:802.

Griffen, George E. 1999. Typhoid fever and childhood vaccine strategies. *The Lancet* 354:698.

Keene, William E., Elizabeth Sazie, M.D., and Janet Kok, et al. 1997. An outbreak of *Escherichia coli* 0157:h7 infections traced to jerky made from deer meat. *Journal of the American Medical Association* 277:1229.

Keller, Jean A. 1999. In the fall of the year we were troubled with some sickness: Typhoid fever deaths, sherman . . . .*American Indian Culture and Research Journal* 23:97.

Kirk, M., R. Waddell, and C. Dalton, et al. 1997. A prolonged outbreak of *Campylobacter* infection at a training facility. *Communicable Disease Intell* 21:57.

Lindsay, James A. 1997. Chronic sequelae of foodborne disease. *Emerging Infectious Disease* 3:474.

Luby S.P., M.K. Faizan, and S.P. Fisher-Hoch, et al. 1998. Risk factors for typhoid fever in an endemic setting, Karachi, Pakistan. *Epidemiology and Infection* 120:129.

Lucas, Beverly D. 1999. Typhoid fever reported in the United States. *Patient Care* 33:13.

Mandrell, R.E., and M.R. Wachtel. 1999. Novel detection techniques of human pathogens that contaminate poultry. *Current Opinion in Biotechnology* 10:273.

Meier, D.E., and J.L. Tarpley. 1998. Typhoid intestinal perforations in Nigerian children. *World Journal of Surgery* 22:319.

Mermin, Jonathan H., John M. Townes, and Michael Gerber, et al. 1998. Typhoid fever in the United States, 1985–1994: Changing risks of international travel and increasing antimicrobial resistance. *Archives of Internal Medicine* 158:633.

Multistate outbreak of *Salmonella* serotype agona infections linked to toasted oats cereal—United States, April–May, 1998. *Morbidity and Mortality Weekly Report* 47:462, 1998.

Neira, Maria. 1997. Cholera: A challenge for the twenty-first century. *World Health* 50:9.

Olson, Rebecca K., Millicent Eidson, and C. Mack Sewell. 1997. Staphylococcal food poisoning from a fundraiser. *Journal of Environmental Health* 60:7.

Outbreak of *Escherichia coli* 0157:H7 infections associated with drinking unpasteurized commercial apple juice—British Columbia, California, Colorado, and Washington, October 1996. *Morbidity and Mortality Weekly Report* 45:975, 1996.

Outbreak of *Salmonella enteritidis* gastroenteritis: investigation by pulsed-field gel electrophoresis. *International Journal of Infectious Disease* 2:159, 1998.

Outbreak of staphylococcal food poisoning associated with precooked ham—Florida, 1997. *Morbidity and Mortality Weekly Report* 46:1189, 1997.

Outbreak of *Vibrio parahaemolyticus* infections associated with eating raw oysters—Pacific Northwest, 1997. *Morbidity and Mortality Weekly Report* 47:457, 1998.

Outbreaks of *Escherichia coli* 0157:H7 infection and cryptosporidiosis associated with drinking unpasteurized apple cider—Connecticut and New York, October 1996. *Morbidity and Mortality Weekly Report* 46:4, 1997.

Outbreaks of *Escherichia coli* 0157:H7 infection associated with eating alfalfa sprouts-Michigan and Virginia, June–July 1997. *Morbidity and Mortality Weekly Report* 46:741, 1997.

Outbreaks of *Escherichia coli* 0157:H7 infection—Georgia and Tennessee, June 1995. *Morbidity and Mortality Weekly Report* 45:249–251, 1996.

Parikh, A.I., M.T. Jay, and D. Kassam, et al. 1997. *Clostridium perfringens* outbreak at a juvenile detention facility linked to a Thanksgiving holiday meal. *Western Journal of Medicine* 166:417.

Pierard, D., et al. 1999. A case control study of sporadic infection with 0157 and non-0157 verocytotoxin in producing Escherichia coli. *Epidemiology and Infection* 122:359.

Preventing zoonotic diseases in immunocompromised persons: the role of physicians and veterinarians. www.cdc.gov/ncidod/eid/vol5no1/grant.htm

Quinonez, Jorge M., Russell W. Steele, Dawn Sokol, et al. 1997. A 4-month-old with hypotonia. (New Orleans Citywide Rounds Index) *Infectious Medicine* 14:30.

Raufman, J.P. 1998. Cholera. *American Journal of Medicine* 104:386.

Roels, T.H., M.E. Proctor, and L.C. Robinson, et al. 1998. Clinical features of infections due to *Escherichia coli* producing heat-stable toxin during an outbreak in Wisconsin: A rarely suspected cause of diarrhea in the United States. *Clinical Infectious Diseases* 26:898.

Rosenberg T., O. Kendall, and J. Blanchard, et al. 1997. Shigellosis on Indian reserves in Manitoba, Canada: Its relationship to crowded housing, lack of running water, and inadequate sewage disposal. *American Journal of Public Health* 87:1547.

Rowan, N.J., et al. 1999. Pulsed-light inactivation of food-related microorganisms. *Applied and Environmental Microbiology* 65:1312.

Salmonella serotype montevideo infections associated with chicks—Idaho, Washington and Oregon, Spring 1995 and 1996. *Morbidity and Mortality Weekly Report* 46:237, 1997.

Sarnighausen, H.E., et al. 1999. Typhoid fever due to salmonella kapemba infection in an otherwise healthy middle-aged man. *Journal of Clinical Microbiology* 37:2381.

Shapiro, R.L., C. Hatheway, and D.L. Swerdlow. 1998. Botulism in the United States: A clinical and epidemiologic review. *Annals of Internal Medicine* 129:221.

Stephenson, Joan. 1997. New approaches for detecting and curtailing foodborne microbial infections. *Journal of the American Medical Association* 277:1337.

Streptococcal toxic-shock syndrome www.cdc.gov/ncidod/eid/volno3/stevens.htm

Vogt, Thomas, and Paul Hasler. 1999. A woman with panic attacks and double vision who liked cheese. *The Lancet* 354:300.

Yang, Samantha. 1998. FoodNet and Enter-net: Emerging surveillance programs for foodborne diseases. *Emerging Infectious Diseases* 4:122.

BACTERIAL INFECTIONS ACQUIRED THROUGH SKIN, MUCOSA, AND BLOODSTREAM FROM HUMAN AND ENDOGENOUS SOURCES

OBJECTIVES

1. *Identify common diseases that may be due to infection from endogenous sources and/or autoinfection.*

2. *Distinguish among folliculitis, boils, and carbuncles.*

3. *Indicate conditions in the host that are conducive for toxic shock syndrome.*

4. *Explain the importance of recognizing impetigo in children.*

5. *Explain the stigma attached to leprosy.*

6. *Discuss reasons for the rise and fall of syphilis and gonorrhea cases over the years.*

7. *Compare chlamydia and gonorrhea.*

8. *Discuss symptoms, treatment, prevention, and control for the following diseases:*

   Folliculitis, boils, and carbuncles
   Impetigo
   Osteomyelitis
   Toxic shock syndrome
   Conjunctivitis
   Meningitis
   Endocarditis
   Leprosy
   Syphilis
   Gonorrhea
   Chlamydia

FOLLICULITIS, FURUNCLES (BOILS), AND CARBUNCLES

Most **furuncles** and **carbuncles** are caused by *Staphylococcus aureus,* as are many cases of **folliculitis.** The basic difference among them is in degree of severity, as can be seen in Figure 6-1. Folliculitis is an infection of a hair follicle. Furunculosis involves deeper layers of the skin, gland, or hair follicle, whereas carbuncles encompass more than one hair follicle and invade deep tissue. *S. aureus* are **pyogenic** (pus-causing) bacteria and are found worldwide. They are common in children, especially in warm weather, and may also occur in places where there is poor personal hygiene and people are crowded. Also, many people who have an initial infection leading to a boil or carbuncle seem to be more susceptible and may develop further infections any time their resistance is lowered sufficiently and other conditions resulting in infection are present. Why some people are more susceptible to *S. aureus* infection than others has not been determined.

Transmission

The hands are the most important mode of transmission. The reservoir of infection is people; *S. aureus* inhabits the nostrils of almost everyone

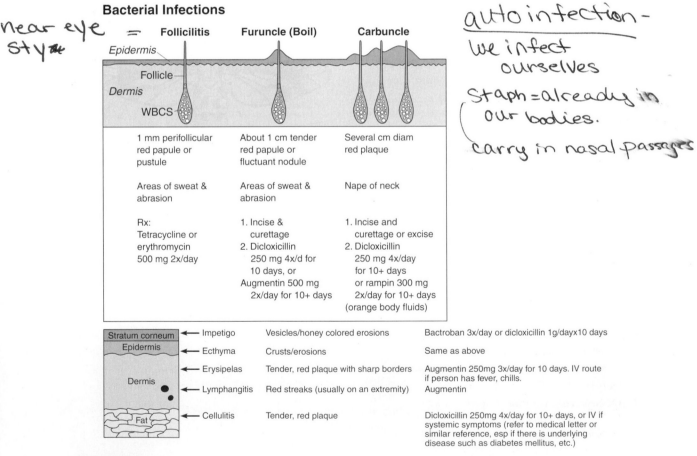

Bacterial Infections

near eye = Sty

auto infection - we infect ourselves
staph = already in our bodies.
carry in nasal passages

Follicilitis	Furuncle (Boil)	Carbuncle
1 mm perifollicular red papule or pustule	About 1 cm tender red papule or fluctuant nodule	Several cm diam red plaque
Areas of sweat & abrasion	Areas of sweat & abrasion	Nape of neck
Rx: Tetracycline or erythromycin 500 mg 2x/day	1. Incise & curettage 2. Dicloxicillin 250 mg 4x/d for 10 days, or Augmentin 500 mg 2x/day for 10+ days	1. Incise and curettage or excise 2. Dicloxicillin 250 mg 4x/day for 10+ days or rampin 300 mg 2x/day for 10+ days (orange body fluids)

Impetigo	Vesicles/honey colored erosions		Bactroban 3x/day or dicloxicillin 1g/dayx10 days
Ecthyma	Crusts/erosions		Same as above
Erysipelas	Tender, red plaque with sharp borders		Augmentin 250mg 3x/day for 10 days. IV route if person has fever, chills.
Lymphangitis	Red streaks (usually on an extremity)		Augmentin
Cellulitis	Tender, red plaque		Dicloxicillin 250mg 4x/day for 10+ days, or IV if systemic symptoms (refer to medical letter or similar reference, esp if there is underlying disease such as diabetes mellitus, etc.)

Figure 6-1
The basic difference among furuncles, carbuncles, and folliculitis is the degree of severity.

at some time. Over sixty percent of the general population carries the organism continuously in any one year. Self-infection is responsible for at least one-third of the infections. Person-to-person transmission is by contact with a person who has a **purulent** (pus-containing) lesion or with an asymptomatic carrier.

Symptoms

The staphylococcal organism may cause an infection wherever there is a break in the skin. Sometimes the infection may occur on an eyelid, and it is then referred to as a stye. When folliculitis occurs, tiny red pustules appear. Most of the time, only one hair follicle becomes infected, but there are conditions under which the result is pustules over a wide area of skin. Boils appear as hard, painful nodules, commonly on the neck, face, axillae (armpits), and buttocks. Boils will generally enlarge and rupture, discharging the pus. A carbuncle is marked by an extremely painful, deep abscess that drains through multiple openings, usually around several hair follicles (Figure 6-2).

Treatment

Folliculitis generally needs no treatment other than keeping the area clean. Use of an antibiotic ointment may aid in healing. For boils and carbuncles, in addition to keeping the area clean and use of antibiotic ointments, pressure should be kept off the site. Hot compresses will facilitate healing. Possible sites of reinfection should be identified and treated. If the infection is severe, it may require antibiotics and surgical drainage, which can be performed in a doctor's office.

Prevention

Good personal hygiene and maintaining a high level of resistance through a positive lifestyle are the best means of preventing staphylococcal infections. Children need to be educated in hand washing and the importance of avoiding common use of toilet articles.

Control

Infants, the ill, and the elderly are the most susceptible to *S. aureus,* and infected persons should avoid contact with them. Education in personal hygiene, with special emphasis on not sharing personal items, even in the family, will help to keep the infection from spreading. Boils are teeming with bacteria, and particular care should be taken in discarding dressings from **lesions** that are draining. Anyone having a boil needs to be cautioned not to try to squeeze it to get the pus out. If the wall of the boil breaks, it can lead to bacteremia (blood poisoning) and deep-tissue infections such as **osteomyelitis,** which will be discussed later in the chapter.

IMPETIGO

Impetigo is especially common in the newborn and children, particularly during hot, humid weather. It is highly contagious and spreads rapidly in families and crowded conditions such as schools. It may be caused by *S. aureus* or *Streptococcus pyogenes.* Poor skin hygiene and skin conditions such as an abrasion or draining wounds are predisposing factors. The infection occurs worldwide and is especially prevalent in

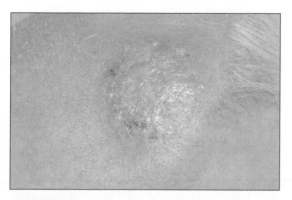

Figure 6-2

A carbuncle is an extremely painful, deep abscess that drains through multiple openings, usually around several hair follicles.

folliculitis	fo-lik-yu-LI-tis
furunculosis	fyu-rung-kyu-LO-sis
Pyogenic	pi-o-JEN-ik
purulent	pur-u-lent

Bacitracin - ointment for Staph & strep

warm weather. People are the reservoir of infection. The incubation period is variable, usually four to ten days. As with other staphylococcal or streptococcal skin infections, communicability lasts as long as there is a discharge of pus or the carrier state is present.

Transmission

Impetigo can be spread quickly through direct and indirect contact. The hands are the main method of transmission, although fomites such as damp towels and other moist objects can also be a means of transmission. As in other staph and strep infections, autoinfection is responsible for about one-third of the cases.

Symptoms

Impetigo starts as a small reddish spot on the skin that develops into a vesicle (a blisterlike small elevation containing fluid) and then becomes **pustular** (filled with lymph or pus). Figure 6-3 is an example of impetigo caused by *S. pyogenes*. The fluid is straw colored, and the pustule ruptures and becomes crusted. Impetigo occurs principally on the face. It is generally localized but can lead to more serious infections deeper in the system.

Treatment

Systemic antibiotics are not used unless fever, malaise, or secondary complications are present. An antibiotic ointment such as bacitracin is gener-

ally prescribed. After the crusts are removed and the skin cleansed, the ointment is applied to the **lesion.**

Prevention *Hand washing*

Education in personal hygiene and a positive lifestyle are the best means of prevention.

Control

Because impetigo is highly contagious, children who have it should be excluded from school or day-care centers and not allowed contact with infants and the chronically ill. Individuals with diabetes and the elderly are also more susceptible and should be protected from infection. There should be an emphasis on frequent hand washing by all who live with or come in contact with the infected individual, and common use of toilet articles should be avoided.

OSTEOMYELITIS

Osteomyelitis is an infection of the bone and bone marrow that may be chronic or acute. The most frequent cause of the infection is *S. aureus*. Bone infections are not as common today as they once were, and with the advent of antibiotics, they are much easier to treat.

The infection occurs more often in children than in adults and more in boys than in girls. The most common sites in children are the lower end of the femur and the upper end of the tibia, humerus, and radius. In adults, osteomyelitis occurs most frequently in the bones of the pelvis and vertebrae. With prompt treatment, the prognosis (outcome) for the acute form is good, but the prognosis for chronic osteomyelitis is poor. Drug users and individuals undergoing trauma to the bone, or surgery, are more susceptible.

Transmission

Because osteomyelitis is an internal infection, person-to-person transmission is unlikely. However, individuals who have the infection may carry *S. aureus* on their skin or mucous membranes or may have a boil or carbuncle from which the infection has traveled to the bone.

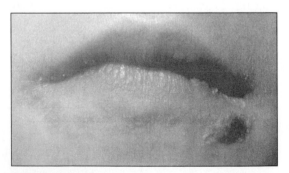

Figure 6-3

Impetigo. This is a superficial strep or staph infection that occurs just beneath the stratum corneum. It generally occurs in the paranasal or perioral area in young people.

clear/straw colored

Symptoms

Osteomyelitis has an abrupt onset with sudden pain in the affected bone, tenderness, heat, swelling, and restricted movement over the bone. There may also be sudden fever, tachycardia (fast heartbeat), nausea, and malaise.

Treatment

Four to eight weeks of antibiotic therapy, surgical **debridement** (removal of dead tissue), and drainage are generally necessary for healing. Analgesics are administered for the pain, which may be severe.

Prevention

Individuals with boils or other pus-containing lesions must refrain from squeezing them to release the pus. As was stated before, this action can break the protecting wall and allow the pathogenic organisms to enter the bloodstream. Risk factors include alcohol abuse, diabetes, malignancy, malnutrition, tobacco use, and other conditions that compromise the immune system.

Control

The individual with osteomyelitis should be checked for a penetration wound from which the organism originated to see whether it is presently infected. Sterile procedures need to be followed in disposal of any bandages from a draining wound.

TOXIC SHOCK SYNDROME

Toxic shock syndrome (TSS) is an acute bacterial infection that usually affects menstruating women under thirty years of age. When cases of the disease suddenly emerged in the early 1980s, an intense investigation took place in an effort to determine the cause of the potentially fatal illness. The infecting organism was identified as *S. aureus.* Unfortunately, the strains that were identified were penicillin resistant, making the infection more difficult to treat. The use of tampons, particularly those that were super absorbent, was soon linked to the majority of cases. There have been a few cases in boys and men and also among nonmenstruating women. Of those cases not occurring in association with menstruation, some have been linked to a cer-

vical cap, diaphragm, sponge, or an infection in another part of the body.

In the late 1980s, six cases of TSS caused by *S. pyogenes* (group A streptococcus [GAS]) were reported. This streptococcal TSS can occur in anyone even without an underlying disease. In spite of treatment, thirty to seventy percent of patients die.

Transmission

Because staphylococcal bacteria are commonly present in the vagina, an infection may occur whenever the right conditions are present to allow the toxin access to the circulatory system. As indicated above, these conditions include use of a tampon during the menstrual period and possibly use of certain birth control methods. There is no person-to-person transmission.

GAS is also a normal inhabitant of the human body and the disease agent can be spread by carriers. In most cases of streptococcal TSS, the portal of entry is not known.

Symptoms Staph Breaks off goes to blood

The symptoms of staphylococcal TSS include fever (generally over 104°F), headache, vomiting, sore throat, diarrhea, muscle aches, sunburnlike rash, low blood pressure, bloodshot eyes, disorientation, reduced urination, and peeling of the skin on the palms and soles of the feet.

Pain is the most common symptom of streptococcal TSS and tends to occur abruptly and severely. The pain usually involves an extremity, but can also mimic other diseases including pneumonia and myocardial infarction. There may be influenza-like symptoms and fever. Confusion is present in over half of the patients. Swelling and redness of tissue occurs in eighty percent of the patients and for most of these, the infection may progress to necrotizing fasciitis ("flesh eating") that requires debridement, fasciotomy, or amputation.

---

lesion   LE-zhun
osteomyelitis   oste-o-mi-e-LI-tis
pustular   PUS-chu-lar
debridement   da-breed-MON
necrotizing fasciitis   NEC-ro-ti-zing fas-ci-IT-is

Treatment

Although the causative organisms are penicillin resistant, other antibiotics such as oxacillin, nafi-cillin, and **methicillin** are effective. Fluid replacement may be necessary to reverse shock.

GAS/TSS is still treatable with penicillin preparations. However, other antibiotics may have to be used with more agressive infections such as necrotizing fasciitis.

Prevention

TSS during menstruation can be avoided by not using tampons. The risk can be reduced by switching to less absorbent tampons and by changing them frequently. Contraceptive devices, which have also been implicated, should not be left in place more than thirty hours or beyond the directions on the package.

Until the actual means of transmission and portal of entry are known, the only prevention for streptococcal TSS is by keeping the immune system as strong and healthy as possible.

Control

Because there is no person-to-person transmission, control is a matter of educating women about safe usage of contraceptive methods and tampons.

More will have to be learned about streptococcal TSS before control measures, other than keeping the immune system strong, can be determined.

CONJUNCTIVITIS

Conjunctivitis is commonly known as "pink eye" from the redness (inflammation) that develops in the white of the eye. The conjunctiva is the mucous membrane that lines the eyelids and also covers the eyeball (Figure 6-4). The condition may be due to allergy or infection by bacteria, viruses, or chlamydia. Most often, conjunctivitis is caused by bacteria or viruses. The most important bacterial agents seem to be *Haemophilus influenzae, Streptococcus pneumoniae,* and *S. aureus. S. pneumoniae* and *H. influenzae* are more common in children whereas *S. aureus* is more common in adults. Incubation is twenty-four to seventy-two hours, and the infection is communicable

as long as it is active. People are the reservoir of infection, and children under five years of age are most susceptible, although those whose resistance is low are also at risk. Although conjunctivitis is usually a mild infection in the United States, other bacteria and also enteroviruses have caused it in other countries, and in Brazil a form known as Brazilian **purpuric** fever, or BPF, has resulted in a seventy percent fatality rate.

Transmission

There are many ways by which an infection of the eye can be transmitted. These include contact with discharges from an infected person, contaminated fingers, fomites, and insect vectors.

Symptoms

Redness, itchiness, purulent discharge, and occasionally photophobia (sensitivity to bright lights) are symptoms of conjunctivitis. Sometimes when the discharge is purulent, the eyelids are stuck together in the morning.

Treatment

Warm water will wash away discharge and crusts on the eyelids. An antibiotic ointment and/or eye drops may be applied, and, depending on the infecting organism, an oral antibiotic may also be used.

Prevention

Attention to personal hygiene is necessary. Sanitary conditions where children play, including the home and day-care centers, need to be enforced at all times.

Control

In addition to preventive methods above, individuals with conjunctivitis should be treated promptly, and contacts watched for possible infection. If an insect vector is involved, then insect control is called for.

MENINGITIS

The meninges are the membranes surrounding the brain and spinal cord, or central nervous system (CNS). Meningitis occurs when these membranes become inflamed as a result of infection with a

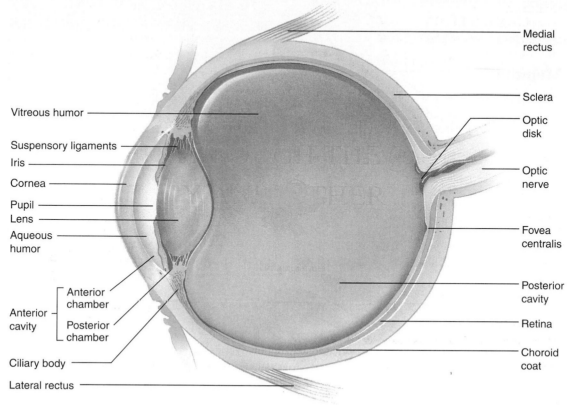

Medial rectus

Vitreous humor

Suspensory ligaments

Iris

Cornea

Pupil

Lens

Aqueous humor

Anterior chamber

Anterior cavity

Posterior chamber

Ciliary body

Lateral rectus

Sclera

Optic disk

Optic nerve

Fovea centralis

Posterior cavity

Retina

Choroid coat

Figure 6-4

Longitudinal section through eyeball and eyelids showing the conjunctiva. Conjunctiva line the posterior surface of the eyelids and cover the cornea.

pathogenic organism. Many times it is a complication of bacterial infection at some other location in the body. There are three organisms that are responsible for most cases of bacterial meningitis: *H. influenzae,* ***Neisseria meningitidis,*** and *S. pneumoniae. H. influenzae* infections (hemophilus meningitis), tend to occur more in children; *N. meningitidis* infections (meningococcal meningitis), occur more in young adults, particularly where there are close quarters such as dormitories or army barracks; and *S. pneumoniae* infections (pneumococcal meningitis) are more frequent in infants, older adults, and alcoholics. Not very many years ago, the case fatality rate was over fifty percent, but with modern and early treatment, the case fatality rate is now between five percent

Can be viral

and fifteen percent. Viruses, fungi, and parasitic worms can also cause meningitis.

Transmission

The mode of transmission varies, depending upon which organism is responsible for the infection. Most forms are transmitted by direct contact with respiratory secretions from the nose and throat of

---

methicillin   meth-i-SIL-in
Haemophilus influenzae   he-MOF-i-lus in-flu-EN-zae
purpuric   pur-PU-rik
Neisseria meningitidis   ni-SEE-re-a men-in-JIT-i-deez

Meningitis

During July and August 1995, the Miami-Dade County Health Department was notified of one probable and four laboratory confirmed cases of meningitis among children vacationing at a local resort area. All of the cases occurred among county residents who either stayed at or visited hotel A. One child died.

The first reported case was in a guest at hotel A who developed a fever on July 8. On July 9, symptoms developed in a sister and brother staying at hotel B who had visited hotel A to play with other children. The sister died shortly after admission to a local hospital. Her brother was admitted with fever, vomiting, leg pain, and a rash.

Investigators noted overcrowding at hotel A, where some rooms had as many as twelve residents. An estimated 730 persons stayed or worked at hotels A and B during the week before onset of symptoms in the first two cases.

After consultation with epidemiologists at Florida Department of Health and CDC, county health officials offered prophylaxis on site to all guests and employees at both hotels. Over a two-day period, 480 persons (66% of the targeted group) received the recommended rifampin dosage. The hotel swimming pool, the site of organized activities for children, was closed.

Approximately five weeks after the first cluster of cases was identified, a case was diagnosed in a seventeen-year-old who provided child care at hotel A during the days before onset of symptoms. A secondary case (occurring at least twenty-four hours after onset in the primary case) was diagnosed in a child who had been in this seventeen-year-old's care and who had resided at the hotel since June. The child and her family had recieved prophylaxis at the time of the first meningitis cluster. The county again offered prophylaxis to all guests and employees at hotel A. No further cases were identified among visitors to the resort area.

Morbidity and Mortality Weekly Report 47:833, 1998.

infected persons. Up to ten percent of the population in countries where the disease is endemic may be asymptomatic carriers.

Symptoms

Symptoms of meningitis also may vary with the infecting agent but generally include fever, intense headache, nausea and/or vomiting, stiff neck, and often a rash. As the meninges become more irritated, other problems occur, such as problems in leg extension after flexion, exaggerated deep tendon reflexes, and back spasm in which the back arches backward so that the body rests on the head and heels. In babies, signs are not so apparent, and the infant may just be fretful and refuse to eat. The infant may vomit a great deal, leading to dehydration. This reduces fluid in the system and keeps the fontanelle (soft spot on top of the head) from bulging, which is one of the signs of intracranial pressure. As the disease progresses, twitching,

seizures, or coma may develop. Children who are older generally have the same symptoms as adults. The onset may be acute or insidious.

Treatment

Usually antibiotics are administered intravenously (IV) for at least two weeks, followed by oral antibiotics. Ampicillin is the drug of choice. However, because of resistant strains of bacteria, ampicillin may not be effective, and it is recommended that **ceftriaxone** or another cephalosporin be used concurrently or by itself until it is known whether the infecting organism is resistant to ampicillin.

Prevention

Antibiotics may be used prophylactically when trauma or surgery invades the area of the brain or spinal cord because infection is always a possibility. A vaccine is available that is effective against

H. influenzae type B and is recommended for children under fifteen months of age. Day-care centers and other places where there is close contact between children need to be monitored when cases are present among those attending. Vaccines are also available and have been shown to be effective for some forms of *N. meningitidis.*

Control

Individuals with meningitis should be isolated for twenty-four hours after start of treatment with antibiotics. Some physicians advise use of **rifampin** prophylactically for all household contacts and in day-care centers when a case has occurred among children.

ENDOCARDITIS

[handwritten: inflamation @ endocardium of the heart]

Endocarditis is inflammation of the endocardium (inner lining) of the heart, particularly the valves. Figure 6-5 shows the three layers of the heart. The infection that causes the inflammation may occur by itself or as a complication of another disease. The disease agent is most often staphylococcal or streptococcal. The disease occurs when bacteria or other organisms are able to enter the bloodstream and infect the heart. There are two types of bacterial

ceftriaxone	sef-tri-AK-son
rifampin	RIF-am-pin

[handwritten: heart doesn't pump as strong - weak blood output]

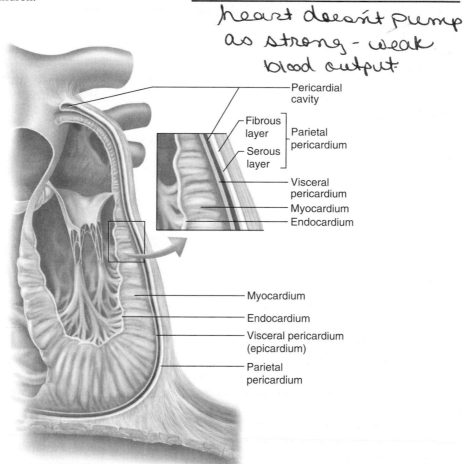

Pericardial cavity

Fibrous layer ⎱ Parietal
Serous layer ⎰ pericardium

Visceral pericardium

Myocardium

Endocardium

Myocardium

Endocardium

Visceral pericardium (epicardium)

Parietal pericardium

Figure 6-5

Section of the heart wall showing the components of the outer heart sac (pericardium), muscle layer (myocardium), and inner lining (endocardium).

endocarditis, acute and subacute. Dental and surgical procedures predispose an individual to this infection, and in those whose hearts have been damaged by some other condition there is greater risk. Drug addicts who inject the drugs are also at risk. Fungal and nonbacterial endocarditis occur, but they are rare. Before antibiotics, ninety-five percent of individuals with bacterial endocarditis died. Today, sixty-five percent to eighty percent recover.

[handwritten margin note: IV Drug Addicts]

Transmission

Bacteria may be introduced into the bloodstream during cardiac surgery, by shared needles, as a result of any kind of intravenous injection, or through a penetrating wound. Because bacteria are common inhabitants on the skin of many people, autoinfection is also possible.

Symptoms

In the subacute form, the infection may be present for months, causing serious damage to the heart but only general and nonspecific symptoms. There may be feverishness, night sweats, vague aches and pains, fatigue, and weakness. Sometimes there is a change in an already present heart murmur or a new murmur. The symptoms for acute bacterial endocarditis are sudden chills, high fever, shortness of breath, and rapid or irregular heartbeat. It is a rapidly progressing infection and may lead to heart failure. Clots may break off from the initial site of the infection and travel to other organs, causing blocking or infection there.

Treatment

High doses of antibiotic drugs are given via IV and continued for as long as six weeks. If a heart valve is damaged, surgical repair or prosthetic replacement may be necessary.

Prevention

Prophylactic treatment with antibiotics is prescribed as a preventive measure for people with heart valve defects. This is especially important before surgical or dental procedures. Those at risk need to be educated as to the signs of endocarditis.

Control

The source should be identified, if possible, to avoid further incidents. The individual does not need to be isolated because endocarditis is not communicable.

LEPROSY (HANSEN'S DISEASE)

Many people are familiar with the stories of lepers in the Bible and the isolation that was imposed upon lepers. If it had not been for the unsightly disfigurations caused by the disease, this segregation of the lepers would not have occurred. There must have been some fear that spread of the disease could be caused by contact with those who had it, even though the true means of disease transmission would not be discovered for centuries. It is now known that although leprosy can be spread through person-to-person contact, it is much less contagious than was once thought. Leprosy, also known as Hansen's disease, is found all over the world (Figure 6-6).

Since WHO set as one of its goals the "elimination of leprosy as a public health problem by the Year 2000," significant advances have been made toward the goal. This does not mean the eradication of leprosy, and the key phrase is "as a public health problem," in which "problem" is defined as a prevalence of one case per 10,000 population.

In 1991 the World Health Organization identified leprosy as a disease that would be eliminated by 2000. This did not happen but the prevalence of leprosy worldwide was reduced 85% from 1984 to the beginning of 1999. The number of new cases remained steady or increased during the same time period due to a number of factors including enhanced reporting of cases. The remaining cases are concentrated in 11 countries, representing 90% of the global burden as shown in Table 6-1.

The infectious organism is *Mycobacterium leprae,* which causes two forms of leprosy, **lepromatous** and tuberculoid; as far as is known now, humans are the only significant reservoir. The incubation period is from eight months to ten years, and the disease is rarely seen in children under three years of age. It is estimated that only three percent of the population is susceptible to the disease.

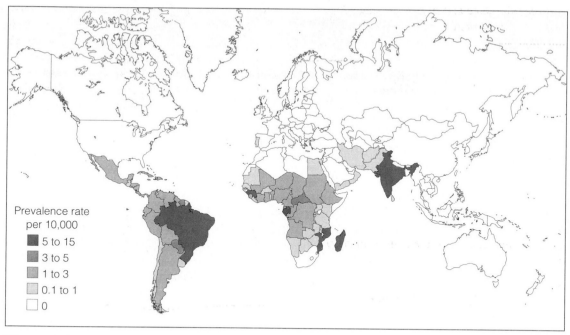

Figure 6-6

The spread of Hansen's disease, also known as leprosy, throughout the world until May 1998. Although not commonly found in the United States, the disease plagues most third world and developing countries.

Transmission

The exact means of transmission is unknown. Only living in prolonged close contact with an infected person puts anyone at risk of contracting the disease. The organisms are present in nasal secretions and probably enter through the upper respiratory tract or a break in the skin.

Symptoms

The organism attacks the peripheral nervous system. In tuberculoid leprosy, there are raised, large **erythematous** (red) plaques or **macules** (discolored spots on skin) with clear borders. These spots become larger, rough, hairless, and gradually colorless, finally leaving painless scars. The disease process occurs particularly on the face, arms, legs, and buttocks. Some typical characteristics of lepromatous leprosy are seen in Figure 6-7. Lepromatous leprosy also causes damage to the upper respiratory tract, eyes, and testes. The lesions eventually form nodules called lepromas on the earlobes, nose, eyebrows, and forehead.

Because individuals with leprosy lose sensation, they are subject to a number of problems. They are unable to tell when something they touch is too hot. An infection may go unnoticed until it has spread so far that amputation is necessary. In undeveloped countries where sanitation is lacking and people sleep on dirt floors, there have been cases of lepers having toes gnawed at by a rat during sleep and actually losing a toe without waking up.

Treatment

Because of increased resistance of *M. leprae* to antibiotics, a number of different drugs are used to treat the disease. Early treatment, before damage has occurred, can lead to a cure. Later treatment

lepromatous	lep-RO-ma-tus
erythematous	er-i-THEM-a-tus
macules	MAK-yuls

Disease itself - doesn't cause disfiguring
attacks periferal nervous system
can't feel anything

TABLE 6-1	Registered Prevalence of Leprosy and Detection Rate in the Top Endemic Countries, 1999[a]			
Country	Registered Cases on January 1	Prevalence (per 10,000)	Newly Detected Cases During the Year	Detection Rate (per 100,000)
India	577,200	5.9	634,901	64.3
Brazil[b]	72,953	4.3	43,933	25.9
Indonesia	23,378	1.1	18,367	8.9
Madagascar	12,989	8.0	8,957	55.2
Myanmar	11,906	2.4	14,357	29.0
Nepal	8,446	3.6	6,570	27.8
Ethiopia	7,764	1.3	4,457	7.4
Mozambique	5,861	3.3	3,764	21.1
Democratic Republic of the Congo	5,853	1.2	3,781	7.9
Guinea	2,388	3.3	3,684	50.3
Total	**734,853**	**4.5**	**748,855**	**46.0**

[a]The top endemic countries included here have the following characteristics: (i) they have a prevalence >1 in 10,000 population; (ii) the number of prevalent leprosy cases is >5,000, or the number of newly detected cases is > 2,000. Ranking of countries is based on the number of registered cases.
[b]1998 information.

WHO Publication—Weekly Epidemiological Record. September 24, 1999. "Global leprosy situation, September 1999" pp. 313–314.

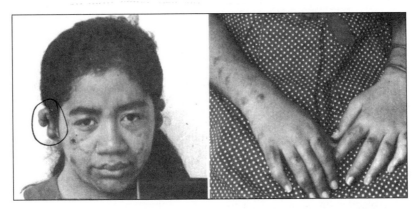

Figure 6-7
Nodules of lepromatous lesions on the face and hands. These photographs show the late stages of the disease.

cannot reverse damage to the skin and other organs that may be involved but can halt the disease. However, increased resistance of the organism to the most effective drugs is causing an intense search for others to be used in treating the disease.

Prevention

According to the *British Medical Journal*,* a vaccine has been developed in India—the first to stimulate the immune system to destroy *M. leprae*.

*BMJ "India Approves Leprosy Vaccine" 2/7/98, v316 Issue 7129, p. 414, 2/3p. By Mudur, Ganapati

[handwritten margin notes: Syphilis ↑ when birth control became popular; Syphilis ↑ drug use]

And in the United States, thalidomide has just been approved to treat one form of leprosy. This drug, which was responsible for children being born with deformities (when used during the mother's pregnancy), has strict rules for its use. However, some in the scientific community feel it is too dangerous to be used at all.

Treatment centers are available so that infected individuals can be away from the family until they are cured. Education of the public concerning the availability of treatment is needed

Control

Investigation of contacts to determine other cases and contact isolation in the case of lepromatous leprosy are the main means of control.

SYPHILIS

Syphilis was present in early Egyptian days; it was described by Hippocrates in 460 B.C.; the Bible refers to syphilis; it was described by a Roman physician in A.D. 25; syphilis is still a problem today. Plagues of syphilis have been the cause of millions of the world's crippled, blind, insane, and dead. It has infected young and old, rich and poor, prince and pauper.

Syphilis has played an important part in shaping the course of history. It is believed that Columbus and his men spread the disease in Spain after their return from the New World. Columbus himself died of the disease. Vasco da Gama carried it to India in 1498, and by 1501 it was in China. It has traveled with armies throughout history. Charles VIII of France died of syphilis, and all his heirs were born dead of syphilis, ending a dynasty. Other kings and emperors acquired syphilis that affected their minds and consequently their actions.

In the United States, syphilis became a very serious problem in the War of 1812. More than 77,000 Union soldiers contracted syphilis during the Civil War. In World War I, about three million cases of syphilis were contracted by the soldiers of all armies. One million men in the U.S. armed services were found to have syphilis between 1940 and 1945.

With the discovery and use of penicillin in the late 1940s, new cases of syphilis began to drop sharply. Almost everyone believed the end of syphilis was in sight, and programs for its control began to be curtailed. Then, in 1958, with the advent of the female contraceptive pill, penicillin-resistant strains, curtailment of programs for control, and a general feeling that the "cure" had been found, the incidence of syphilis began to rise again. In 1982, a sharp decrease in the number of cases began, probably as a result of less and "safer" sex because of the AIDS scare, but by 1986, a new epidemic of syphilis had begun (Figure 6-8). According to the CDC, three factors contributed to that epidemic. First, the use of cocaine and other drugs tends to promote high-risk sexual behaviors, and those who use it are hard to find (their illegal activity means they do not want to be found). Second, the individuals with the highest risk do not have access to health care, do not know where or when to find help, or do not consider health care a high priority. Third, those most involved with drug use are often jobless, uneducated, come from dysfunctional families, and have many sex partners.

In 1991, the rates started to decline again and continue to decline. Primary and secondary syphilis cases declined by eighty-four percent from 1990 to 1997. In a report in the *Morbidity and Mortality Weekly Report**, four factors were identified that may have contributed to this most recent decline. First, because of the epidemic in the mid-1980s, increased state and federal resources were invested in syphilis control programs. Second, the implementation of HIV prevention activities since the mid-1980s probably contributed to declines in all sexually transmitted diseases (STDs) although exact figures are not yet available. Third, a decline in crack cocaine use could have resulted in a decrease in syphilis because addicts exchanged sex for drugs. And finally, immunity in the population from exposure during the last epidemic may have contributed to the decline. The syphilis rate is now at its lowest

*"Primary and Secondary Syphilis—United States, 1997" *Morbidity and Mortality Weekly Report* 47:483, 1998.

[handwritten note at bottom: latent - no symptoms dormant]

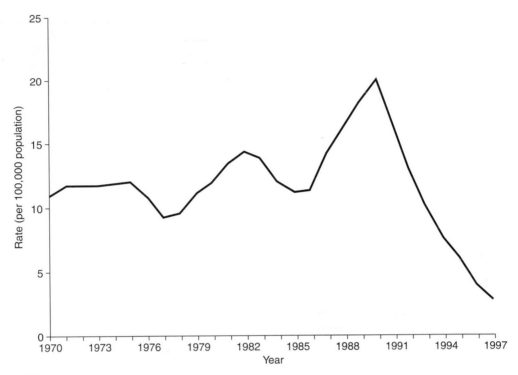

Figure 6-8

Primary and secondary syphilis rates per 100,000 population, United States, 1970–1997.

level nationwide since reporting began in 1941, but blacks and people in the South still have unusually high rates (Figures 6-9 and 6-10).

Syphilis and other diseases transmitted mainly through sexual relations were initially called venereal diseases after Venus, the Roman goddess of love. As it became clear that there were other means of transmission of these diseases, and to erase some of the stigma attached to the term venereal disease, a new term, *sexually transmitted diseases,* has come into use.

Syphilis is caused by a spirochete, **Treponema pallidum,** which is capable of entering the body through the mucous membrane. The infection spreads throughout the body in progressive stages: primary, secondary, latent, and late, or tertiary, syphilis. The incubation period for syphilis can run from ten days to three months but is usually three weeks. The disease is communicable during the first three stages and can be transmitted to the fetus in the womb. Susceptibility is general, although only thirty percent of those exposed become infected.

Transmission

Direct contact with body fluids containing the organism, during sexual or other intimate contact, is the major means of transmission. Infection of the fetus occurs through the placental membrane. The organism can be transmitted through blood transfusion from a victim in the early stages. It is possible to contract syphilis by contact with contaminated articles but highly unlikely because the organism can only exist in moist body fluids. Exposure to air, drying, and soap and water will all destroy *T. pallidum.*

Symptoms

The first sign of syphilis is a painless sore or **chancre** at the point at which the organism invaded the body (Figure 6-11). This sore is teeming with **spirochetes,** but because it is painless, because it may be in the rectum or on the cervix, and because

mother has = baby born w/ it

Cant catch it off toilet seat

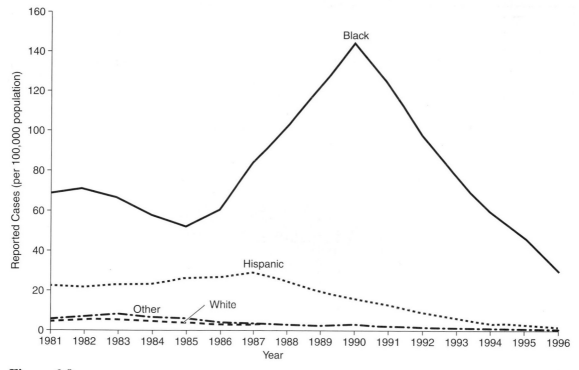

Figure 6-9

Primary and secondary syphilis rates, United States, 1981–1996.

it disappears in four to six weeks, it generally goes untreated and undiagnosed. This is the primary stage.

The secondary stage, which may develop within a few days to eight weeks, most often includes a rash, lymph node enlargement, headache, aches and pains in the bones, loss of appetite, fever, and fatigue. Hair may fall out in clumps, and meningitis may occur. Secondary syphilis disappears without treatment in a matter of weeks or months. This is the beginning of the latent stage.

For many, there will be no more symptoms, but about thirty percent will go on into the late, or tertiary, stage. It is at this time, after traveling deep within the body and into many areas that the spirochete does its great damage. The first symptoms appear in one to twenty-five years. The basic lesion of tertiary syphilis is known as a **gumma** (Figure 6-12). There are no spirochetes in this lesion, and it is painless.

Among the more serious effects in the late stages are cardiovascular syphilis, which affects the aorta and leads to **aneurysms** and heart valve disease; neurosyphilis, leading to progressive brain damage and general paralysis; and **tabes dorsalis,** which affects part of the spinal cord. The disease is no longer communicable in the late stage.

Treatment

Syphilis can be cured with penicillin in all three stages, but organ damage caused by the disease cannot be reversed. The fetus can be cured in the womb if the mother is treated soon enough.

Treponema pallidum   trep-o-NE-ma PAL-i-dum
chancre   SHANG-ker
spirochetes   SPI-ro-keets
gumma   GUM-a
tabes dorsalis   TA-bes dor-SAL-is

Prevention = Monogamus Relationships

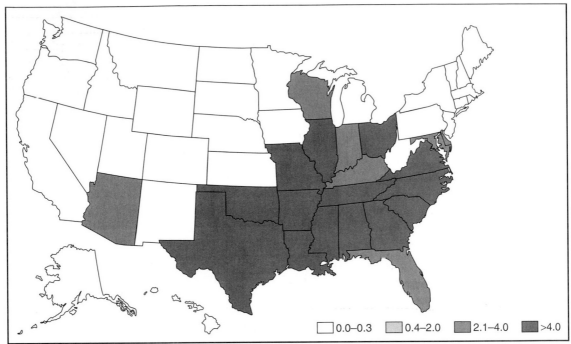

NOTE: The Year 2000 Objective is ≤4.0 per 100,000 population.

Figure 6-10

Primary and secondary syphilis reported in the United States, by population and state for 1996.

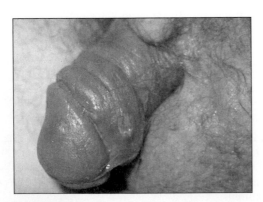

Figure 6-11

Chancre on penis.

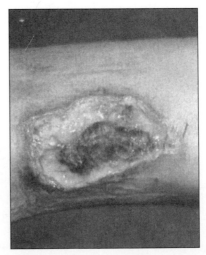

Figure 6-12

The basic lesion of syphilis, a gumma.

Prevention

The best means of prevention is by maintaining monogamous relationships. Condoms offer some protection. Immunity develops slowly after infection with *T. pallidum,* but if treatment occurs early, in the first or second stage, and/or HIV is present, the amount of immunity is reduced.

Control

Contact investigation is the most important feature of syphilis control. Interviews with diagnosed cases by professional interviewers and a concerted effort to track down and screen all reported contacts help to control the disease.

GONORRHEA   *The Clap*

Gonorrhea, like syphilis, is a very old disease. It was described nearly 5000 years ago by the Chinese and later by the Egyptians. There are also references to it in the Bible. Gonorrhea is caused by the gonococcus *Neisseria gonorrhoeae,* and Galen gave it its name, which means "flowing seed." The most common nickname is "the clap." Not long ago, gonorrhea was the most common sexually transmitted disease, but it is now second to chlamydia. The incubation period is two to seven days. In the last twenty years, the number of cases have increased all over the world; in the United States, the number of cases was still going down as of 1996 but the number of women with the disease has continued to move closer to the number of men who have it (Figure 6-13). Communicability may be present for months, and there is general susceptibility to the disease.

Transmission

Transmission is by contact with body fluid of an infected individual and almost always through sexual activity. In children older than one year of age, it is generally a result of sexual molestation.

Treatment Difficult = 3 strands = resistant to Penicillin

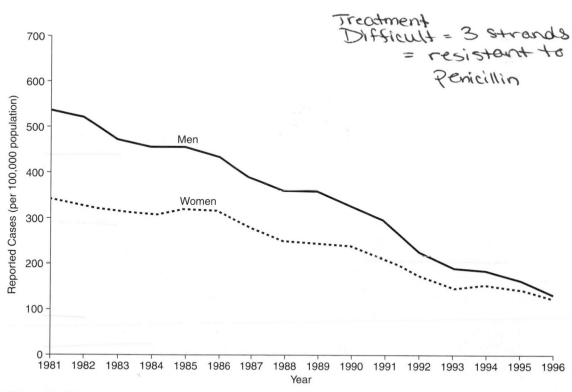

Figure 6-13

Gonorrhea, by sex, United States, 1981–1996.

Symptoms

In eighty percent of women, there may be no symptoms until the disease has infected the fallopian tubes. If there are symptoms, they usually consist of a vaginal discharge or a burning sensation on urination.

Figure 6-14 shows a sign of gonorrhea in men, a purulent urethral discharge. There is also redness and swelling at the site of infection, and many have painful urination. Men may also be asymptomatic. If the disease is untreated, other symptoms occur, depending upon the site of infection. These may include frequent urination, itching and pain of the vulva, redness, swelling, and discharge from the vagina.

Infection through anal sex causes inflammation of the rectum and anus; gonococcal pharyngitis may result from oral sex. Babies may acquire a severe eye infection during childbirth. If they are born in a hospital, silver nitrate drops in their eyes to prevent infection are required.

Untreated gonorrhea may lead to inflammation of the prostate or testes in men, affecting fertility, and to pelvic inflammatory disease (PID) in women, leading to the possibility of ectopic pregnancy and infertility.

For both sexes, there is the chance of gonococcal arthritis, septicemia, and heart disease.

Treatment

Gonorrhea is usually treated with penicillin or ampicillin. Three strains of *N. gonorrhoeae* are resistant to antibiotics. These are penicillinase-producing *N. gonorrhoeae* (PPNG), chromosomally mediated resistance to penicillin (CMRNG), and plasmid-mediated high-level tetracycline resistance (TRNG). Although treatment has become more difficult because of these resistant bacteria, the disease still can be cured by other antibiotics, sometimes in combination. However, if damage has occurred (scar tissue and/or sterility) it may not be possible to correct.

Prevention

The best means of prevention is to have sex in a monogamous relationship only. Condoms offer some protection. There is no immunity after infection with gonorrhea, and no vaccine is available to date. *You can get it again*

Control

Contact investigation and treatment of infected individuals are the best means of control. No vaccine has been developed.

CHLAMYDIA GENITAL INFECTIONS
→most common

With the improvement of laboratory equipment has come the discovery of new organisms and strains. When **chlamydiae** were first discovered, there was a question as to what class of microorganisms they were, because, like viruses, they multiply in cells or other organisms but otherwise have many of the characteristics of bacteria, including susceptibility to antibiotic treatment. At present, they are generally classified as bacteria. Chlamydiae are a cause of nonspecific urethritis (NSU), sometimes called nongonococcal urethritis (NGU). Chlamydia causes more STD in the United States than any other organism. The reported rates in the United States for 1984 to 1996 are shown in Figure 6-15. The map in Figure 6-16 shows the reported cases of chlamydia in women in the United States for 1996. In addi-

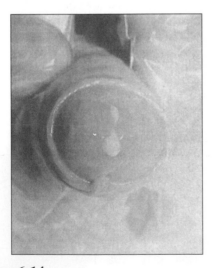

Figure 6-14

A purulent urethral discharge is the commonest presentation of gonorrhea in males.

7-14 Day incubation

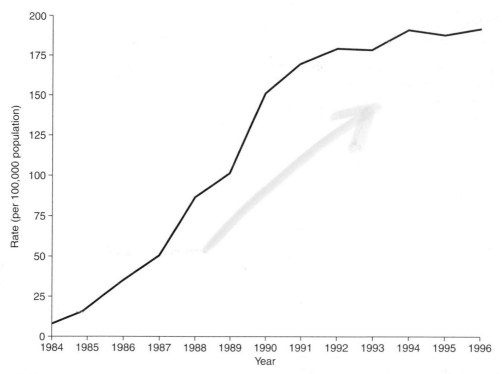

Figure 6-15

Chlamydia, reported rates, United States, 1984–1996.

tion to causing urethritis in men and cervicitis in women, *Chlamydia trachomatis* is also responsible for trachoma and lymphogranuloma. Chlamydial infections can be found all over the world, and recognition of them has been increasing in the United States, Australia, Canada, and Europe. The incubation period is thought to be seven to fourteen days but has not been clearly identified yet. Everyone is susceptible to the chlamydia organism.

Transmission

C. trachomatis is transmitted by sexual intercourse and during childbirth to babies in the birth canal, causing eye infection and pneumonia in the newborn.

Symptoms

Both men and women may be asymptomatic. When there are symptoms, these may include a discharge from the penis or vagina, swelling of the testes for men, or painful urination for women. If the disease is not treated, it can lead to infertility in men and women.

Treatment

Antibiotics are usually very successful for treatment of chlamydia.

Prevention

The best method of prevention is to have sexual relations only within a monogamous relationship. Condoms offer some protection.

Control

Testing of partners and other contact investigation are the means of control.

chlamydia   chla-MYD-ia

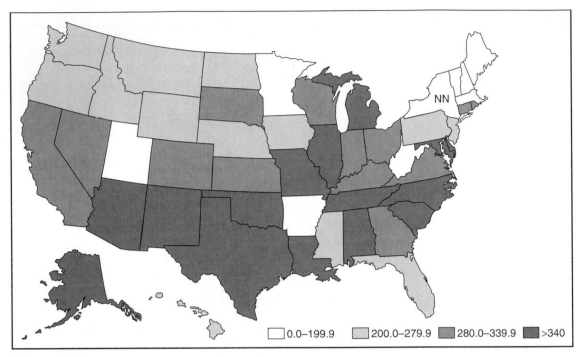

Figure 6-16
Chlamydia cases in women, United States, 1996.

DID YOU KNOW?

Pause for Thought

Animals are susceptible to syphilis too, and for a long time it was thought that shepherds got the disease from their sheep, thereby causing its occurrence and transmission in humans. Now, because of a discovery in 1987 of the remains of a bear over 11,000 years old that showed signs of having syphilis, it is thought that humans got the disease from the bite of a bear or through contact with the bear's meat after killing it for a meal.

SUMMARY

Table 6-2 summarizes the principal information related to infectious diseases acquired through the skin, mucous membranes, and bloodstream.

TABLE 6-2	Bacterial Diseases Acquired Through Skin, Mucosa, and Bloodstream			
Disease	**Special Characteristics**	**Transmission**	**Major Symptoms**	**Prevention/ Control**
Folliculitis, boils, and carbuncles	All are caused by *S. aureus.* Pressure or squeezing of boil or carbuncle can lead to complications	Person-to-person or autoinfection	Inflammation, pain, Boils— hard, painful nodule, discharge of pus, one opening, Carbuncle— extremely painful deep abscess, discharge of pus, multiple openings	Good personal hygiene, education of children in hand washing, healthy lifestyle
Impetigo	Especially common in newborn and children, highly contagious	Direct and indirect contact	Fluid-filled vesicles that rupture and become crusted; mostly around mouth and nose	Good personal hygiene and a positive lifestyle
Osteomyelitis	Infection of bone and bone marrow	No person-to-person transmission	Abrupt onset, sudden pain in bone, tenderness, heat, swelling and restricted movement	Refrain from squeezing boils; healthy lifestyle
Toxic shock syndrome	Usually affects menstruating women under 30 years of age	No person-to-person transmission	Fever, headache, vomiting, sore throat, diarrhea, muscle aches, rash, bloodshot eyes, low blood pressure, disorientation, reduced urination, peeling of skin on palms and soles of feet	No tampons, or less absorbent tampons changed frequently; contraceptive devices not left in place more than 30 hours or beyond directions on package
Conjunctivitis	Also called "pink eye"	Direct and indirect contact	Redness, itchiness, purulent discharge	Good personal hygiene and a positive lifestyle

TABLE 6-2	*Continued*			
Disease	**Special Characteristics**	**Transmission**	**Major Symptoms**	**Prevention/ Control**
Meningitis	Caused by several different bacteria and other organisms	Direct and/or indirect, depending on infecting organism	Fever, chills, malaise, headache, vomiting, stiff neck, back spasms	Prophylactic antibiotics for high risk individuals; vaccine for some bacteria
Endocarditis	Exists in two types: acute and subacute. It is a risk in dental and surgical procedures, drug addicts. Caused by different strains of bacteria and other organisms	Bacteria introduced into bloodstream by IV, surgery, shared needles, wound; no person-to-person transmission	Acute: sudden chills, high fever, shortness of breath, rapid or irregular heatbeat	Prophylactic treatment with antibiotics for those at risk
Leprosy	Also called Hansen's disease, has low contagion, incubation is 9 months to 20 years. Exists in two types: tuberculoid and lepromatous	Exact means unknown; probably through upper respiratory system or break in skin; prolonged close contact with infected individual necessary	Large, red plaques or macules on skin that become nodules; affects the nervous system	Organism resistant to antibiotics; other drugs being used
Syphilis	Has caused much suffering and death for thousands of years. Has affected history. Four stages are: primary, secondary, latency, and tertiary (late); First two stages disappear without treatment. Fetus can be	Direct contact with body fluids containing the spirochete	Primary: chancre Secondary: more chancres, rash, lymph node enlargement, headache, aches and pains in bones, fever, fatigue, loss of hair Latency: none Tertiary: cardiovascular, brain damage,	Monogamy, condoms, contact investigation, and treatment of infected individuals

| **TABLE 6-2** | *Continued* | | | |

Disease	Special Characteristics	Transmission	Major Symptoms	Prevention/ Control
Syphilis—Cont'd	infected through placenta. All three stages and fetus can be cured with penicillin. Incubation 10 days to 3 months, usually 3 weeks		paralysis, and many more	
Gonorrhea	Is an ancient disease, second most common STD. Babies may acquire eye infection passing through birth canal; Incubation is usually 2–7 days	By contact with infected body fluids, generally through sexual activity	Women often, men sometimes, asymptomatic; if symptoms, they usually include discharge from the vagina or urethra, painful urination, redness and swelling at site of infection	Treatment of sexual partners, contact investigation, and treatment of infected individuals
Chlamydia	*C. trachomatis* is an intracellular organism, but other characteristics resemble bacteria. The organism is susceptible to antibiotics; Causes more STD than any other organism; Incubation is probably 7–10 days or longer	By sexual intercourse; to babies in birth canal	Both men and women may be asymptomatic; a discharge from penis or swollen testicles may be present in men, painful urination in women; in a pregnant woman, baby can have eye infection and pneumonia	Monogamous sexual relations and use of condoms

Antibiotics used topically (in an ointment), orally, or intravenously are the primary treatment for bacterial infections.

QUESTIONS FOR REVIEW

1. What are the differences among folliculitis, furuncles, and carbuncles?

2. Why does autoinfection play such a big part in contracting folliculitis, furuncles, and carbuncles?

3. What dangers are there in squeezing a boil?

4. Describe the lesion caused by impetigo.

5. What treatment is effective for impetigo?

6. What increases susceptibility to osteomyelitis?

7. What conditions seem to predispose an individual to TSS?

8. What are the symptoms for TSS?

9. How can TSS be avoided?

10. What causes "pink eye"?

11. How is an eye infection transmitted?

12. How does meningitis usually occur?

13. What are some specific symptoms of meningitis?

14. What factors predispose an individual to endocarditis?

15. What is the difference between acute and subacute endocarditis?

16. In what states has leprosy been reported?

17. What is one of the main problems with eradication of leprosy?

18. What is the difference between tuberculoid and lepromatous leprosy?

19. In what way has syphilis affected history?

20. Why has the incidence of syphilis fluctuated so over the years?

21. Identify the four stages of syphilis and symptoms for each stage.

22. Why is syphilis sometimes not identified until the late stage?

23. What happens to the baby in the womb if its mother has syphilis?

24. Why is it unlikely that syphilis will be contracted by means other than sexual intercourse?

25. What are the most important ways to prevent and control syphilis?

26. Why has treatment of gonorrhea become difficult?

27. What is generally the cause of gonorrhea in children?

28. What are the symptoms and complications of gonorrhea?

29. In what ways can chlamydia be transmitted?

FURTHER READING

Ahmad, Khabir. 1999. WHO initiates global leprosy health care alliance. *The Lancet* 354:1802.

Aral, S. O., et al. 1999. Sexual mixing patterns in the spread of gonococcal and chlamydial infections. *American Journal of Public Health* 89:825.

Asoesberro, F., et al. 1999. Fungal endocarditis in critically ill children. *European Journal of Pediatrics* 158:275–80.

Ault, Alicia. 1998. Thalidomide makes a return to US health care. *The Lancet* 352:298.

Boyles, Salynn, and Sandra W. Key, "New strains of bacterial Meningitis may be emerging." *Tuberculosis & Airborne Disease Weekly,* 98–9.

Brandt, E. R., and M. F. Good. 1999. Vaccine strategies to prevent rheumatic fever. *Immunologic Research* 19:89.

Calhoun, Jason H., Richard T. Laughlin, Jon T. Maher, et al. "Osteomylitis: Diagnosis, staging, management." *Patient Care,* 32(2):93–101.

Chamot, E., et al. 1999. Gonorrhea incidence and HIV testing and counseling among adolescents and young adults seen at a clinic for sexually transmitted diseases. *AIDS* 13:971.

Cimerman, M., et al. 1999. Femur osteomyelitis due to a mixed fungal infection in a previously healthy man. *Journal of Clinical Microbiology* 37:2106.

Cluster of syphilis cases linked to the internet. *Modern Medicine.* 67:14, 1999.

Cohen, Deborah A., and Malanda Nsuami. 1999. Repeated school based screening for sexually transmitted diseases: a feasible strategy. *Pediatrics* 104:1281.

Diang'a, Alex. 1998. Beating back leprosy. *World Press Review* 45:40.

Dyson, C., et al., 1999. Infective endocarditis: an edidemiological review of 128 episodes. *Journal of Infection* 38:87.

Gregory, Tanya, and Gary L. Darmstadt. 1998. Scarlet fever and its relatives. *Patient Care* 32:109.

Groseclose, Samuel L., and Akbar A. Saidi. 1999. Estimated incidence and prevalence of genital chlamydia trachomatis infections in the US. *Sexually Transmitted Diseases* 26:339.

Han, Yangsook, and Bruce F. Coles. 1999. Assessment of geographically targeted field intervention on gonorrhea incidence in New York. *Sexually Transmitted Diseases* 26:296.

Holtom, P. M., and A. M. Smith. 1999. Introduction to adult posttraumatic osteomyelitis of the tibia. *Clin Orthop* 360:6–13.

Hook III, Edward W. 1998. Is elimination of endemic syphilis transmission a realistic goal for the USA? *The Lancet* 351:19.

Howell, Rene M., et al. 1999. Control of chlamydia trachomatis infections in female army recruits: cost effective screening and . . . *Sexually Transmitted Diseases* 26:519.

Incident Chlamydia trachomatis infections among inner-city adolescent females. *Journal of the American Medical Association* 280:521, 1998.

Jacobson, Robert R., and James L. Krahenbuhl. 1999. Leprosy. *The Lancet* 353:655.

Kirchner, Jeffrey T. 1998. Changes in the incidence of bacterial meningitis. *American Family Physician* 57:1121.

Kuznar, Wayne. 1998. Hot tubs: Reservoirs for infection. *Dermatology Times* 19:80.

Leprosy beyond the year 2000. *The Lancet* 350:1717, 1998.

Leprosy vaccine approved in India. *Southern Medical Journal* 91:691, 1998.

Mader, Jon T. 1999. Bone and joint infections in the elderly: practical treatment guidelines. *Drugs and Aging* 16:67–80.

Mohle-Boetani, J. C. 1999. Virtal meningitis in child care center staff and parents; an outbreak of echovirus 30 infections. *Public Health Reports* 114:249–256.

Morrow, Gary L., and Richard L. Abbott. 1998. Conjunctivitis. *American Family Physician* 57:735.

Norrby-Teglund, A., et al. 1999. Risk factors in the pathogenesis of invasive group A streptococcal infections. *Infection and Immunity* 67:1871.

Preventing spread of meningeal disease. *American Family Physician* 57:860, 1998.

Primary and secondary syphilis. *Morbidity and Mortality Weekly Report* 47:493, 1998.

Primary and secondary syphilis—United States, 1998. *Journal of American Medicine.* 282:1715, 1999.

Remez, L. 1999. Independent predictors of chlamydia and gonorrhea do not identify adolescents at high risk of infection. *Family Planning Perspectives* 31:101.

Roder, Bent L., and Dorte A. Wandall. 1999. Clinical features of staphylococcus aureus endocarditis. *Archives of Internal Medicine* 159:462.

Rotbart, H. A. 1999. Clinical significance of enteroviruses in serious summer febrile illnesses of children. *Pediatric Infectious Disease* 18:869–74.

Sadovsky, Richard. 1998. Tobacco smoke exposure and meningococcal disease risk. *American Family Physician* 57:2848.

Stollerman, Gene H., and Alan L. Bisno. 1999. Is dentistry a risk factor for endocarditis? *Hospital Practice* 34:30.

Swain, Geoffrey R., Stephen J. Kowalewski, et al. 1998. Reducing the incidence of congenital syphilis in Milwaukee: A public/private partnership. *American Journal of Public Health* 88:1101.

Taubert, Kathyryn A., and Adnan S. Dajani. 1998. Preventing bacterial endocarditis: American Heart Association guidelines. *American Family Physician* 57:457.

Taylor-Robinson, D., and A. Renton. 1999. Diagnostic tests that are worthwhile for patients with sexually transmitted bacterial infections in industrialized countries. *International Journal of STD and AIDS* 10:1.

Tomaszewski, D., and D. J. Avella. 1999. Vertebral osteomyelitis in a high school hockey player: a case report. *Journal of Athletic Training* 34:29–33.

Walling, Anne D. 1999. Impetigo. *American Family Physician* 59:1042.

7

BACTERIAL DISEASES ACQUIRED THROUGH SKIN AND MUCOSA FROM ARTHROPOD VECTORS, ANIMAL SOURCES, AND THE SOIL

O B J E C T I V E S

1. *Discuss the dangers of bioterrorism and the organisms that might be used as weapons.*

2. *State ways by which disease is transmitted to humans from animals.*

3. *Identify some of the arthropod vectors responsible for disease transmission.*

4. *Recognize the importance of pest control and sanitation.*

5. *Describe preventive measures to be taken to avoid infection with zoonoses.*

6. *Compare Lyme disease, Rocky Mountain spotted fever, and Ehrlichiosis.*

7. *Explain why tetanus shots and boosters are important.*

8. *Discuss characteristics, transmission, symptoms, prevention, and control for the diseases in this chapter.*

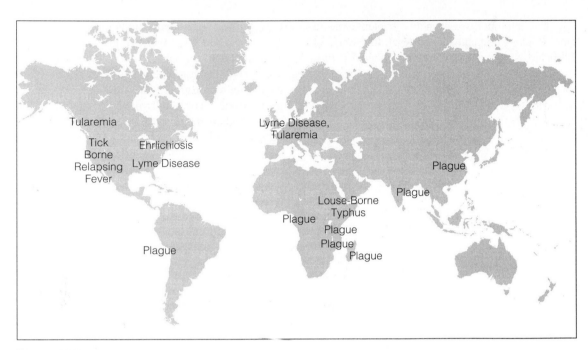

Figure 7-1

Distribution of tularemia, Lyme disease, Ehrlichiosis, and the plague, worldwide.

Adapted from Duane J. Gubler, Centers for Disease Control and Prevention, Fort Collins, Colorado.

PATHOGENIC BACTERIAL RESERVOIRS AND ZOONOSES

Humans are the chief reservoir for most pathogenic bacteria. Animals, insects, and the soil also serve as reservoirs for these disease agents. The infectious diseases of animals that can be transmitted to humans are called **zoonoses.** Arthropod vectors (insects that carry disease) are often involved in the transfer of organisms from one reservoir to another. Most of these arthropod vectors are parasitic (living on other species) and, while securing a blood meal from an animal or human, may pick up infectious microorganisms and later infect another animal or human by inoculation. Some of these arthropods act only as mechanical carriers and are not true reservoirs, because the vector does not maintain the organism. Other arthropods become reservoirs for an organism if it infects them and is able to develop and multiply.

Infection by arthropod vector is not the only way that bacterial and rickettsial diseases of animals can be transmitted to humans. They may also be transmitted through other direct and indirect means, depending upon the nature of the disease and the animal involved. And some of these diseases have potential as biologic weapons—either in a terrorist attack or in warfare.

Animals also carry other pathogenic organisms in addition to bacteria that can cause disease in humans. In this chapter we will discuss zoonotic diseases caused by bacteria and rickettsia and acquired most often through the skin and mucosa. If any of these organisms is developed as a weapon, the mode of transmission could be by inhalation.

Some of the vectorborne diseases are among those identified as Resurgent or Reemerging diseases (see Chapter 1). Epidemics of many of these diseases have occurred recently in many parts of the world, including the United States (Figure 7-1).

---

zoonoses   zo-o-NO-sis

The first four diseases in this chapter, Lyme disease, Rocky Mountain spotted fever, tularemia, and Ehrlichiosis are most often transmitted by ticks. Plague is fleaborne, whereas the transmission of leptospirosis, brucellosis, tetanus, and anthrax is by contact with some part of an animal's body or excreta.

LYME DISEASE

In 1975 a group of children in Lyme, Connecticut, developed symptoms of an infection that was identified as tickborne, spirochetal, and zoonotic. It was called Lyme disease, and since that time it has appeared in every state except Montana. Figure 7-2 shows the number of cases reported to the CDC in 1997. The increase in cases in the United States in recent years can be seen in Figure 7-3.

The disease agent is a spirochete called **Borrelia burgdorferi,** which is carried by the tiny tick, **Ixodes scapularis,** pictured in Figure 7-4. This tick is found on deer, wild rodents, and other animals. These animals can act as secondary reservoirs. The incubation period is three to thirty-two days after exposure to the tick. All people are probably susceptible to Lyme disease, and indications arc that immunity does not result from one infection, because repeated infections have occurred. Highest rates of the disease are in children five to nine years of age and adults over thirty years of age. Although people don't generally die from Lyme disease, the sequelae pose a serious threat to the health and lifestyle of the victim. The white-footed mouse is the most important reservoir for *B. Burgdorferi* in North America.

Transmission

The disease is acquired through the bite of an infected tick. The spirochete can also be transmitted to the fetus if a pregnant woman gets the dis-

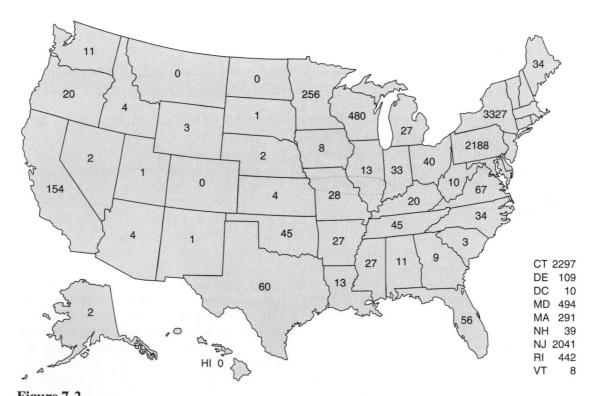

CT 2297
DE 109
DC   10
MD 494
MA 291
NH 39
NJ 2041
RI 442
VT   8

Figure 7-2

Reported number of Lyme disease cases, by state, United States, 1997.
Center for Disease Control and Prevention.

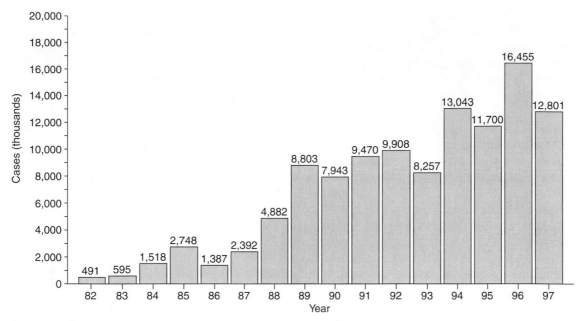

Figure 7-3

Number of reported cases of Lyme disease, United States, 1982–1997.

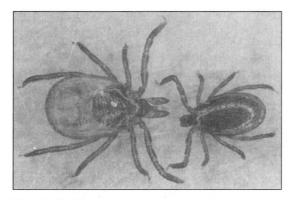

Figure 7-4

The deer tick (*I. dammini*), partly engorged (left) and unengorged (right).

ease. There is no evidence of person-to-person transmission.

Symptoms

There has been great difficulty in diagnosing Lyme disease in the early stages because the symptoms are variable and sometimes not noticed. Most patients do not remember being bitten or seeing a tick.

Lyme disease typically occurs in three stages. The first is marked by a distinctive lesion, **ery-thema migrans** (EM), which appears as a red macule or papule, often at the site of the tick bite (Figure 7-5). This lesion may expand to over fifty cm in diameter and often feels hot and sticky. Similar lesions may erupt within a few days if there was more than one tick bite. The lesion or lesions is accompanied by malaise, fatigue, fever, headache, stiff neck, muscle aches, aching in various joints, rash, and swollen lymph glands. Preceding the appearance of EM, the victim sometimes has a persistent sore throat and dry cough. The second stage appears weeks to months later, with neurologic abnormalities that may last days or months. Cardiac abnormalities may also develop. In the third stage, which may be weeks to years later, swelling and pain in the knees and

Borrelia   bor-RE-le-a
Ixodes scapularis   iks-O-dez skap-U-lar-is
erythema   er-i-THE-ma

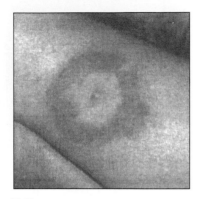

Figure 7-5

Large, red, slowly spreading rash characteristic of Lyme disease called erythema migrans.

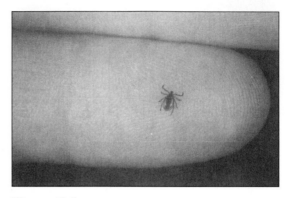

Figure 7-6

The deer tick (*I. dammini*). Its tiny size is demonstrated when shown in its unengorged stage on the tip of a finger.

other large joints occur, which may lead to the development of chronic arthritis.

One of the more serious side effects of Lyme disease is fibromyalgia. This syndrome is not fatal but has no cure, and in many cases the victim is unable to continue working. Fibromyalgia will be discussed with other musculoskeletal disorders in Chapter 16.

Treatment

Lyme disease can be cured by antibiotics in all three stages. If arthritis has become established, symptoms are reversed only half of the time. In the EM stage, penicillin is the treatment of choice for children, tetracycline for adults. Other antibiotics are also effective if victims are unable to take or do not respond to the initial treatment. Ten to twenty days of treatment with antibiotics in the early stages will minimize later symptoms. In the later stages, antibiotics given in high doses intravenously may be effective.

Prevention

The Food and Drug Administration (FDA) recently approved a vaccine for Lyme disease. However, the manufacturer has been told to keep testing its safety. The FDA does not usually give approval before results of final testing but because Lyme disease is a serious threat that can have devastating effects, the immediate benefits of the vac-

cine outweigh the possible problems with long-term use.

Individuals who camp, hunt, or walk in areas inhabited by deer need to take special precautions. Long-sleeved shirts and long pants should be worn, with the pants tucked into socks or boots. Wearing light-colored clothing makes it easier to see the ticks. Insect repellants should be used. After leaving the areas, individuals should shower and towel down briskly, because the tick is tiny and difficult to see (Figure 7-6). Each person should be inspected for ticks, and if you are alone, use a mirror to inspect yourself. If a tick is discovered, it should be grasped gently, at the head, with tweezers, and pulled off firmly but gently. Removing it promptly may prevent transferral of the bacteria. Domestic animals that have been in deer-inhabited areas should also be checked for ticks.

Control

When cases occur in areas where the disease is not endemic, studies should be conducted to determine the source of the infection.

ROCKY MOUNTAIN SPOTTED FEVER

This typhus infection was initially identified in the Rocky Mountain region of the United States but is

Vaccine!
given in 3 doses
over a year.

Children=more suseptible

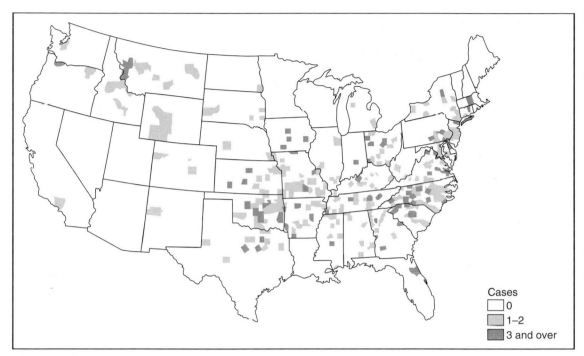

Cases
☐ 0
▨ 1–2
▧ 3 and over

Figure 7-7
Reported cases of Rocky Mountain spotted fever by county, United States, 1990.

now found in many parts of the country as seen in Figure 7-7. The number of reported cases rose sharply in the 1970s and then decreased over the next twenty-five years. However, in 1998 there was a significant increase in cases (Figure 7-8). The disease can be fatal without proper treatment. The infectious agent is *Rickettsia rickettsiae* and the reservoir of infection is in ticks. The incubation period is from three to about fourteen days. The infection is not spread person to person. Susceptibility is general, and one attack confers immunity for life.

Transmission
Figure 7-9 is a picture of the tick that transmits Rocky Mountain spotted fever. The tick needs to be attached for several hours before the rickettsiae become infective. Individuals may also become infected if crushed tissues or feces of the tick are rubbed into a bite or an abrasion.

Symptoms *Flu-like symptoms*
Mild fever, loss of appetite, and a slight headache may develop gradually about a week after the bite, or there may be a sudden onset of severe symptoms including high fever, prostration, aching, tender muscles, severe headache, nausea, and vomiting. In about half the cases, small pink spots appear on the wrists and ankles and spread over the body. The spots darken, enlarge, and may bleed. They even occur on the soles of the feet and palms of the hands. The individual in Figure 7-10 has a well-developed rash on the legs and feet.

Treatment
Antibiotics are effective as treatment.

Prevention/Control
People who live or go into tick-infested areas should examine their bodies and their pets regularly for the presence of ticks (see discussion under Lyme disease).

Tick needs to be attached for several hrs.

3-14 day incubation period
Shorter incubation = worse symptoms

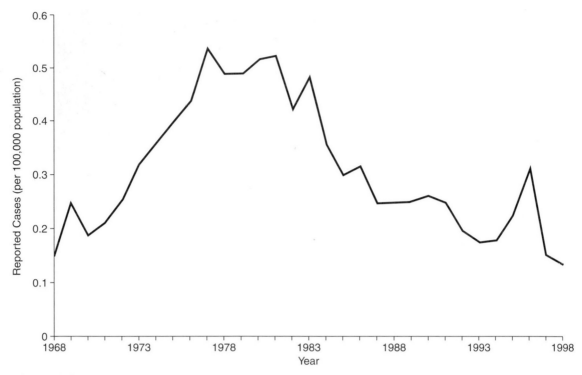

Figure 7-8

Rocky Mountain spotted fever, by year, United States, 1968–1998.

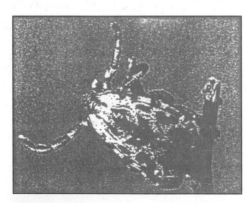

Figure 7-9

The Rocky Mountain wood tick, carrier for Rocky Mountain spotted fever.

TULAREMIA

A number of wild animals harbor the bacterium *Francisella tularensis,* the cause of tularemia, but hares and rabbits are the main source for the infection in humans. The disease received its name from Tulare, California, where it was first discovered. Figure 7-11 shows the counties where cases were reported in 1993. The incubation period is from one to fourteen days, but in most cases it is three to five days. All ages are susceptible to the disease, but cases of reinfection are rare. With appropriate treatment, there are few fatalities.

Tularemia, plague, brucellosis, anthrax, and other infectious diseases have been identified as potential biologic weapons. The threat of bioterrorism is real and attempts to use biologic weapons have occurred or been suspected. Although so far the attempts have had little success, many experts still believe the threat to be real and imminent. Microbiologist Raymond Zilinskas of the University of Maryland Biotechnology Institute has said, "It is really a matter of time. I don't understand why it hasn't happened already."* For this reason, these diseases are included in this chapter—so there might be some

*Robert Taylor, "The bio-terrorist threat," *New Scientist* May 11, 1996.

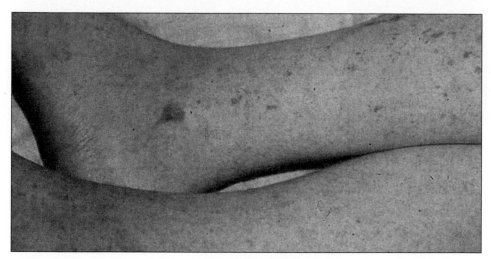

Figure 7-10

The rash of Rocky Mountain spotted fever.

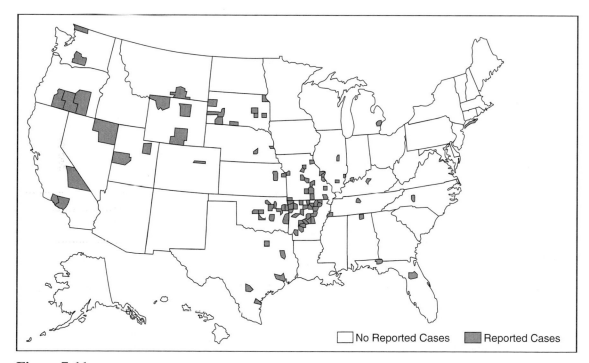

☐ No Reported Cases   ▨ Reported Cases

Figure 7-11

Tularemia, counties reporting cases, United States, 1993.

Franciscella tularensis   FRAN-si-SEL-a TOO-la-REN-sis

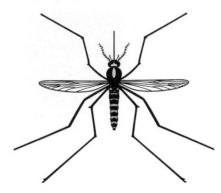

Figure 7-12

Arthropod vector that can transmit tularemia—mosquito.

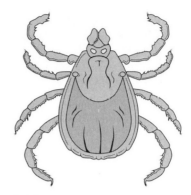

Figure 7-14

Arthropod vector that can transmit tularemia—tick.

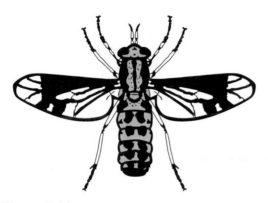

Figure 7-13

Arthropod vector that can transmit tularemia—fly.

recognition of the symptoms by people, including medical and health professionals, who have never seen them before.

Transmission

Humans may become infected with *F. tularensis* by inoculation while cleaning or working with the skins of infected animals; by fluid from infected flies, ticks, or other animals; by the bite of insects carrying the organism; by eating insufficiently cooked rabbit or hare meat; by drinking contaminated water; or by inhalation of dust from contaminated soil, grain, or hay. Figures 7-12, 7-13, and 7-14 show three of the arthropods that can transmit tularemia. There is no person-to-person transmission.

Symptoms

The infection may be limited to tissues surrounding the portal of entry, with the formation of an ulcer and involvement of regional lymph glands. If the infectious material is inhaled, this may be followed by a pneumonic or typhoidal disease. If infection comes from eating meat containing the organism, there may be pharyngitis, intestinal pain, diarrhea, and vomiting. Some strains of the organism are more virulent than others. Occasionally the disease begins with a fever and systemic illness.

Treatment

Tularemia can be treated with any number of antibiotics, including streptomycin. Early treatment leads to a cure, but antibiotics are administered until the temperature of the victim has been gone for several days to avoid a chronic low-grade infection that may occur.

Prevention

Gloves should be used when skinning or handling wild animals, especially rabbits. The meat of rabbits and wild rodents must be cooked thoroughly. In areas where there is known infection among the rodent population, people need to be educated in methods that will protect them. Vaccines are available, but their use in the United States is restricted to high-risk populations, particularly laboratory workers.

Control

There is no need to isolate individuals who have been infected, because tularemia is not a communicable disease. Open lesions need to be protected, and any materials contaminated with discharge from ulcers disinfected.

EHRLICHIOSIS

Ehrlichiosis has been recognized for many years as a disease in dogs and some other animals. In the United States, the first human case was described in 1987. By 1996, over 500 cases had been confirmed by the CDC. Because the symptoms can range from mild to life-threatening, and because it is an emerging disease that might not be recognized, the total number of victims infected by the organism is thought to be much higher. *Ehrlichia chaffeensis* (discovered at Fort Chaffee, Arkansas)

was identified as the pathogen and the disease was named human monocytic Ehrlichiosis (HME) because it was known to target the monocytes. Not until 1994 was it discovered that there were actually two similar but distinct diseases caused by two different bacteria. The second was caused by an *Ehrlichia* equilike organism and called human granulocytic Ehrlichiosis (HGE) because it was known to infect granulocytes. By April 1996, 142 cases of HGE had been identified. The distribution of HME and HGE in the United States is shown in Figure 7-15.

These illnesses can be very mild or, with no treatment, fatal. The incubation period for Ehrlichiosis is seven to twenty-one days.

Ehrlichiosis	Ehr-LICH-e-osis
Ehrlichia chaffeensis	AR-lik-e-A cha-FEEN-sis

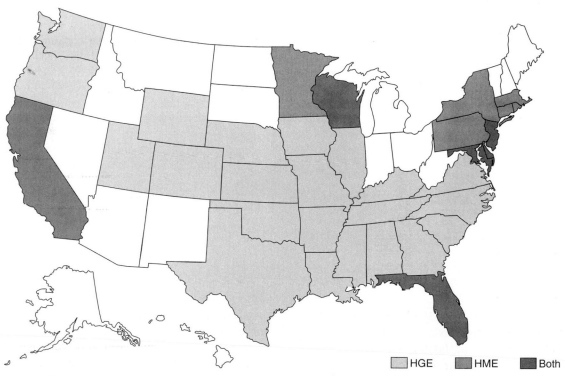

HGE　HME　Both

Figure 7-15

Spread of HGE and HME in the United States.

Center for Disease Control and Prevention, Atlanta, Georgia.

Transmission

There is no evidence of person-to-person transmission. Possible vectors for human Ehrlichiosis are the American dog tick, lone star tick, and *I. scapularis,* the deer tick that also transmits Lyme disease.

Symptoms

The most common symptoms are fever, malaise, myalgia, headaches, and rigors (alternating chills and fever). There may also be nausea, vomiting, cough, diarrhea, abdominal pain, pharyngitis, arthralgias, and mental confusion. A rash may occur, but not right away. When it does occur, its location is usually unrelated to the site of the tick bite. It erupts most often on the trunk, legs, or arms, but can be on the face, palms, or soles. If untreated, the symptoms can progress until there is multiorgan failure and ultimately death.

Treatment

The treatment of choice is tetracycline. It is uncertain which drugs will be effective if tetracycline fails because HME, and HGE particularly, are emerging diseases and not enough studies have been completed to identify other drugs that are effective.

Prevention

Avoidance of tick bites is the best means of prevention for all tickborne diseases. Refer to the information for Lyme disease for details.

Control

Educating the public is the only means of control at the present time. The correct way to remove a tick to reduce the chances of infection is illustrated in Figure 7-16.

PLAGUE

Bubonic plague, or the Black Death, spread through Europe and Asia during the Middle Ages and came closer to annihilating the human race than any other disease in the history of the world. The disease is caused by a bacillus, *Yersinia pestis,* which resides in wild rodents. In areas where famine exists, rodents move closer to

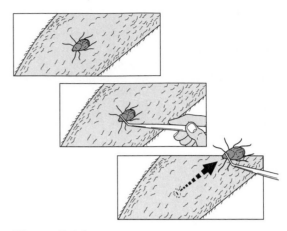

Figure 7-16
The proper method of removing a tick to avoid infection.

humans to find food. When they die, their infected fleas leave the rodents and move to humans, thus spreading the disease.

Plague is still dangerous today, existing in rodent populations in the western third of the United States, large areas of South America, north-central, eastern, and southern Africa, the Near East, and other parts of the world (Figure 7-17). Figure 7-18 shows the number of reported cases per year from 1966 to 1996 in the United States.

Plague comes in several forms. Bubonic plague is the most common. Pneumonic plague can occur as a primary infection but often is an extension of the bubonic form. Septicemic plague may develop as a progression of bubonic or pneumonic plague but also manifests as a severe, rapid, systemic infection with no apparent signs of bubonic or pneumonic plague. Pneumonic plague is highly communicable from person to person, whereas the other two forms are not generally communicable except in unusual circumstances. The incubation period varies from one to seven days. Without treatment, bubonic plague has a mortality rate of about fifty percent to sixty percent. The mortality rate for both pneumonic and septicemic plague approaches 100 percent without treatment. With treatment, the mortality

CASE STUDY

Plague

On August 17, 1996, a sixteen-year-old resident of western Colorado had onset of pain followed by numbness in her left arm and left axillary pain. During August 18 and 19, she had chills, fever, and several episodes of vomiting. On August 19, she was evaluated at a local hospital emergency department. After examination and testing, she was discharged with a diagnosis of possible brachial plexus injury related to a fall from a trampoline on August 14. She was prescribed analgesics, and an appointment with a neurologist was scheduled.

On August 21, she was found semiconcious at home and taken to the same hospital. She was confused and complained of neck pain and generalized soreness. Within an hour of arrival at the hospital, she experienced respiratory arrest and was intubated. A chest radiograph revealed bilateral pulmonary edema. She was given an antibiotic intravenously and trans-ferred to a referral hospital with diagnoses of septicemia, disseminated intravascular coagulation, adult respiratory distress syndrome, and possible meningitis. Her condition rapidly deteriorated, and she died later that day.

Postmortem testing of blood and respiratory aspirate confirmed *Y. pestis* as the disease agent. An environmental investigation by health officials revealed evidence of an earlier extensive prairie dog die-off adjacent to the patient's residence. Four family dogs and one cat tested positive for *Y. pestis*. Investigators concluded that the girl was probably exposed to *Y. Pestis* by direct contact with infectious material while handling the cat. Because the diagnosis was established after the standard seven-day maximum plague incubation period had elapsed, antibiotic prophylaxis of family members and medical personnel was not instituted.

From *Morbidity and Mortality Weekly Report* 46:617, 1997.

rate for all three forms of plague is approximately eighteen percent and is dependent on the victim's age, physical condition, and the time between onset and treatment. There is general susceptibility to plague, with the immunity acquired from infection offering the only form of resistance to the disease.

Transmission

Plague is usually transmitted to humans through the bite of a flea from an infected rodent host (Figure 7-19). Rats, squirrels, prairie dogs, and hares are common carriers, and domestic pets may carry plague-infected fleas into homes. Other sources of exposure resulting in human infection include the handling of tissues of infected animals, airborne droplets from humans or pets with pneumonic plague, and careless handling of laboratory cultures.

Symptoms

Symptoms vary for the three forms of plague. The symptoms for bubonic plague include fever, chills, headache, and exhaustion, and swelling, pain, and hemorrhage in the lymph nodes. The swellings are called "buboes," and the dark color from the hemorrhaging led to the term "Black Death." Primary pneumonic plague generally has an acute onset, with high fever, chills, severe headache, fast heartbeat, rapid, labored breathing, and a productive cough. The sputum is at first yellowish and later turns to frothy pink or red. A cough producing bloody sputum is the first sign of secondary pneumonic plague. Primary and secondary pneumonic plagues rapidly cause severe distress and may lead

---

Yersinia pestis   yer-SIN-e-a pes-TIS

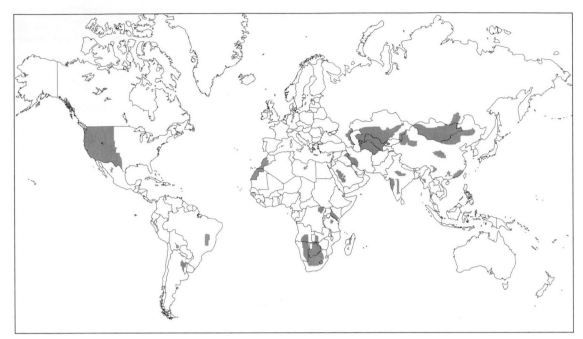

Figure 7-17

World distribution of the plague in 1998.

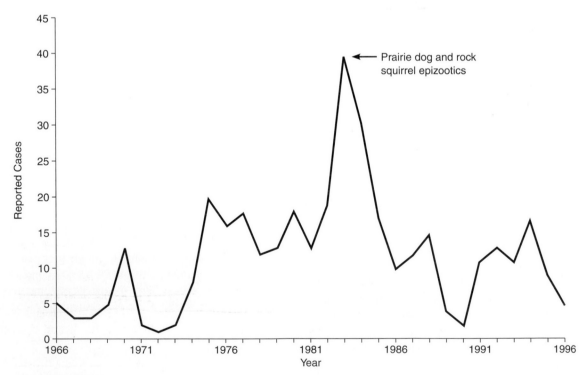

Figure 7-18

Plague among humans, by year, United States, 1966–1996.

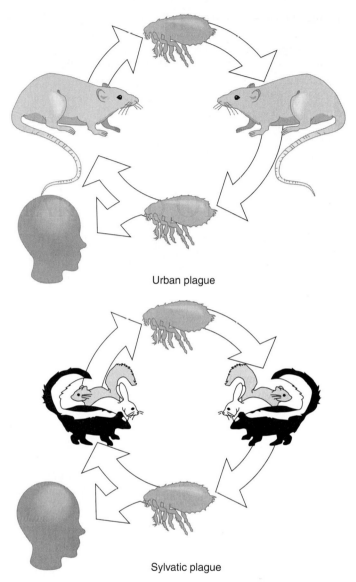

Urban plague

Sylvatic plague

Figure 7-19

Transmission of plague from fleas to animal hosts and to humans.

to death. When septicemic plague occurs, the symptoms include extreme elevation of temperature (above 106°F), convulsions, prostration, shock, and blood clotting. Septicemic plague is rapidly fatal unless promptly treated.

Treatment

Streptomycin has proved to be the most effective drug against *Y. pestis.* Penicillin is ineffective against plague. Treatment must begin within eight to twenty-four hours of onset, and, in the case of septicemic and pneumonic plagues, treatment must start within eighteen hours to prevent death. Other drugs are used as supportive therapy, depending on symptoms.

Prevention

The most effective measure for preventing plague is the destruction of rats and their fleas. Elimination of unsanitary conditions that encourage rat breeding is necessary. The elimination of rats and their fleas must take place simultaneously to keep the hungry insects from invading human populations in the vicinity. People who live in or near plague areas should be warned not to camp near rodent burrows and to report dead or sick rodents to authorities. Seaports and buildings nearby are of particular concern because of the possibility of infected animals being brought in from other countries.

A killed bacteria vaccine is available but lasts only a few months and is not always effective. Some countries use live attenuated vaccine, but the side effects are worse, and there is no evidence that it provides better coverage. Individuals in high-risk areas and those who work in laboratories and have to handle the bacillus should be vaccinated, but other preventive methods should be taken also.

Control

International health regulations require the reporting of suspected or confirmed cases of plague. The report first goes to the local health authority and from there on up. Isolation of victims and destruction of all insects on their person or clothing or in their baggage are necessary. Any soiled articles (from sputum or infected discharge) need to be disinfected. In the case of pneumonic plague, contacts should be given prophylactic treatment and isolated for seven days. In an epidemic of bubonic plague, contacts need to be protected. Contact investigations should take place to identify the source of the infection and measures taken to eliminate any rat and flea populations so identified.

LEPTOSPIROSIS

There are many different types of **Leptospira,** the spirochete responsible for **leptospirosis.** Infection with these organisms is more common in parts of the world other than the United States, with the exception of an infection caused by *Leptospira interrogans,* which is quite widespread in the United States. When the infection caused by *L. interrogans* is severe, it is called "Weil's disease," after a German physician. Weil's disease is an acute infection in which the organisms localize in the kidneys, producing kidney dysfunction. The spirochete may spread through the blood to other parts of the body such as the liver and nervous system. Fatalities may occur as a result of **hepatorenal** (liver and kidney) failure or because of myocardial involvement. The reservoir for leptospirosis is in domestic and wild animals, including rats and other rodents. The average time for developing symptoms is ten days after exposure, with a range of four to nineteen days. Excretion of the spirochete in the urine may continue up to eleven months after the illness. Human susceptibility appears to be universal, but immunity follows infection.

Transmission

Transmission is by contact of the skin, especially if the surface is broken by abrasion or a cut, and by water, moist soil, or vegetation contaminated with the excreta of infected animals. Infected animals secrete large numbers of the spirochete in their urine and may contaminate water used for drinking, swimming, or irrigation. Some individuals such as sugarcane workers, those who work in rice fields, sewer workers, and miners are at higher risk of contracting the infection. Veterinarians, farmers, and slaughterhouse workers are also at greater risk. Children have been known to contract this infection after swimming in farm ponds.

Symptoms

Symptoms are variable and include fever, headache, chills, malaise, vomiting, muscle aches, and watery eyes. Sometimes, meningitis, rash, jaundice, renal insufficiency, anemia, and hemorrhages in the skin and mucous membranes occur. Deaths are rare, but increase with age, particularly among individuals who have jaundice and untreated kidney insufficiency. Death is generally due to liver failure, kidney failure, and/or heart problems.

Treatment

Several forms of penicillin and other antibiotics are effective in destroying the organisms. Kidney dialysis may have to be performed in some cases.

Prevention

Workers in hazardous professions need to be educated to the danger of infection. Protective clothing should be worn, particularly on the hands and feet. The public needs to be educated about the dangers of swimming in potentially contaminated waters, such as farm ponds. Infected animals need to be kept out of human living, working, and recreational areas. Any rat or rodent population should be exterminated. Vaccines are available for livestock and dogs but are strain specific.

Control

The source of infection, such as a swimming pool or farm pond, needs to be found and the contamination eliminated or use prohibited if decontamination is not possible.

BRUCELLOSIS

Another name for brucellosis is **"undulant** fever," a term that describes the variable nature of the disease. The word "undulant" means "rising or falling like waves," and brucellosis is a disease that does this. It is a disease that affects cattle and other animals and is transmitted to humans directly or indirectly. Brucellosis occurs worldwide but is more prevalent in other countries than it is in the United States. There was a slight upswing in cases in the United States at the end of 1996 (Figure 7-20). In North America, the most common infecting organism is *Brucella abortus,* which is found in cattle. The incubation period is

Leptospira	lep-to-SPI-ra
leptospirosis	LEP-to-spi-RO-sis
hepatorenal	HEP-a-to-RE-nal
undulant	UN-du-lant

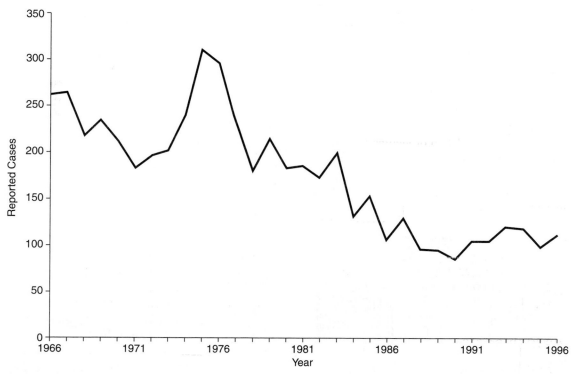

Figure 7-20

Brucellosis, by year, United States, 1966–1996.

difficult to determine because the onset of the disease is slow and insidious, but is estimated to be five days to several months. Individuals who recover from brucellosis acquire immunity to it, but the duration of the immunity is uncertain. Most individuals who drink contaminated milk become infected, and it is believed that a majority of human beings are susceptible to brucellosis infection.

Transmission

There is ordinarily no person-to-person transmission. Humans become infected with brucellosis through direct contact with animal tissues, inhalation of contaminated dust of barns or slaughterhouses, or ingestion of unpasteurized dairy products from infected animals. Figure 7-21 shows some of the ways that brucellosis can be transmitted.

Symptoms

The onset of brucellosis is usually slow and insidious, with an irregular fever, chills and sweating, myalgia (muscle aches and pains), weakness, and malaise. If the onset is acute, the symptoms are more pronounced, and there may be severe headache, backache, and exhaustion. There may be other generalized symptoms such as gastrointestinal discomfort, enlarged lymph nodes and spleen, hepatitis with jaundice, and mental depression. These symptoms may gradually become milder and eventually disappear, but the disease often becomes chronic and recurs over years. Some individuals develop endocarditis, osteomyelitis, or pyelonephritis (inflammation of kidney and pelvis), and endometritis (inflammation of the lining of the uterus) may occur in women.

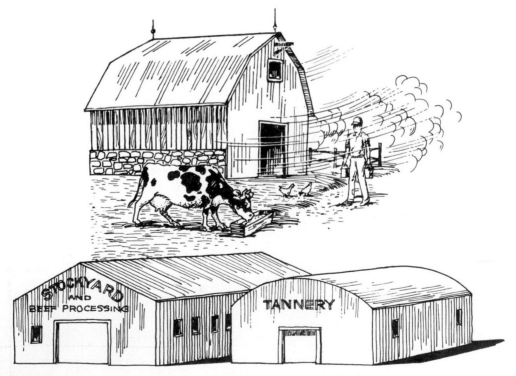

Figure 7-21
Sources of infection for brucellosis.

Abscesses may also form in the testes, ovaries, kidneys, and brain. Fatality is rare, but even with recovery, there is often residual allergy or damage to bones and other tissues.

Treatment

Prolonged treatment with antibiotics is necessary to eradicate the organism in protected intracellular sites. Tetracycline and streptomycin are used for three- and two-week periods, respectively, and in severe cases corticosteroids may be given by IV for three days, followed by oral corticosteroids. Bed rest is advised as long as there is a fever.

Prevention

There is no vaccine for brucellosis. Farmers and workers in slaughterhouses, packing plants, and butcher shops need to be educated as to the nature of the disease and the risk in the handling of carcasses or products of potentially infected animals. Milk should be pasteurized, and if not, boiling is effective in destroying brucella organisms.

Control

Control depends on thorough investigation to find the source of the infection and setting up appropriate controls on infected animals and their products.

TETANUS

Clostridium tetani is one of the strains of bacteria sometimes found in the intestinal tract of humans and other mammals, where it does no harm. Folklore has attributed the cause of tetanus to a rusty nail, and because the type of deep puncture anaerobic wound caused by a rusty nail provides the best growing conditions for the bacteria, tetanus may well develop from this source. However, the spores of *C. tetani* can be introduced into any wound, and if anaerobic conditions prevail, then the spores will germinate, multiply, and produce the deadly tetanus toxin.

The organism is found worldwide, but the disease is more common in agricultural regions and in underdeveloped areas. The number of cases in the United States has decreased steadily since 1966 (Figure 7-22). Tetanus is a significant cause

of death in many countries where contact with animal excreta is more likely and immunization is inadequate. It is one of the most common causes of neonatal (newborn) death in these countries. In these deaths, the unhealed umbilical cord is the portal of entry. The reservoir of infection is the intestine of animals, including humans.

The incubation period is influenced by the type of wound and the number of infecting organisms. With the right conditions, tetanus toxin can be produced within a few days, but incubation sometimes requires three weeks or longer. The average is ten days. Nonimmunized individuals are all susceptible to tetanus. As people get older and are no longer protected by the shots (see under Prevention), they become more susceptible. Individuals who recover from tetanus may not have immunity. The fatality rate ranges from thirty percent to ninety percent depending on age, length of incubation, and treatment. In the United States, in experienced intensive care centers, the mortality rate has dropped from sixty percent to thirty percent.

Transmission

Spores of the tetanus bacillus are found everywhere and are common in the dust of streets as well as in soil. Anything or any place that has been contaminated with fecal matter may contain spores. When tetanus spores are introduced into the body, usually through a puncture wound, but also through lacerations, burns, and trivial or unnoticed wounds, and begin to multiply, then the deadly toxin is produced. The presence of dead tissue and/or foreign bodies favors the growth of the pathogen in the wound.

Surveillance of tetanus in the United States from 1995 to 1997 disclosed a disproportionate number of cases in the twenty to fifty-nine year old age group. This was related in part to an increased number of cases among intravenous drug users (IDUs). The high risk among IDUs is related to (1) the high prevalence of abscesses, which favor anaerobic conditions for bacterial

---

Clostridium tetani   klo-STRID-e-um te-TA-ne

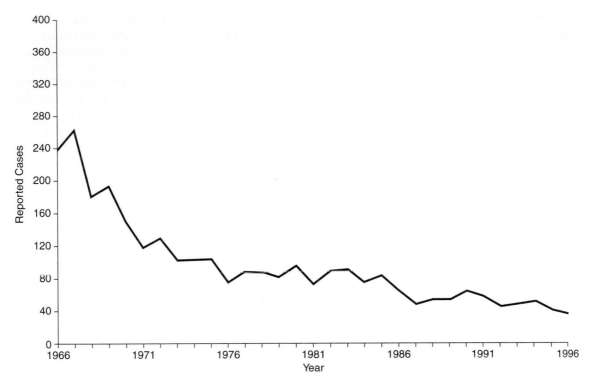

Figure 7-22

Tetanus, by year, United States, 1966–1996.

growth, secondary to nonsterile injection practices; (2) subcutaneous injection; (3) contamination of the drug supply and (4) low prevalence of immunity.*

Symptoms

The first symptom may be rigidity in the abdomen or the area of the wound. The tetanus toxin attacks the central nervous system and results in painful, involuntary muscle contractions. These contractions affect the neck and facial muscles, leading to locked jaw (lockjaw is another name for tetanus), and a grinning expression known as **risus sardonicus.** Somatic muscles may become involved, leading to arched back rigidity and boardlike abdominal rigidity. Other symptoms include tachycardia, profuse sweating, and low-grade fever.

*Barbara Bardenheier, Rebecca D. Prevots, Nino Khetsuriani, et al., 1998, "Tetanus surveillance—United States, 1995–1997," *Morbidity and Mortality Weekly Report* July 3, 1998/47 (SS-2); 1-13.

Treatment

If tetanus antitoxin is administered before the toxin becomes attached to nerve tissue, the toxin will be neutralized. If a nonimmunized individual receives a puncture wound, tetanus antitoxin or tetanus immune globulin (TIG) must be given as soon as possible (within seventy-two hours). After this, they need active immunization with the tetanus toxoid. If the patient has not had tetanus immunization for five years, a booster injection needs to be given. If tetanus develops, then the individual will require airway maintenance and a muscle relaxant. Tracheotomy and mechanically assisted respiration may also be used. High-dose antibiotics are administered, preferably penicillin, for ten to fourteen days.

Prevention

Active immunization with tetanus toxoid gives certain and durable (ten-year) protection. Infants should be immunized at two to three months with the DTP vaccine, which protects against diphtheria, tetanus, and pertussis (whooping cough). Booster doses are given at regular intervals. After the initial series, boosters are recommended at ten-year intervals.

The public needs to be educated on the need for complete immunization, the hazards of puncture wounds, and the potential need for a booster after injury.

Control

Identification of the source of infection (in a situation in which others could become infected because of lack of sanitary conditions or some environmental hazard) is the only measure necessary for control. Cases of tetanus should be reported to the local health authority (required in most states and countries).

ANTHRAX - Chemical Warfare

Anthrax is a disease of domestic animals, mainly sheep, cattle, goats, and horses. It has been known since antiquity and was described in Homer's *Iliad.* Anthrax is caused by *Bacillus anthracis,* which Robert Koch identified in 1876. Human anthrax thus became the first human disease proved to be of bacterial origin. Human anthrax occurs in workers who process animal products or in farmers or veterinarians who work directly with infected animals. The spores of *B. anthracis* can survive for years after the infected animal has died, in soil and in the hide, hair, and wool.

Immunization and other measures to protect workers who might be exposed have made anthrax infrequent and sporadic in the United States, but it is endemic in areas of the Middle East, Asia, Africa, and South America. The disease usually appears within a week after exposure. Indications are that animals and humans surviving an attack of the disease are resistant to reinfection. Some individuals have inapparent infections and may have some natural resistance.

With a death rate of ninety-nine percent for any who are exposed to anthrax and unvaccinated, it is one of the most feared biologic weapons.

During the height of the Persian Gulf conflict, there were reports that Saddam Hussein was preparing capsules laden with the anthrax bacillus to drop on the United Nations troops. Anthrax develops quickly and if the bacteria are inhaled, death occurs quickly. Fortunately the war was comparatively brief, and either the Iraqis decided not to break international laws against germ warfare or the mechanism for releasing the bacteria was not in place. Because of the continuing threat of biologic weapons, American troops deployed to Southwest Asia and Korea are now vaccinated for anthrax.

Transmission

Figure 7-23 shows the way in which anthrax is transmitted. *Infection of the skin* (cutaneous infection) is caused by contact with tissues of animals dying of the disease, or by a great variety of animal products, including bone meal, shaving-brush bristles, hair or wool used in textile industries, and hides processed for leather goods. Cutaneous anthrax also may result from contact with soil associated with infected animals. An additional source of skin infection may

risus sardonicus   RI-sus sar-DO-nik-us

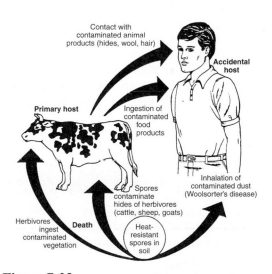

Figure 7-23

Transmission of anthrax.

News = Military getting immunized

inhalation - causes lesions

be biting flies that feed on a diseased animal. *Intestinal anthrax* is caused by eating undercooked, contaminated meat. There is no evidence that the spores are transmitted by milk from infected animals. Inhalation of the spores leads to *inhalation anthrax*. The spore source can remain infective for years. There is no person-to-person transmission.

Symptoms

In cutaneous anthrax, itching begins first at the site of entry. A papule (red, elevated area) appears within a day or so and quickly becomes a vesicle. Figure 7-24 shows the lesion and vesicles of anthrax in the early stages. There is generally no pain in the early stages. In a few days, the vesicle becomes larger and turns black and is referred to as a malignant pustule. There is swelling around the ulcer, caused by the multiplication of the bacilli and production of a cell-damaging toxin.

If untreated, the infection spreads to nearby lymph nodes and to the bloodstream, causing overwhelming septicemia (blood poisoning) that leads to shock and death in a few days. The case fatality rate is five percent to twenty percent when untreated. Inhalation anthrax produces only mild symptoms at first, similar to those of an upper respiratory infection. In three to five days, the symptoms become more severe, with respiratory distress, fever, and shock. Death occurs soon after the symptoms become worse in almost every case of inhalation anthrax. Intestinal anthrax is rare and difficult to recognize, with typical symptoms of abdominal distress, fever, and signs of septicemia. Death occurs in most cases.

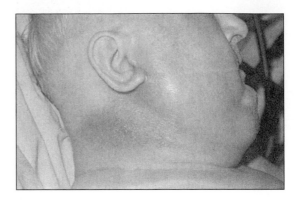

Figure 7-24
Early anthrax lesion.

Treatment

Because anthrax develops so quickly, early diagnosis and treatment are essential. Penicillin is the drug of choice, and tetracycline has also been found to be effective.

Prevention

A vaccine is available that provides active immunization to animals and persons at high risk. Education in sanitary measures, in means of anthrax transmission, and in care of minor abrasions for those working with animals or animal products also helps to prevent infection.

Control

Special precautions need to be taken with dead or dying animals. Animal products for commercial processing should be sterilized whenever possible. Protective clothing and gloves should be used by workers in at-risk occupations. Dust control may also be necessary in contaminated areas.

SUMMARY

Table 7-1 summarizes relevant data on bacterial diseases acquired through the skin and mucosa from arthropod vectors, animal sources, and soil.

TABLE 7-1	Bacterial (Including Rickettsial) Diseases Acquired Through Skin and Mucosa from Arthropod Vectors, Animal Sources, and the Soil			
Disease	**Special Characteristics**	**Transmission**	**Major Symptoms**	**Prevention/ Control**
Lyme disease	Identified originally in Lyme, Connecticut. Found in other parts of country and spreading. Disease agent is a spirochete	Transmitted by the bite of an infected tick. Can be transmitted to fetus if a pregnant woman gets the disease. Deer carry ticks	Three stages: first—EM, malaise, fatigue, muscle aches, fever, stiff neck, joint aches, rash, swollen lymph glands; sore throat and dry cough may precede EM. Second— Neurologic and cardiac abnormalities Third— Arthritis	Special clothing precautions need to be taken by individuals who camp, hunt, or walk in areas inhabited by deer. Inspection of animals and humans for ticks after being in such areas and prompt removal of any ticks found
Rocky Mountain spotted fever	Initially found in Rocky Mountains, now in many parts of country. Few cases in fall or winter. Men infected most often in West, children in Eastern part of U.S.	Tick attaches itself and injects rickettsiae. Also feces of tick rubbed into bite or abrasion	Fever, anorexia, slight headache about a week after bite or sudden fever, prostration, myalgia, severe headache, nausea and vomiting; in 50% of cases small pink spots on wrists and ankles that spread over body; spots darken, enlarge, and may bleed	Same as other typhus diseases and Lyme disease
Tularemia	Hares and rabbits are main source of infection in humans. Low fatality with	Inoculation while working with infected animal or from flies or ticks. Ingestion of insufficiently	Formation of sore at site of entry and swollen lymph glands in region; if inhaled, pneu-	Should use gloves when skinning or handling wild animals. Thorough cooking of *Continued*

| | **TABLE 7-1** | *Continued* | | | |

Disease	Special Characteristics	Transmission	Major Symptoms	Prevention/ Control
Tularemia— Cont'd	proper treatment	cooked meat or contaminated water. Inhalation of dust from contaminated soil, grain, or hay. No person-to-person transmission.	monic or typhoidal disease; if from ingestion, sore throat, intestinal pain, diarrhea, and vomiting	meat of wild rodents. Vaccination for high-risk groups
Ehrlichiosis	This emerging disease has two forms, monocytic and granulocytic. It is fatal with no treatment. Incubation is 7–21 days.	No evidence of person-to-person transmission. Tick is vector	Fever, malaise, myalgia, headaches, rigors; rash may occur unrelated to location of tick bite	Avoid tick bites. Education of public
Plague	Bubonic known as the "Black Death." Also pneumonic and septicemic forms. Mortality 60%–100% without treatment	Transmitted to humans by bite of a flea from an infected rodent. Pneumonic transmitted by airborne droplets from pets to humans or person to person	Bubonic: headache, fever, chills, and exhaustion; swelling, pain, and hemorrhage in the lymph nodes. Pneumonic: high fever, chills, severe headache, fast heartbeat, rapid, labored breathing, productive cough. Septicemic: chills, fever, prostration, convulsions, shock	Destruction of rats and fleas. Elimination of unsanitary conditions. Isolation of victims and destruction of all fleas on person, clothes, or baggage. Soiled articles disinfected. Vaccine for one year available. Contact investigation is necessary
Leptospirosis	Also called Weil's disease. Excretion of spirochete in urine may continue up to 11 months after the illness	Skin contact with water, moist soil, or vegetation contaminated with excreta of infected animals	Fever, headache, chills, malaise, vomiting, muscle aches and watery eyes	Education of workers in hazardous areas, education of public about swimming in contaminated waters such as

TABLE 7-1	*Continued*			
Disease	**Special Characteristics**	**Transmission**	**Major Symptoms**	**Prevention/ Control**
	More prevalent in men— occupational hazard			farm ponds, control of infected animals
Brucellosis	"Undulant fever" affects cattle and other animals. Most individuals are susceptible to brucellosis	Transmitted by ingestion of unpasteurized milk or milk products; contact with tissues of infected animals; inhalation of contaminated dust	Fever, chills, sweating, muscle aches and pains, weakness, and malaise	Education of individuals who work with cows or their products; pasteurizing or boiling milk
Tetanus	Puncture wounds provide best growing conditions. Spores will produce toxin in any wound with anaerobic conditions. Incubation takes 10 days. Most cases caused by minor injury; 30% to 90% fatal without immunization. More prevalent in rural and tropical areas. Recent increase among IDUs	Anything contaminated with fecal matter may contain spores. If they are introduced into the body and begin to multiply, the deadly toxin is produced	Rigidity in abdomen, painful, involuntary muscle contractions	Active immunization with tetanus toxid with periodic boosters
Anthrax	Spores survive for years after animal is dead. Occurs in workers who process animal hides or	Contact with tissues or products of an infected animal, contaminated soil, biting flies,	Cutaneous: itching at site of entry, vesicle that turns black. Inhalation: mild at first, like	Vaccine for animals and people at high risk. Education of those working with animals

TABLE 7-1   Continued

Disease	Special Characteristics	Transmission	Major Symptoms	Prevention/ Control
Anthrax—Cont'd	farmers or vets who work with animal hides. Infrequent in U.S. but endemic in Middle East, Asia, Africa, and South America. Death rate for unvaccinated exposed individuals is 99%. One of most feared biologic weapons	may produce cutaneous anthrax. Eating undercooked infected meat causes intestinal anthrax. Inhalation of spores leads to inhalation anthrax. No person-to-person transmission	upper respiratory infection, 3–5 days— severe respiratory distress, fever, shock. Intestinal: abdominal distress, fever, septicemia	Special precautions with dead or dying animals, sterilization of animal products when possible, protective gloves and clothing for workers in at-risk occupations, dust control in contaminated areas

QUESTIONS FOR REVIEW

1. What is an arthropod vector?
2. What is the difference between an insect vector that is a reservoir for an organism and an insect vector that acts as a mechanical carrier?
3. What term is used to denote infectious diseases of animals that can be transmitted to humans?
4. What hosts are used by *Ixodes scapularis?*
5. Describe the three stages of Lyme disease.
6. What treatment is generally used for Lyme disease?
7. In what part(s) of the country is Rocky Mountain spotted fever found?
8. How can Rocky Mountain spotted fever be avoided?
9. What is the main source of tularemia?
10. In what ways can *F. tularensis* be transmitted?
11. How and why do the symptoms of tularemia vary?
12. What measures need to be taken to prevent tularemia?
13. Distinguish between the two types of Ehrlichia.
14. Identify three forms of plague and the symptoms for each.
15. How is plague transmitted?
16. What is the most effective way to prevent plague?
17. How is plague controlled?
18. What dangerous complications may occur in leptospirosis?
19. Where might children easily be exposed to leptospirosis? Why?
20. What occupations pose the greatest risk for being infected with leptospirosis?
21. What are the methods for control of leptospirosis?
22. In what ways can brucellosis be transmitted?
23. Where does the highest rate for tetanus occur and why?
24. What is the procedure for treating tetanus?
25. What regimen is recommended for tetanus shots?
26. Explain what is meant by the statement that anthrax is an occupational disease.
27. What is distinctive about the anthrax lesion?
28. Discuss the control methods suggested for anthrax.

FURTHER READING

Abramson, J. S. 1999. Rocky Mountain spotted fever. *Journal of Pediatric Infection Disease.*

Azad, Abdu F., and Charles B. Beard. 1998. Rickettsial pathogens and their arthropod vectors. *Emerging Infectious Diseases,* 4:179.

Bardenheier, Barbara, Rebecca D. Prevots, Nino Khetsuriani, et al. 1998. Tetanus surveillance— United States, 1995–1997. *Morbidity and Mortality Weekly Report* 47:1.

Barlett, John G. 1999. Applying lessons learned from anthrax case history to other scenarios. *Emerging Infectious Diseases* 5:561.

Barnard, J. P., and A. M. Friedlander. 1999. Vaccination against anthrax with attenuated recombinant strains of bacillus anthracis that produce protective antigen. *Infection and Immunity* 67:562.

Baskin, Yvonne. 1998. Home on the range. *Bioscience* 48:245.

Blaser, Martin J. 1998. Passover and plague. *Perspectives in Biology and Medicine* 41:243.

Borer, A., et al. 1999. Massive pulmonary haemorrhage caused by leptospirosis successfully treated with nitric oxide inhalation and haemofiltration. *Journal of Infection* 38:1.

Brown, S., et al. 1999. Role of serology in the diagnosis of lyme disease. *Journal of American Medical Association* 282:62.

Cairney, Richard. 1999. Antivaccine advocates line up to support airman. *Canadian Medical Association Journal* 160:883.

Childs, James, Robert E. Shope, et al. 1998. Emerging zoonoses. *Emerging Infectious Diseases* 4:453.

Cieslak, Theodore J., and Edward M. Eitzen, Jr. 1999. Clinical and epidemiologic principles of anthrax. *Emerging Infectious Diseases* 5:552.

Conaty, Susan M., and Raymond J. Dattwyler. 1999. Experts tick off caveats on lyme vaccination. *Consultant* 39:1.

Diphtheria and tetanus toxoids and whole cell pertussis vaccine. Clinical Reference System, 1998.

Dixon, Terry C., et al. 1999. Anthrax. *New England Journal of Medicine* 341:815.

Dos Santos, Claudia C., et al. 1999. Two tick-borne diseases in one: a case report of concurrent babesiosis and lyme disease in Ontario. *Canadian Medical Association Journal* 160:1851.

Drage, L. A. 1999. Life threatening rashes: dermatologic signs of four infectious diseases. *Mayo Clinic Procedures* 74:68–72.

Ember, Louis. 1998. Anthrax events hike scientific interest. *Chemical and Engineering News* 76:12.

Emerging infections on center stage at first international meeting. *Journal of the American Medical Association* 279:1055, 1998.

Essert, S. D., et al. 1999. The protective effect of immunization against diphtheria, pertussis and tetanus in relation to sudden infant death syndrome. *FEMS Immunology and Medical Microbiology* 25:183.

First lyme disease vaccine available. *Canadian Medical Association Journal* 160:1814, 1999.

Friedlander, Arthur M., and Phillip R. Pittman. 1999. Anthrax vaccine. *Journal of the American Medical Association* 282:2104.

Godsmith, Ann. 1999. The plague. *Quarterly Review of Literature* 37/38:41.

Golden, Frederic. 1998. The ticks are back: And thanks to el Nino, there may be more than ever. The good news: that new vaccine works. *Time* 151:60.

Gubler, Duane J. 1998. Resurgent vector-borne diseases as a global health problem. *Emerging Infectious Diseases* 4.

Henderson, D. A. 1998. Bio-terrorism as a public health threat. *Emerging Infectious Diseases,* 4:488.

Holden, Constance. 1999. Typhus reemerges as plague suspect. *Science* 283:1111.

"Human ehrlichiosis update." Hygienic Laboratory, The University of Iowa. www.uhl.uiowa.edu/Publicatins/ Hotline/1995All.

Ibrahim, K. H., et al. 1999. Bacillus anthracis: medical issues of biologic warfare. *Pharmacotherapy* 19:690.

Inglesby, Thomas V. 1999. Anthrax: a possible case history. *Emerging Infections Diseases* 5:556.

Inglesby, Thomas V., et al. Anthrax as a biological weapon. *Journal of the American Medical Association* 281:1735.

Jones, T. F. 1999. Family cluster of Rocky Mountain spotted fever. *Journal of Clinical Infectious Disease* 12:529–33.

Josefson, Deborah. 1998. Scientists uncover how anthrax works. *British Medical Journal* 316:1482.

Klinman, D. M., et al. 1999. Immune recognition of foreign DNA: a cure for bioterrorism. *Immunity* 11:123.

Ko, Albert I., et al. 1999. Urban epidemic of severe leptospirosis in Brazil. *The Lancet* 354:820.

Lucas, Beverly D. 1999. Now you can prevent lyme disease. *Patient Care* 33:180. Lyme disease. Geriatrics 54:15, 1999.

MacKenzie, Debora. 1998. Bioarmageddon. *New Scientist,* 159:2152.

Marwick, Charles. 1999. Scary scenarios spark action at bioterrorism symposium. *Journal of the American Medical Association* 281:1071.

Morris, Kelly. 1999. US military face punishment for refusing anthrax vaccine. *The Lancet* 353:130.

Nadelman, Robert B., and Gary P. Wormser. 1998. Lyme borreliosis. *The Lancet* 352:557.

Niegbylski, M. L., et al. 1999. Lethal effect of rickettsia rickettsii on its tick vector. *Applied and Environmental Microbiology* 65:773. Parasitic diseases. Health Letter CDC, 1999.

Oksi, J, and L. -M. Voipio-Pulkki, J. Uksila, et al. 1997. Borrelia burgdorferi infection in patients with suspected acute myocardial infarction. *The Lancet* 350:1447.

Outbreak of epidemic typhus associated with trench fever in Burundi. *The Lancet* 352:353, 1998.

Pinto, Larry. 1999. Get ticked off at lyme disease! *Pest Control* 67:10.

Ratsitorahina, Mahery, Suzanne Chanteau, et al. 1999. Epidemiological and diagnostic aspects of the outbreak of pneumonic plague in Madagascar. *The Lancet* 355:111.

The Rhode Island Tick Pickers, Tick Research Laboratory, University of Rhode Island, "Ehrlichiosis," [www.uri.edu/artsci/zool/ticklab].

Rose, Verna L. 1999. Interim guidelines for anthrax exposure. *American Family Physican* 59:2655.

Rosen, Peter. 2000. Coping with bioterrorism. *British Medical Journal* 7227:71.

Sexton, Daniel J., Ralph G. Corey, Christopher Carpenter, ct al. 1998. Dual infection with *Ehrlichia chaffeensis* and a spotted fever group rickettsia: A case report. *Emerging Infectious Diseases* 4(2).

Shimoni, Zvi, Anatoly Dobrousin. 1999. Tetanus in an immunised patient. *British Medical Journal* 7216:1049.

Statewide surveillance for Ehrlichiosis—Connecticut and New York, 1994–1997. *Morbidity and Mortality Weekly Report* 47:476, 1998.

Strobino, Barbara, Syed Abid. 1999. Maternal lyme disease and congenital heart disease: a case control study in an endemic area. *American Journal of Obstetrics and Gynecology* 180:711.

Tetanus among injecting-drug users—California, 1997. *Journal of the American Medical Association* 279:987, 1998.

Tick-borne diseases. *Emerging Infectious Diseases* 4:137, 1998.

Update: leptospirosis and unexplained acute febrile illness among athletes participating in triathlons—Illinois and Wisconsin. *Journal of American Medical Association* 280:1474.

Varde, Shobha, John Beckley, et al. 1998. Prevalence of tick-borne pathogens in *Ixodes scapularis* in a rural New Jersey county. *Emerging Infectious Diseases* 4:97.

Wei, Ty. 1999. Acute disseminated encephalomyelitis after Rocky Mountain spotted fever. *Pediatric Neurology* 21:503.

VIRAL DISEASES ACQUIRED THROUGH THE RESPIRATORY ROUTE

O B J E C T I V E S

1. *Identify common viral diseases acquired through the respiratory route.*

2. *State means of transmission for the diseases in this chapter.*

3. *Differentiate between influenza and the common usage of the term* **flu**.

4. *Explain the high death rate among the elderly in influenza epidemics.*

5. *Identify those who should have the influenza vaccine.*

6. *Explain why infectious mononucleosis is called the college disease or the kissing disease.*

7. *State complications that may occur with mononucleosis.*

8. *Describe the symptoms for chickenpox.*

9. *Relate herpes zoster to chickenpox.*

10. *Distinguish between measles and rubella.*

11. *Identify complications for mumps.*

12. *Explain the significance of smallpox as a communicable disease.*

THE COMMON COLD

This most common of all communicable diseases has been responsible for more lost days on the job and has had more time and effort spent on it to find a cause than all the other communicable diseases in history. For all the misery a cold can cause, it will end without treatment and is never fatal. However, if an individual's resistance is compromised for some reason, a cold can lead to serious illness. Some of the more common complications are laryngitis, bronchitis, sinusitis, and otitis media. Over 100 different types of rhinovirus cause colds, and nearly 100 other "cold-causing" viruses have been identified. The incubation period for a cold is usually about forty-eight hours, and symptoms generally last two to seven days. Colds occur in all parts of the world. They are more frequent in children, becoming fewer with age. However, there is a greater chance for complications when an older person gets a cold. The infection is communicable from at least twenty-four hours before the onset of symptoms to five days or more after onset. Everyone seems to be susceptible to colds.

Transmission

Colds are transmitted by direct or indirect contact (Figure 8-1). Studies conducted at the Cold Laboratory in Salisbury, England, have indicated a greater chance of infection by handling contaminated articles and then rubbing the eyes than by droplet spread. The organism is capable of entering the mucous membrane of the eyes. Close personal contact is necessary for the virus to spread and this occurs most frequently at home and in the school. Rhinoviruses are not spread by simple kissing. They are able to exist for some time on various objects.

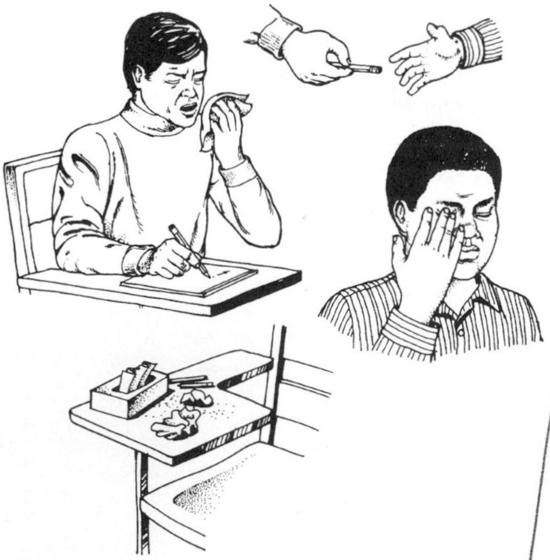

[handwritten: #1 way to get a cold.]

Figure 8-1
Transmission of the common cold.

Using a pencil that was used by someone with a cold or licking your fingers as you go through papers received from someone who was working on them and had a cold, can transmit the virus if you then rub your eyes. Actually, covering your mouth and nose when you cough or sneeze (which is considered polite) means that you can spread a cold to the next objects or people you touch.

Symptoms

Most colds start with a tickle in the throat, a watery discharge from the nose, and sneezing. Many times the nasal discharge is copious and causes irritation to the nose and skin around it. Some colds will gradually clear up at this point, but others produce more severe symptoms usually caused by a secondary bacterial infection. The discharge thickens and becomes yellowish or green, eyes water, and fever, sore throat, headache, malaise, myalgia, and a nonproductive cough occur. Included in the secondary infections that can occur are laryngitis, tracheitis, acute bronchitis, sinusitis, or otitis media.

Treatment

There is no known cure for the common cold. Treatment is for symptoms only. Drinking plenty of liquid and getting extra rest can help the victim feel better but will not shorten the duration of the cold. Because of the possibility of Reye's syndrome*, analgesics and cold remedies should not be used for children unless prescribed by the doctor. Although over-the-counter (OTC) remedies may alleviate some of the symptoms temporarily, overuse may be counterproductive. Most antibiotics have no effect on a viral disease but may be used prophylactically for individuals at risk for developing a secondary bacterial infection.

Prevention

There is no scientific evidence that extra vitamins, orange juice, or avoiding drafts and chilling will

*Because of the danger of Reye's syndrome, only acetaminophen or ibuprofen (Tylenol or Advil/Nuprin) should be given to an infant or child who is ill. Reye's syndrome is a very serious illness involving the liver and central nervous system. It has been a rare complication in children who are given salicylates (aspirin) for upper respiratory viral infections. Although this complication has occurred mostly in influenza or chickenpox, young children should not be given aspirin for any upper respiratory infection unless recommended by a physician.

[handwritten: no aspirin acetaminophen Tylenol & advil/ok.]

prevent colds. A high degree of fitness, socially, mentally, physically, and spiritually, may help to limit the number of colds a person has.

There is much evidence that there is a link between a recent history of psychologic stress and general resistance to infection. Stress seems to suppress resistance. Learning and using ways to handle stress can increase resistance to disease.

Also good hygiene, particularly frequent hand washing, around infected individuals will help decrease a person's degree of exposure. But sooner or later, most people develop one or more colds a year. Individuals who are over sixty-five years of age or at risk because of heart or respiratory problems may be counseled by their doctor to have a "cold shot," but the protection given is for only a few of the 200 or so viruses that can cause a cold.

Control
Education of the public in personal hygiene, sanitary disposal of tissues used in control of discharges from mouth or nose, and in frequent hand washing will help in the control of colds. Individuals with a cold should be isolated from

patients in a children's hospital. Ill persons should avoid direct and indirect contact with young children, the debilitated or aged, and people with another illness. People should also avoid smoking in a home where there are children or older people. Smoking causes enough air contamination to increase the chances of pneumonia and some other respiratory diseases developing in the very young or very old.

INFLUENZA

Most people refer to influenza as "the flu." The only problem with this term is that it is used to cover so many different illnesses, some of which are not even upper respiratory, as influenza is. Influenza can be a very dangerous disease, developing rapidly, spreading quickly, and leading to complications, most often pneumonia, which can be fatal.

A comparison of symptoms for a cold and influenza can be seen in Table 8-1.

Influenza occurs in all parts of the world, and the greatest death toll from the disease, twenty

TABLE 8-1	**Comparison of Symptoms of a Cold and Influenza**	
Symptoms	**Cold**	**Influenza**
Fever	Rare	Characteristic, high (102–104°F), lasts 3–4 days
Headache	Rare	Prominent
General aches, pains	Slight	Usual; often severe
Fatigue, weakness	Quite mild	Can last up to 2–3 weeks
Extreme exhaustion	Never	Early and prominent
Stuffy nose	Common	Sometimes
Sneezing	Usual	Sometimes
Sore throat	Common	Sometimes
Chest, discomfort, cough	Mild to moderate; hacking cough	Common; can be severe
Complications	Sinus congestion or earache	Bronchitis, pneumonia; can be life-threatening
Prevention	None	Annual vaccination; amantadine or rimantadine (antiviral drugs)
Treatment	Only temporary relief of symptoms	Amantadine or rimantadine within 24–48 hours after onset

[handwritten: avg. year kills 20,000 people]

[handwritten: Vaccine = based on last years virus]

million, was a result of the pandemic of 1918. In the last 100 years, pandemics also occurred in 1957 and 1968. Epidemics occur in the United States almost every year, principally in the winter, whereas in the tropics they often occur in the rainy season. In both cases people move from outdoor activities to indoors, and close quarters usually are a factor in the transmission of influenza. The months of highest influenza activity in the United States can be seen in Figure 8-2. The incubation period is one to five days, and the disease is communicable for three to five days from the first sign of symptoms in adults but up to seven days in children.

[handwritten left margin: 3 different Strands]

Influenza viruses change all the time, and for this reason everyone is susceptible to new forms. The viruses are classified into three groups. Type A is the most prevalent and responsible for most epidemics of influenza. Type B has been associated with widespread or regional epidemics and pandemics every two to three years. There are also "mixed" A and B epidemics. Type C is endemic and has been identified in scattered cases and minor localized outbreaks. The different strains of A and B have been named according to where they were first identified, so there is Hong Kong flu, Russian flu, etc. (The forms of influenza also have

identifying numbers and letters.) Infection with one strain results in immunity to that strain but not to others that may develop.

Another strain of influenza was identified in Hong Kong in May 1997. Chickens were the host. It was the first time humans had been infected with influenza by an **avian** (from birds) virus. Although only seventeen people ranging from two to sixty years of age were infected, six died. The concern with a new strain is great because no one will have built up antibodies. So far there is no evidence of person-to-person transmission but if this does occur with a new strain, there is a possibility of an influenza pandemic.

Transmission

The influenza virus is spread through the air from person to person, particularly in places where a lot of people are in close quarters. It is also transmitted by airborne droplets and indirect contact with contaminated objects. The virus is able to survive for hours in dried mucus.

[handwritten right margin: 1918 war: infermiery boats]

Symptoms

Typical symptoms for influenza are sudden onset of chills, temperature from 101 to 104°F, headache, malaise, muscle aches, and a nonproductive cough. Sometimes other symptoms

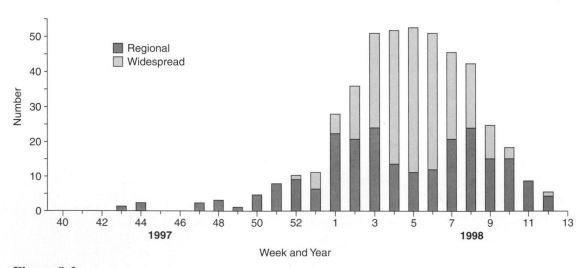

Figure 8-2

Number of state and territorial epidemiologists reporting widespread or regional influenza activity, by week and year, United States, Sept. 28, 1997 through March 28, 1998.

[handwritten: Epidemics = Every 50 yrs — Epidemic Strain changes so much from the previous year that the vaccine is ineffective]

*most common complication =
bacterial & secondary pneumonia* | *Kids ages 5-14
School - closed quarters
Spread*

CHAPTER 8 Viral Diseases Acquired through the Respiratory Route **163**

develop, such as sore throat, hoarseness, conjunctivitis, and inflammation and congestion of the nasal mucosa. The symptoms generally last three to five days, but cough and weakness may last for several weeks.

Treatment

Bed rest, analgesics (acetaminophen for children), and plenty of liquid are the best treatment. For individuals in a high-risk category for developing pneumonia, the drugs, **amantadine** or rimantadine, can be used to reduce the severity of the disease if given within twenty-four hours. Two new drugs, **zanamivir** (trade name, **Relenza**) *inhaled* and GS4104 have been effective in treating influenza Types A and B in trials. Antibiotics may also be given to combat secondary bacterial infections.

Prevention *Tamiflu = pill/w/in 24 hrs.*

For people over sixty-five years of age and those with respiratory disease or circulatory diseases vaccination is recommended. It must be given every year and is sixty percent to seventy percent effective. Even if it does not keep the individual from getting the disease, it will lessen the severity of the symptoms. A nasal vaccine has been in human trials and is awaiting FDA approval. It is hoped that the nasal spray, when used for children, will help reduce the number of cases in adults. Influenza is generally a mild disease in children. However, they take it home and pass it on to the rest of the family including the elderly, for whom it is a severe disease—sometimes with fatal secondary infections, most often pneumonia.

Control

Closing of schools generally occurs too late to do any good. Education of the public in basic personal hygiene is the best means of control.

INFECTIOUS MONONUCLEOSIS

Epstein-Barr virus (EBV), a member of the herpes group, is the infecting agent for infectious mononucleosis, which mainly affects young adults and children. Only a laboratory test can determine whether a person has the disease, because the symptoms are all nonspecific. Incubation is four to six weeks, and mononucleosis may be communicable for a year or more after infection. "Mono" occurs worldwide. Most people are susceptible, but infection confers a high degree of immunity.

Transmission

Because the victim carries the EBV in the throat, transmission is generally by the **oral-pharyngeal** route. Mononucleosis has been called the kissing disease or the college disease because spread often occurs among courting teenagers and frequently in colleges. It may also be spread by transfusion, but apparent disease rarely develops from this source. Close contact such as sharing a can of soda is necessary for transmission (Figure 8-3).

Symptoms

Typically, there are prodromal symptoms of headache, malaise, and fatigue. After three to five days, fever, swollen lymph glands, and sore throat develop. There may also be an enlarged spleen, liver involvement, and tonsillitis or pharyngitis. A rash and jaundice occur in a small percentage of victims. Complications may include ruptured spleen, meningitis, encephalitis, hepatitis, and anemia. *↗ Worst*

avian	a-vi-un
amantadine	a-MAN-ta-den
zanamivir	ZAN-a-mi-VIR
Relenza	re-LEN-za
oral-pharyngeal	o-ral far-IN-je-al

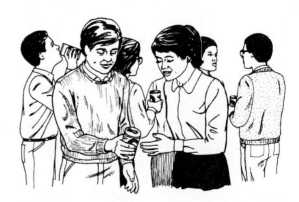

Figure 8-3
Transmission of mononucleosis.

[handwritten top margin: WBC's = over 50%]

[handwritten: Diagnosis = Blood Test]

Treatment

Treatment is symptomatic. Individuals with the disease are restricted from any contact sports because of the danger of a ruptured spleen. Individuals with mono should also be restricted in activity because their resistance is low. Fatalities have been recorded of people dying of a blow to the spleen when they participated in sports before complete recovery from mono. If a secondary bacterial infection is present, antibiotics may be used. In severe cases, steroids may be used.

Prevention

There is no known way to prevent mono, but basic personal hygiene and avoidance of close contact with infected individuals will decrease the risk.

Control

There is also no way to control the infection except for education of the public concerning the means of transmission.

VARICELLA (CHICKENPOX)

[handwritten: for test know incubation time]

Most people throughout the world have had chickenpox by ten years of age. It is a mild but very contagious disease of childhood. In adults, the disease can have severe effects. Congenital chickenpox may cause birth defects. Chickenpox is caused by human herpes virus 3 (**varicella zoster**). The incubation period may be two to three weeks but is generally thirteen to seventeen days. The disease may be communicable from five days before to five days after the appearance of the first vesicles. Infection confers long immunity. The organism stays in the body after the disease has run its course and years later may cause herpes zoster, or shingles.

[handwritten left margin: contagious usually 1-2 days before rash - 5 days after]

Transmission

Herpes zoster is communicable to individuals who have not had chickenpox, but they get chickenpox—not shingles. The disease lasts from ten days to five weeks.

Chickenpox can be spread by direct contact with respiratory secretions and fluid from lesions of the infected person or by indirect contact with fomites.

Symptoms

The first symptoms are fever, malaise, and anorexia. Within twenty-four hours, the rash typically begins as small red spots on the trunk or scalp that eventually become clear vesicles on a red base. This has been referred to as the "dewdrop on a rose petal"(Figure 8-4). The vesicles are extremely pruritic (itchy) and break easily, forming a scab. The rash spreads to the face and sometimes to the extremities. New vesicles develop every three or four days, so there are different stages of development present—red spots, vesicles, and scabs—at the same time. Some children even have lesions on the mucous membranes of the mouth, conjunctivae, and genitalia. If a child scratches the rash persistently, infections, scarring, impetigo, and boils may occur. In some cases, symptoms are so mild and the lesions so few that they escape notice. Figure 8-4 shows the different lesions that can occur in chickenpox, and Figure 8-5 shows all of the stages of the rash on one child.

Treatment

[handwritten: Baths - calamine lotion]

Relief of symptoms is the main goal of treatment because there is no cure for chickenpox. Bicarbonate of soda baths or calamine or antihistamine lotions help to relieve the pruritis. In severe cases, an antiviral agent, acyclovir, may be used.

Prevention

A vaccine was licensed for use in the United States in 1995 that lasts for at least six years. The vaccine is recommended for all children at twelve to eighteen months of age. If records show that a child has had chickenpox then the vaccine is not necessary. Varicella vaccine is also recommended for immunization of all children by their thirteenth birthday unless there is a reliable history of having had chickenpox. After that age, the disease is more severe, complications occur more frequently, and two doses of vaccine are needed.

Varicella-zoster immune globulin (VZIG) is effective in decreasing the severity of symptoms or preventing the disease if given within ninety-six hours after exposure. It is available for high-risk individuals.

[handwritten bottom: Like herpes — Virus stays dormant in body, & may come back out as shingles]

[handwritten: Don't give shingles person to person]

CASE STUDY

Varicella

On April 3, 1997, a thirty-two-year-old woman with Crohn's disease sought medical evaluation at a local emergency department because of onset of abdominal and back pain. On March 7, therapy had been initiated with 40 mg prednisone daily. On physical examination, she had mild, generalized abdominal tenderness with no specific signs or abdominal guarding. She was afebrile, and a white blood cell (WBC) count was normal. A benign syndrome was presumptively diagnosed, and she was discharged.

Her symptoms persisted, and on April 4, she sought medical evaluation at the office of her health care provider. Findings on physical examination were unchanged, but because of her underlying medical condition, she was referred for surgical consultation.

On April 5, the abdominal pain persisted, and she returned to the ED for evaluation. Her WBC count was elevated, and she was admitted to the hospital. Diagnoses of colitis and ileitis with possible perforation and intraabdominal abscess were considered, and treatment was initiated with broad-spectrum antibiotics. On physical examination, a maculopapular, vesicular rash with crusted lesions was observed on her trunk, head, and neck. Varicella was presumptively diagnosed, and she was placed in isolation. The patient reported that she had had onset of a mild macular, nonpruritic rash on her back on April 3 and that she had been exposed on March 12 and 13 to her four-year-old unvaccinated niece with varicella.

On April 6, the vesicles became hemorrhagic, and she began bleeding from intravenous sites. She rapidly developed hypotension and disseminated intravascular coagulation (DIC), and died from shock the same day. On autopsy, evidence of viral inclusion bodies in multiple organs was consistent with varicella, and varicella was determined to be the cause of death.

Morbidity and Mortality Weekly Report 46(19); 409–412, 1997.

Control

Children should be excluded from school for at least five days after the first lesion appears or until all vesicles are dry. Articles of clothing that may have been contaminated by discharge need to be disinfected.

HERPES ZOSTER (SHINGLES)

There are few infectious diseases capable of causing the excruciating pain of herpes zoster. This infection usually occurs in adults and is caused by reactivation of the chickenpox virus, which has lain dormant in sensory nerves for years. It is believed that a decline in the defenses of the immune system allows the virus to reemerge and cause shingles. The attack often follows a stressful incident that also lowers resistance. It is a very common disease in older people and others whose immune systems have been weakened.

Transmission

Herpes zoster is not as easily transmitted as chickenpox, but nonimmune individuals can be infected by contact with fluid from the vesicles. However, they get chickenpox, not shingles.

Symptoms

The prodromal symptoms are fever and malaise. Within two to four days, severe deep pain, pruritis, and paresthesia (numbness or tingling) or **hyperesthesia** (increased sensitivity) develop in the area affected. The eruptions usually occur on the trunk, arms, or legs, along a nerve pathway (Figure 8-6). The rash generally occurs about five days after the pain and other symptoms appear and sometimes not at all. When it does appear, it begins as small,

zoster   ZOS-ter
hyperesthesia   HI-per-es-THE-ze-a

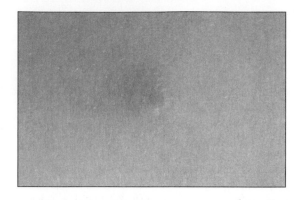

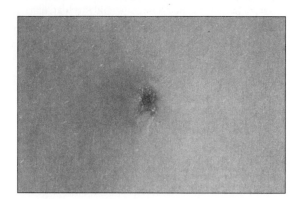

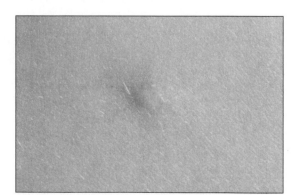

Figure 8-4   The evolution of the lesion in chickenpox.

(Top) "Dew drop" on a rose petal: a thin-walled vesicle with clear fluid forms on a red base.

(Middle) Vesicle becomes cloudy and depressed in the center, the border is irregular.

(Bottom) A crust forms in the center and eventually replaces the remaining portion of the vesicle at the periphery.

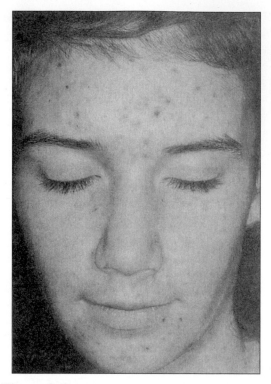

Figure 8-5

Chickenpox lesions on the face in all stages of development.

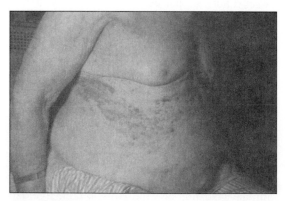

Figure 8-6

The lesions of shingles often follow a nerve pathway in an irregular pattern around the waist.

pain can come & go for years - nerve damage

slightly raised red spots that turn into blisters. Within three days, the blisters turn yellow, flatten, and scab over, sometimes leaving a pitted scar. Pain following the attack can be very severe but varies in different individuals from none at all to intermittent attacks for months or years. It is generally worse in older patients.

Treatment

Treatment can be palliative only, and although many different measures have been tried, none is consistently effective. Analgesics provide temporary partial relief.

Prevention

No means of prevention are known.

Control

No control measures are necessary except for personal hygiene and avoidance of those at risk.

MEASLES (RUBEOLA, RED MEASLES, HARD MEASLES)

Before the advent of the vaccine in 1963, measles was one of the most common communicable diseases throughout the world. The incidence in developed countries has dropped considerably, and in the United States, where vaccination is now required for children before they enter school, the number of cases dropped from over 450,000 in 1960 to 138 in 1997. The line graph and inset bar graph in Figure 8-7 vividly demonstrate the success of immunization programs. Some cases in this country are the result of importation. Measles, although most of the time comparatively mild, has the potential for complications that can be fatal. For this reason, it is a disease that needs to be controlled. In developing nations it is responsible for more than one million deaths each year. The incubation period is seven to eighteen days, usually fourteen days to onset of the rash. The disease is communicable from slightly before symptoms appear until four days after the rash appears. Everyone who has not had the disease or been immunized is susceptible. Rubeola does not cause congenital defects as rubella (German measles) does. Rubella will be covered in the next section.

Transmission

Measles is one of the most communicable of all diseases. It is spread through airborne droplets, direct contact with nasal or throat secretions of infected individuals, and by articles that have been freshly contaminated.

Symptoms

Early symptoms of measles include fever, photophobia (light sensitivity), malaise, anorexia, conjunctivitis, runny nose, and cough. A unique characteristic of the disease, Koplik's spots, appears four to five days after the initial symptoms. Koplik's spots are on the oral mucosa opposite the molars and look like tiny, bluish grey specks surrounded by a red halo. About five days after these spots appear, the temperature rises sharply, and a slightly itchy rash appears. This rash starts behind the ears and gradually spreads over the whole body. Once the rash reaches the feet, it begins to fade in the same order it appeared, leaving a brownish discoloration that disappears in seven to ten days. During the worst of the disease, about two to three days after the rash appears, there is a temperature of 103 to 105°F, severe cough, puffy red eyes, and runny nose. The face has a distinctive appearance. Encephalitis is the most serious complication.

Treatment

Plenty of fluids, acetaminophen for fever, and other remedies to relieve symptoms are usual treatment. Antibiotics are only used in case of secondary bacterial infection. Aspirin is no longer recommended for children because of the chance of developing Reye's syndrome.

Prevention

Routine vaccination during the second year of life is the best method of prevention.

Control

If live vaccine is given within seventy-two hours of exposure, it may provide protection. Immunoglobulin (IG) may be used for individuals in the household or who have had contact if they are at risk for complications. There should be contact investigation to determine the source and to vaccinate those who have not been vaccinated.

can't get it again

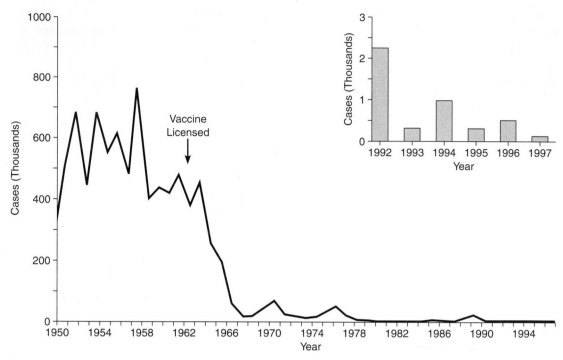

Figure 8-7
Reported measles cases by year, United States, 1950–1997.

(Rubeola)

RUBELLA (GERMAN MEASLES, THREE-DAY MEASLES)

This normally mild disease in children and adults is extremely dangerous for an unborn child when a pregnant woman is infected during the first trimester of pregnancy. Rubella was once common worldwide, but since the vaccine was developed, it is less prevalent in most developed countries. In the United States, reported cases dropped from over 12,000 in 1976 to an annual average of 183 from 1992 to 1996. Figure 8-8 shows the number of rubella and congenital rubella syndrome cases from 1980 to 1996. The reported number of rubella cases by state is shown in Figure 8-9.

The incubation period is fourteen to twenty-three days, and the disease is communicable for about one week before and at least four days after onset of the rash. Active immunity is acquired by having the infection or by vaccination. Infants receive antibodies from immune mothers, which protect them for six to nine months.

Transmission

Droplets or direct contact with throat and nasal secretions of infected individuals leads to infection. Infants who have acquired rubella congenitally shed the virus in their pharyngeal secretions and urine for months after birth and are a source of the infection for their contacts.

Symptoms - *URI symptoms*

In children, symptoms are mild, with a rash on the face that spreads to the body. After a few days the rash disappears. There may also be a slight fever and enlargement of the lymph nodes. In up to half of the cases the symptoms are inapparent, and the infection is never recognized. Adolescents and adults may have more pronounced symptoms.

• vaccine - not given to pregnant women
• get titer - to determine if you are immune
• if pregnant women gets Rubella - Birth Defects ↑

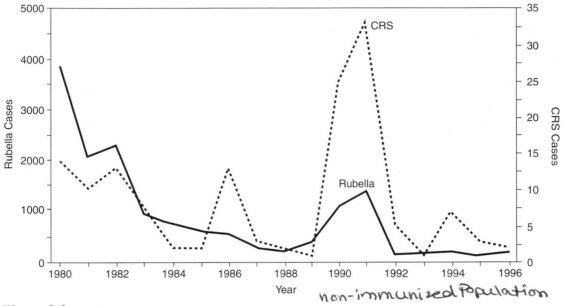

non-immunized Population

Figure 8-8

Number of reported rubella and congenital rubella syndrome (CRS) cases, by year, United States, 1980–1996.

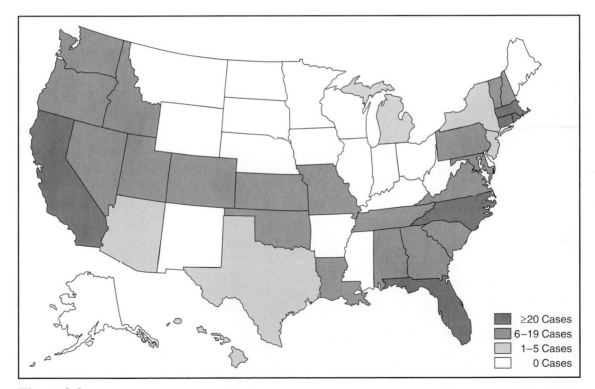

Figure 8-9

Number of reported rubella cases, United States, 1994–1996.

[handwritten, top margin] Mumps = more/most painful in adult male
– scrotum inflamation

Treatment

No specific treatment is available. Acetaminophen may be used to reduce fever.

Prevention

Vaccination of infants is highly effective in preventing the disease.

Control

Any known cases of rubella should be isolated from pregnant women. Contact investigation and identification of pregnant contacts is necessary to test for infection and to advise them regarding the possibilities for the unborn infant.

MUMPS (INFECTIOUS PAROTITIS)

Before the development of the mumps vaccine, it was commonly believed that male children should be exposed to the virus and allowed to get mumps. The belief had good reason behind it because, in the adult male, mumps could be an excruciatingly painful disease because of orchitis (inflammation of the testes). Today, with the vaccine, the wisest course of action is for everyone to be protected from the disease because, at any age, there can be serious complications. Mumps is most prevalent in the five- to nine-year-old age group. Mumps is caused by **paramyxovirus,** which infects the parotid gland. The incubation period is commonly eighteen days, and it is communicable from six days before symptoms appear and up to nine days after they appear. Many individuals have inapparent infections, but they can still communicate the disease. Immunity to the disease (lasting about one year) is transferred from mother to baby. Having the disease confers lifelong immunity. Most adults born before 1967 (when vaccine became available) were probably infected and had the disease even though there were no recognizable symptoms.

Transmission

Mumps is spread by airborne droplets and by direct contact with the saliva of an infected person.

Symptoms

It is estimated that about thirty percent of mumps sufferers have no symptoms. When symptoms do

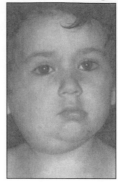

Figure 8-10

Mumps (infectious parotitis) in a child. In 70% of patients with mumps, both sides become infected. For this child only the right side is involved.

occur, they vary widely and may include myalgia, anorexia, malaise, headache, and low-grade fever, followed by an earache that is aggravated by chewing, and parotid gland tenderness and swelling (Figure 8-10). The temperature is 101 to 104° F, and there is pain during chewing or drinking sour or acidic liquids. In addition to orchitis, which has already been mentioned, complications include **epididymitis,** meningitis, and, rarely, a number of other serious illnesses. All complications occur more frequently in males.

Treatment

As with most viral diseases, antibiotics are ineffective. Analgesics, plenty of fluids, and rest are the main forms of treatment. Antipyretics may be used if the fever remains high, and intravenous fluid replacement if the victim has difficulty swallowing.

Prevention

A safe, effective vaccination is available and should be administered to all children. Fifteen months of age is the recommended time for the vaccination along with that for measles and rubella.

Control

Individuals with mumps should be excluded from school for nine days after the onset of the disease. Contact investigation and immunization of any contacts is advised.

[handwritten, bottom margin] disease spreads in children quickly
– children put everything in their mouths.

SMALLPOX

Smallpox is included in this text because of its historical significance as the first communicable disease recognized officially as eradicated. On October 26, 1979, the WHO declared smallpox eradicated two years after the last reported case, which was in Somalia. A case has not been reported in the United States since 1949. Smallpox was a highly infectious viral disease that was extremely common in the nineteenth century and before. It was spread by respiratory discharges and less often by contact with lesions. The symptoms began with chills, high fever, headache, backache, severe malaise, and vomiting. Sometimes symptoms were more severe, with convulsive seizures, delirium, or coma. Two to three days after symptoms appeared, victims began to feel better, but then lesions appeared around the mouth and throat, and a rash spread over the body and eventually developed into pus-filled blisters. These "pox" ruptured, became crusted, and sometimes left deep, pitted scars. No treatment was available, and the disease killed up to forty percent of those affected.

Cooperation in a vaccination program by countries all over the world led to eradication. There were certain characteristics of smallpox that aided in eradication. First, although spread person to person, it was infectious for only a short period. Second, it was easily recognized. Finally, it occurred only in humans. There are only two places in the world where the virus exists at the present time as far as is known: the CDC in Atlanta and at a research institute in Moscow. The virus is kept in these laboratories so that it will be available to make vaccine on the chance that the disease could break out again.

paramyxovirus pa-ram-IKS-o-v-I-rus
epididymitis ep-i-DID-i-MI-tis

SUMMARY

Table 8-2 summarizes relevant data on viral diseases acquired through the respiratory route.

	Special		**Major**	**Prevention/**
Disease	**Characteristics**	**Transmission**	**Symptoms**	**Control**
Common cold	Caused by close to 200 different viruses. In 50%, strain of virus is unknown. Most common communicable disease	Direct or indirect; hand to eye most likely, also by droplets	Runny nose, watery eyes, headache Secondary infection: bronchitis, laryngitis, otitis media, sinusitis (usually bacterial)	Personal hygiene, frequent washing of hands, general fitness, avoidance of direct contact with infected individuals

TABLE 8-2 Viral Diseases Acquired by the Respiratory Route

Continued

TABLE 8-2	*Continued*			
Disease	**Special Characteristics**	**Transmission**	**Major Symptoms**	**Prevention/ Control**
Influenza	Respiratory tract disease Fatalities from complications, often pneumonia. Epidemics evolve slowly	Direct or indirect contact; airborne droplets	Sudden onset of chills, temperature, headache, malaise, muscle aches, cough	Vaccination for at-risk individuals
Infectious mononucleosis	Epstein-Barr virus, herpes group. Lab test necessary to confirm diagnosis. Serious complications are possible. High school and college age most commonly affected	Oral-pharyngeal route	Headache, malaise, fatigue, fever, swollen glands, sore throat, enlarged spleen, possibly hepatitis	Basic personal hygiene and avoidance of close contact with infected persons; do not share pop cans, drinking glasses, or utensils
Varicella (Chickenpox)	Varicella zoster virus. Mild in children; severe in adults. Virus stays in body, may cause herpes zoster years later	Direct or indirect contact, airborne droplets from respiratory tract, discharge from vesicles	Fever, malaise, anorexia, rash, vesicles	IG for high-risk individuals, vaccine in Japan; exclusion of children from school
Herpes zoster (Shingles)	Reactivation of chickenpox virus in adults. Occurs with lowered resistance from stress or other causes	Communicable through fluid from vesicles	Fever, malaise, severe pain, pruritis, numbness, tingling, increased sensitivity in affected area; blisters, scab pitted scar; may be intermittent severe pain for years	Palliative only, no remedy has proved to be consistently effective
Measles	A comparatively mild disease with	Direct and indirect transmission through	Fever, photophobia, malaise, anorexia,	Vaccination, IG for at-risk household

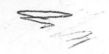

TABLE 8-2	Continued			
Disease	**Special Characteristics**	**Transmission**	**Major Symptoms**	**Prevention/ Control**
Measles—Cont'd	potentially fatal complications	airborne droplets, nasal or throat secretions, fomites; communicable before rash and 4 days after	conjunctivitis, coryza, cough, Koplik's spots, temperature, rash Complication: encephalitis	contacts, contact investigation
Rubella	Birth defects in child of pregnant woman who acquires disease, especially during first 4 months of pregnancy. Incubation of 2–3 weeks. Most often occurs among children	Droplets or direct contact with nose or nasal secretions of infected person; infection of fetus; infants with congenital rubella also spread infection	Mild, with a rash, slight fever, swollen lymph nodes possible; up to 50% of cases inapparent	None known; acetaminophen to ease discomfort; pregnant women should be isolated from known cases; contact investigation
Smallpox	Declared eradicated by WHO, October 1979. Cause of much suffering and death (40% of victims). Infective when first lesion appears for about 3 weeks or until scabs are gone	Most often through respiratory discharges; also contact with lesions and fomites; rarely airborne	Chills, high fever, headache, backache, severe malaise, vomiting; sometimes seizures, delerium, coma; sudden onset, lesions on face first; rash, pus-filled blisters that broke, sometimes leaving deep pitted scars	Worldwide vaccination program led to eradication. Only selective vaccination now
Mumps	Extremely painful disease in adult males	Airborne droplets and direct contact with saliva of infected person	None in 30%; malaise, anorexia, myalagia, headache, lowgrade fever;	Vaccination; exclusion from school for 9 days after onset; contact investigation

TABLE 8-2	*Continued*			
Disease	**Special Characteristics**	**Transmission**	**Major Symptoms**	**Prevention/ Control**
Mumps—Cont'd			earache, parotid gland swelling and tenderness; complications may include orchitis, epididymitis, meningitis	

There are some antiviral drugs that can be used to treat these diseases: amandadine and rimantadine for influenza and acyclovir for viruses in herpes family. Penicillin and most other antibiotics are ineffective.

Ans. Ques 1-9 (Due Thurs)

① Describe common cold virus - Know for Thurs

QUESTIONS FOR REVIEW

H.W

1. What are some complications that can occur with the common cold?
2. What is the most likely way by which a cold is acquired?
3. What symptoms indicate a secondary bacterial infection?
4. What is the best treatment for a cold?
5. What is the best way to avoid a cold?
6. What is the difference in meaning between influenza and the term *flu* as it is commonly used?
7. Why is influenza a dangerous disease?
8. Why has influenza been a difficult disease to prevent?
9. How are amantadine and rimantadine used in treating influenza?
10. What is the disease agent for infectious mononucleosis?
11. Why is mono called the college disease?
12. What complications may occur with infectious mononucleosis?
13. In what ways can chickenpox be a severe disease?
14. What is meant by the term "dewdrop on a petal"?
15. What complications may occur if a child scratches the lesions of chickenpox?
16. What is the goal of treatment in chickenpox?
17. When is VZIG used for chickenpox?
18. What is the cause of shingles?
19. How is shingles transmitted?
20. Where do the lesions for herpes zoster occur?
21. What may happen to an individual years after having an attack of shingles?
22. What are the unique characteristics among the symptoms of measles?
23. What danger is there to the fetus if a pregnant woman acquires rubella?
24. How can measles and rubella be prevented?
25. What is the historical significance of smallpox?
26. What characteristics of smallpox aided in its eradication?
27. What are the symptoms of smallpox?
28. What complications may occur with mumps?

FURTHER READING

Bardi, Jason. 1999. Aftermath of a hypothetical smallpox disaster. *Emerging Infectious Diseases* 5:547.

Bonn, Dorothy, and Alan McGregor. 1998. H5N1 influenza investigation eases fears of pandemic. *The Lancet* 351:115.

Clover, Richard. 1999. Influenza vaccine for adults 50 to 64 years of age. *American Family Physician* 60:1921.

Cohen, Jeffery L., and Philip A. Brunell. 1999. Recent advances in varicella-zoster virus infections. *Annals of Internal Medicine* 130:922.

Doepel, Laurie K. 1997. "Nasal flu vaccine proves effective on children." *Dateline:NIAID,* National Institute of Allergy and Infectious Diseases. www.niaid.nih.gov.

Epidemiology of measles—United States, 1998. *Journal of the American Medical Association* 282:1323.

Frankel, David. 1999. Eradicating measles in the Americas. *The Lancet* 353:1424.

Gensheimer, K. F., et al. 1999. Preparing for pandemic influenza: the need for enhanced surveillance. *Emerging Infectious Diseases* 5:297.

Grose, Charles. 1999. Varicella-zoster virus: less immutable than once thought. *Pediatrics* 103:1027.

Influenza and pneumococcal vaccination rates among persons with diabetes mellitus—United States, 1977. *Journal of the American Medical Association* 283:48, 1999.

Is smallpox history? *The Lancet* 353:1539, 1999.

Katz, Jonathan. 1999. Smallpox vaccine. *Science* 285:2067.

Kimmel, Sanford R., and Sandra Puczynski. 1999. Practices of family physicians and pediatricians in administering poliovirus vaccine. *Journal of Family Practice* 48:594.

Kobayashi, Makoto, et al. 1999. Can we stop national immunization days before global eradication of poliomyelitis: *The Lancet* 353:2129.

Lewandowski, Donna M. 1999. Myocarditis. *American Journal of Nursing* 99:44.

Maeda, A., et al. 1999. An immunocompetent child with herpes zoster following post-exposure prophylaxis of varicella by oral acyclovir. *Acta Paediatrica* 88:1161–2.

Marwick, Charles. 1999. Scary scenarios spark action at bioterrorism symposium. *Journal of the American Medical Association* 281:1075.

Maudlin, Robert K. 1999. First pill to treat flu approved. *Modern Medicine* 67:53.

Meier, Christopher R., Susan S. Jick, Laura E. Derby, et al. 1998. Acute respiratory tract infections and risk of first time acute myocardial infarction. *The Lancet* 351:1467.

Meltzer, Martin I., and Nancy J. Cox. 1999. The economic impact of pandemic influenza in the United States: priorities for intervention. *Emerging Infectious Diseases* 5:659.

Merrer, J., et al. 1999. Rubella encephalitis in young adults: arguments for a better vaccination policy. *Presse Medicale* 28:395.

Mitchell, Peter. 1999. WHO starts final campaign against polio. *The Lancet* 354:230, 1999.

National Institute of Allergy and Infectious Diseases. 1998. [www.niaid.nih.gov]. Nasal spray vaccine prevents both the flu and flu-related earaches. *NIAID News.*

Omer, M. I. A. 1999. Measles: a disease that has to be eradicated. *Annals of Tropical Paediatrics: International Child Health* 19:125.

Plotkin, Stanley A., et al. 1999. The eradication of rubella. *Journal of the American Medical Association* 281:561.

Poliomyelitis prevention: revised recommendations for use of inactivated and live oral poliovirus vaccines. *Pediatrics* 103:171, 1999.

Pougatcheva, S. O., et al. 1999. Development of a rubella virus DNA vaccine. *Vaccine* 17:2104.

Prevention and control of influenza. *Morbidity and Mortality Weekly Report,* 4/30/99 48/No.RR4 pp. 1–49.

Sadovsky, Richard. 1999. Varicella-zoster virus infection: recent advances. *American Family Physician* 60:1518.

Shimada, Atsuyoshi, et al. 1999. Amyotrophic lateral sclerosis in an adult following acute paralytic poliomyelitis in early childhood. *Acta Neuropathologica* 353:478.

Taylor, Brent, and Elizabeth Miller. 1999. Autism and measles, mumps, and rubella vaccine: no epidemiological evidence for a causal association. *The Lancet* 353:2026.

Walter, R., et al. 1999. Reactivation of herpes virus infections after vaccinations? *The Lancet* 353, 1999.

Waters, C., et al. 1999. New recommendations for adult immunization. *Journal of the American Medical Association* 282:2199.

Zimmerman, Richard Kent. 1999. Poliovirus vaccine options. *American Family Physician* 59:113.

Viral Diseases Acquired through the Alimentary and Other Routes

OBJECTIVES

1. *Explain the importance of the polio vaccine.*

2. *Distinguish among hepatitis A, B, C, D, E, and G.*

3. *State steps to take when someone is bitten by a wild or domestic animal.*

4. *Describe the effects of rabies without treatment.*

5. *Identify possible symptoms of encephalitis.*

6. *Distinguish between herpes simplex virus Type I and II.*

7. *Indicate when warts need to be treated.*

8. *Discuss the history of AIDS.*

9. *Identify means of transmission, symptoms, treatment, prevention, and control for diseases in this chapter.*

POLIOMYELITIS (INFANTILE PARALYSIS, POLIO)

One of the most dramatic medical events in the 1950s was the development of a vaccine for polio. Dr. Jonas E. Salk (Figure 9-1) devised the first vaccine for polio, and six years later, Dr. Albert Sabin developed the second, which has almost entirely replaced Salk vaccine. Polio was first recognized in 1840 and became epidemic in Norway and Sweden in 1905. During the first half of this century, the disease became pandemic, and the word *polio* produced more fear in the American people and people all over the world than the word *AIDS*

(handwritten, top margin) Paralytic Polio ↑ w/ age (FDR)

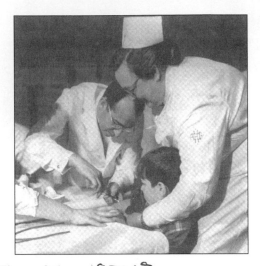

Figure 9-1   *(handwritten)* 1950's

Dr. Jonas Salk, developer of the first vaccine for poliomyelitis.

does today. AIDS is mostly a danger to a segment of the population who practice a certain lifestyle, whereas polio was (and is) a threat to all. Paralysis and death were synonymous with polio, or infantile paralysis as it was called in the early days. Symbolic of the paralyzing form of the disease was the dreaded "iron lung," a monstrous armor of iron into which the victims were slid until only their heads were free. This machine was an artificial respirator, the forerunner of the much simpler apparatuses used in hospitals today. Polio can range from asymptomatic illness to paralysis and *(handwritten: to death)* major illness, depending upon the course of the infection. It is caused by poliovirus, an *enterovirus.* Originally, polio was a disease of children, but in recent years it has occurred more often in people older than fifteen years of age. Minor outbreaks still occur, usually among nonimmunized segments of the population, such as the Amish of Pennsylvania, among whom there was an outbreak in 1979. Figure 9-2 shows the decrease in paralytic cases following the development of the vaccines. Polio usually has an incubation period of seven to fourteen days, although incubation has been known to range from three to thirty-five days. The period of communicability is not accurately known, but the disease is most

infectious during the first few days before and after the onset of symptoms. The virus exists in the feces for three to six weeks or longer. Most people are susceptible to the disease, but susceptibility to the paralytic form increases with age at time of infection. There are three types of the polio virus, and immunity following infection is type specific.

Many years after having polio, some of the survivors develop symptoms similar to those they had with the acute illness—unexpected fatigue, pain, and weakness in the muscles. In the early 1980s, the medical community recognized the symptoms as "post-polio syndrome." It was defined as "a neurological disorder that produces a cluster of symptoms in individuals who had recovered from paralytic polio many years earlier."*

In 1988 WHO identified polio as a disease to be eradicated by 2000. By 1994, North and South America were certified free from the illness. Three major foci of the efforts now are South Asia, West Africa, and Central Africa. However, with air travel moving people from areas where the disease is present in a day or less, nobody is "safe." Polio, like all infectious diseases, must be eradicated all over the world for anyone to be safe from transmission by travelers and immigrants.

Transmission

Direct contact through close association with someone who has the disease is necessary for infection with the poliomyelitis virus. The main means of transmission is the fecal-oral route when there are poor methods of sanitation. Where sanitation is good, it is spread more by pharyngeal secretions. The organism is easier to detect and lasts longer in feces than in secretions from the throat.   *(handwritten)* Fecal-oral

Symptoms

The symptoms for poliomyelitis vary, depending upon the progression of the disease. Although the word *polio* brought fear to all at one time, it was only due to hearing about the worst cases. For most, polio is a comparatively mild disease. There are four possible outcomes of infection:

*Lauro S. Halstead, 1998, "Post-polio syndrome," *Scientific American* 278:42.

(handwritten, bottom margin)
1950's Polio Vaccination
Paralytic Polio — paralyzed from neck down (Paralized vital organs) = death

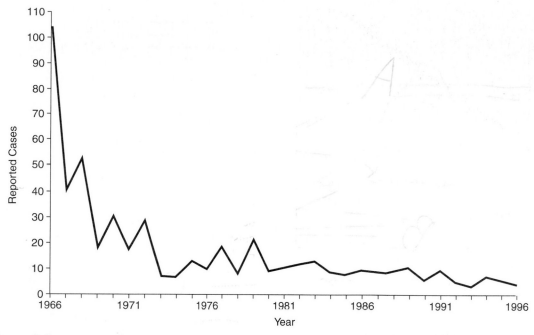

Figure 9-2

Poliomyelitis (paralytic), by year, United States, 1966–1996.

(1) Asymptomatic illness occurs in at least ninety percent of poliovirus infections. (2) Minor illness with fever, headache, malaise, sore throat, and vomiting occurs in approximately five percent of patients. (3) Nonparalytic poliomyelitis with back pain and muscle spasms in addition to the symptoms of minor illness occurs in one percent to two percent of patients. (4) Paralytic polio with spinal and/or cranial paralysis occurs three to four days after minor illness has subsided. This form occurs in one-tenth of one percent to two percent of infected individuals. The extent of paralysis varies, depending upon how many nerves are affected. Only one leg may be involved, or the individual may have progressive paralysis that eventually affects vital organs and leads to death.

[handwritten margin notes: 90% ①, 5% ②, 1-2% ③, ④ ⅟₁₀ – 2%]

Treatment

Other than analgesics to relieve pain, there is no treatment for polio. Physical therapy is used to counteract muscle atrophy.

Prevention

Immunization for polio should begin at two months of age. Routine immunization of adults is not recommended except those at risk because of occupation or travel to high-risk areas.

Control

Because the greatest risk of infection is during the prodromal period, isolation is unnecessary. Identifying contacts to identify individuals who are ill and provide appropriate treatment is recommended.

VIRAL HEPATITIS

[handwritten: A, B, & C (5 types) 6th (G) identified]

There are at least five different viruses that cause hepatitis (inflammation of the liver). The most common are hepatitis A (HAV), hepatitis B (HBV), and hepatitis C (HCV), which will be discussed in

poliomyelitis	POL-e-o-MI-el-I-tis

[handwritten at bottom: ✻ Prodromal ✻ (2nd stage)]

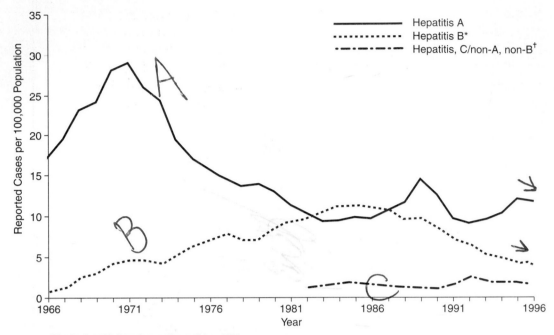

Figure 9-3

Hepatitis, by year, United States, 1966–1996.

this chapter. Non-A, non-B hepatitis, now referred to as hepatitis C, is a form transmitted by unclean needles and found frequently among drug users. Figure 9-3 shows the comparative number of reported cases for the first three types of hepatitis. Figures 9-4 and 9-5 show the reported cases of hepatitis A and hepatitis B by state. Hepatitis D, formerly delta hepatitis, occurs only in someone who has hepatitis B, because it needs the B virus for its own survival. No outbreaks of hepatitis E have been reported in this country. It is similar to hepatitis A. In 1996, a sixth virus was identified and named hepatitis G. However, its relationship to hepatitis is still being studied.

Hepatitis A (Infectious Hepatitis)

Hepatitis A, formerly called infectious hepatitis, occurs in all parts of the world. In developed countries, it occurs frequently in day-care centers where there are diapered children, among intravenous drug users, individuals who practice

unprotected sexual intercourse, and among travelers to countries where it is endemic. Epidemic cycles have not occurred in the United States since 1971, but in 1983, the number of reported cases started to increase and reached a peak by 1989 before slowing down as shown in Figure 9-3. The primary reservoir of infection is people, although the virus has been found in chimpanzees and other nonhuman primates. The average incubation period is twenty-eight to thirty days. Hepatitis A is communicable during the last part of the incubation period to a few days after the onset of jaundice. (Jaundice does not occur in some cases, particularly children—see under Symptoms.) Susceptibility is general, and the low incidence of reported cases among children suggests that some infections are asymptomatic.

Transmission
The virus is present in the **feces** of infected persons and transmitted person to person by the fecal-oral route. Most often this occurs when the

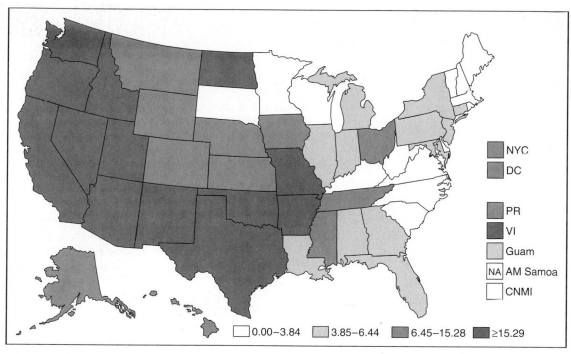

Figure 9-4

Hepatitis A, reported cases per 100,000 population, United States and territories, 1996.

infected person handles food and contaminated food is eaten by others. The virus may also be present in shellfish from contaminated water and, if not cooked at a high enough temperature, transmitted to humans. Transmission of hepatitis A by blood is rare, but individuals who have had it should not donate blood.

Symptoms

There is usually a sudden onset with fever, malaise, anorexia, nausea, and abdominal discomfort, followed within a few days by jaundice (in some cases). The illness is usually mild, lasting one to two weeks. The severity of the illness generally increases with age. Children are often asymptomatic or have flulike symptoms but no jaundice. A diagnosis can only be made with liver function tests. The few fatalities that occur are in older patients.

Treatment   None

There is no specific treatment for hepatitis A.

Prevention/Control

The public needs to be educated about good sanitation and personal hygiene. There should be particular emphasis on proper hand washing and sanitary disposal of feces. Individuals working in day-care centers need to use proper methods to minimize the possibility of fecal-oral transmission. Thorough hand washing after changing diapers and before meals is mandatory. Immunoglobulin (IgM) should be given to staff and attendees at any center where a case occurs. Administration of IgM to families of attendees should also be considered. Travelers to high-risk areas should be given prophylactic doses of IgM. Oysters, clams, and other shellfish from contaminated areas should be heated at a high temperature for four minutes or steamed for ninety seconds. In case of an epidemic, the source of the infection needs to be identified by epidemiologic

feces FE-sez

CONTEMPORARY CONCERNS

Better Safe than Sick

Microwaving food bought at a fast-food place can reduce the risk of catching hepatitis A. When a worker who routinely picked up food for his fellow employees came down with hepatitis A that was traced to a cook at a local fast-food restaurant, scientists could not understand why he became ill with the infection and the other twelve workers who ate the same food did not. Further investigation showed that he ate his food on the way back to the plant, but the others reheated theirs in the microwave, evidently at a temperature high enough to destroy the organism.

studies. Any common source of infection should be eliminated.

Hepatitis B (Serum Hepatitis)

This viral hepatitis has a slower onset than infectious hepatitis. The average incubation period is sixty to ninety days, and blood from the victim is thought to be infective weeks before the symptoms appear and to remain infective through the carrier stage, which may be for life. The disease is milder and sometimes asymptomatic in children.

Transmission

Blood, saliva, semen, and vaginal fluids have shown to be infectious. Contaminated needles, syringes, and other intravenous equipment are important vehicles for spreading the disease. The infection may also be spread by contamination of sores or exposure of mucous membranes to contaminated blood or blood transfusion. Donated blood that has been screened is considered relatively safe. Since the advent of AIDS, screening of blood for hepatitis (and other) antibodies has become routine. The chance of receiving contaminated blood through transfusion is one "in a million" today. The infection can also be acquired through homosexual or heterosexual intercourse.

Symptoms

The symptoms of hepatitis B include insidious onset of anorexia, vague abdominal discomfort, nausea, vomiting, and sometimes rash and jaun-

[handwritten: mutates]

dice. Type B has a higher mortality rate than type A, particularly in people over forty years of age.

Treatment

Interferon is used to treat chronic hepatitis B. It has been shown to slow the progress of the disease in about forty percent of patients treated.

Prevention/Control

Vaccines are available, but their high cost prohibits general use. Vaccination is recommended for those at increased and continuing risk of infection and for all newborns. Blood must be continually screened, and all needles and syringes sterilized, or if they are disposable, proper methods of disposal must be used.

[handwritten: now = scheduled vaccine for children]

Hepatitis C (Non-A or Non-B)

The CDC estimates that 36,000 to 230,000 Americans are infected with hepatitis C each year. Of these, twenty-five percent to thirty percent have symptoms. Approximately 3.9 million Americans are currently infected with the virus. Groups at risk include injecting drug users, hemodialysis patients, health care workers, sexual contacts of infected persons, persons with multiple sex partners, and infants born to infected women. Most new infections are due to high-risk drug use (60%) or sexual behaviors (20%). The incubation period is five to nine weeks.

Transmission

Generally, hepatitis C is transmitted through blood, although there is evidence that it can be

[handwritten: • spread like B • as many deaths as aids • 2nd cause of liver disease behind alcoholism]

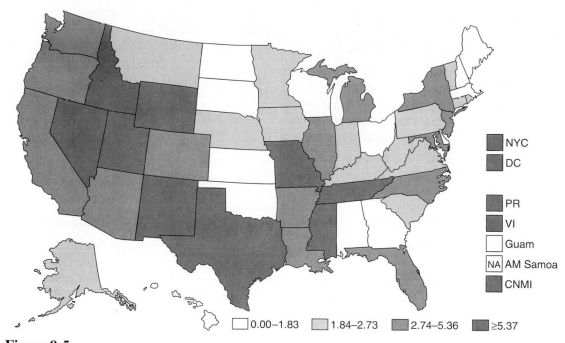

Figure 9-5

Hepatitis B, reported cases per 100,000 population, United States and territories, 1996.

passed from mother to unborn child at the time of birth or through breast feeding.

Symptoms

The symptoms of hepatitis C are slow in manifesting or the person may be asymptomatic. Symptoms may not appear until the liver disease has progressed to cirrhosis or cancer. If there are symptoms, they are similar to the symptoms of hepatitis A and hepatitis B: fatigue, abdominal pain, loss of appetite, intermittent nausea, vomiting, and jaundice.

Treatment *More useful for C than B*

Interferon has been used when the disease becomes chronic but has slowed the progress of the disease only fifteen percent to thirty percent of the time.

Prevention/Control

Prevention and control measures are the same as for hepatitis B.

RABIES (HYDROPHOBIA)

Rabies is a disease of animals, especially bats, skunks, foxes, raccoons, dogs, cats, and cattle. Since 1990, the number of cases of rabies in the United States has increased significantly. This increase is due largely to the emergence of bat-associated rabies (Figure 9-6). The disease is communicated to humans by the bite of a rabid animal. Without treatment, it is almost always fatal. Figure 9-7 shows the number of cases in the United States and Puerto Rico by year. It is estimated that 30,000 deaths from rabies occur worldwide each year, mostly in developing countries.

The incubation period is usually two to eight weeks, depending on a number of factors. Incubation periods have been known to be as little as five days to a year or more. The period of communicability varies, depending on the mammal involved. Dogs and cats are communicable for three to ten days before the onset of symptoms and

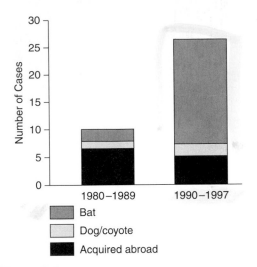

Figure 9-6

Emergence of bat-associated rabies in humans in the United States.

for as long as the disease lasts. All warm-blooded mammals are susceptible, and there is no known natural immunity in humans.

Although there have been few or no human deaths in the United States from rabies recently, the number of animal deaths reported has almost doubled in the last few years. Individuals who work with the animals that can carry rabies and those who camp, hike, or otherwise spend time outdoors need to know the procedure to follow if bitten by an animal—especially if the bite is unprovoked. Also, those traveling to other countries should be immunized if they will be in developing countries where the prevalence of rabies is high.

Transmission

Transmission is most often by introduction of the saliva of an infected animal by a bite or scratch into the muscle tissue. A few cases have resulted from

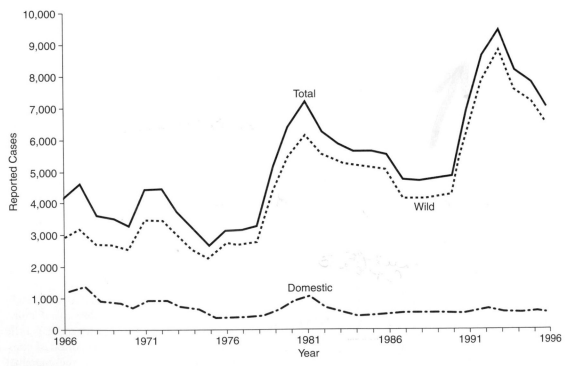

Figure 9-7

Rabies in wild and domestic animals, by year, United States and Puerto Rico, 1966–1996.

corneal transplants when the organs were removed from individuals with undiagnosed CNS disease. No other person-to-person transmission has ever been documented. Transmission by air has been demonstrated in caves, and in Latin America transmission from bats to domestic animals is common.

Symptoms

The severity of the wound site in relation to nerve supply, distance from the brain, the amount of virus introduced, and layers of clothing are all factors in determining how quickly symptoms appear. The initial symptoms are local or radiating pain or burning and a sensation of cold, itching, and tingling at the bite site. There are also typical symptoms of fever, malaise, headache, anorexia, nausea, sore throat, and persistent loose cough. Then the patient will begin to show nervousness, anxiety, irritability, **hyperesthesia** (increased sensitivity to sensory stimuli), pupillary dilation, tachy-

cardia, shallow respirations, and excessive salivation, tears, and perspiration. About two to ten days after onset of these symptoms, the victim experiences restlessness, hyperactivity, disorientation, and in some cases, seizures. There is often an intense thirst, but attempts to drink induce violent, painful spasms in the throat (the reason for the name *hydrophobia*). Eye and facial muscles may become paralyzed. Coma and death follow three to twenty days after the onset of symptoms. Figure 9-8 shows the sequence of events following inoculation with rabies virus.

Treatment

Rabies is generally fatal if not treated promptly. Wound treatment and immunization must be given as soon as possible after the bite occurs. Any animal

hyperesthesia	HI-per-es-THE-ze-a

leave wound open

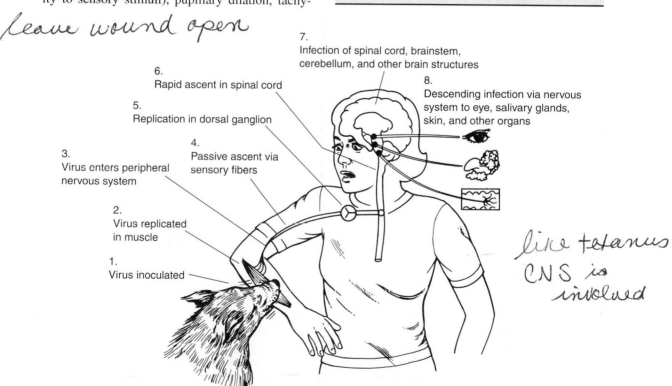

7.
Infection of spinal cord, brainstem, cerebellum, and other brain structures

6.
Rapid ascent in spinal cord

8.
Descending infection via nervous system to eye, salivary glands, skin, and other organs

5.
Replication in dorsal ganglion

4.
Passive ascent via sensory fibers

3.
Virus enters peripheral nervous system

2.
Virus replicated in muscle

1.
Virus inoculated

like tetanus CNS is involved

Figure 9-8

Progression of rabies virus infection; numbered steps describe sequence of events.

cleaned w/ soap & water (handwritten)

bite should be washed thoroughly (cleaned and flushed with water). The wound should not be sutured or closed. Although a person's own defenses may keep him or her from developing rabies even after being bitten by an infected animal, wound treatment must be given as soon as possible after the bite occurs. Vaccines that are used in the United States at this time are rabies vaccine, human diploid cell vaccine (HDCV), rabies vaccine adsorbed (RVA), and rabies immune globulin, human (HRIG). When or if these vaccines are administered depends upon the circumstances of the case involved.

Prevention

For prevention of rabies, registration, licensing, and vaccination of all dogs and cats is recommended. Stray, ownerless animals should be impounded and vaccinated or destroyed as necessary. An animal of any species that is acting strange or sick should not be picked up or handled. These animals should be reported to the police and/or local health department. Any pet animal that has bitten a person with no provocation should be caged and observed for ten days for signs of rabies. If a wild animal bites a person, it should be destroyed immediately and the head kept (on ice) and turned in for testing. Individuals at high risk (those who work with animals) should receive vaccinations. *work w/ Bats* (handwritten)

Control

Respiratory secretions of someone bitten by a rabid animal may contain the virus, and contacts must be protected from them until it is determined that the victim does not have the disease. Any animal known to have bitten someone needs to be held for observation for ten days. Valuable dogs and cats should not be killed unless it is established that they do have the disease. Unwanted dogs and cats and wild animals should be killed immediately and the brain checked for rabies.

ENCEPHALITIS *West-Nile* (handwritten)

Encephalitis is a severe inflammation of the brain usually caused by a mosquito-borne or tick-borne virus. In addition, encephalitis may be a sequela of another viral infection, such as polio, rabies, or mumps. This discussion will confine itself to arthropod-borne viral **encephalitides** (plural of encephalitis). There are four main viral agents in the United States. Eastern equine encephalitis (EEE) is recognized in the eastern and north-central sections of the United States; western equine encephalitis (WEE) in the western and central states; LaCrosse encephalitis in the east and central states, and St. Louis encephalitis in most of the states (Figure 9-9). These and other kinds of viral encephalitis occur in other parts of the world also.

Encephalitis occurs more in summer and early fall, particularly when conditions have been right for breeding many mosquitoes. The winter reservoir for most of these viruses is unknown. The incubation period is usually five to fifteen days. There is no person-to-person transmission. People are more susceptible in infancy and old age.

Transmission

These viral encephalitides are transmitted by the bite of an infected mosquito.

Symptoms

For most viral encephalitis infections there are few or no symptoms. When symptoms do occur, they begin suddenly with fever, headache, and vomiting and progress to include stiff neck and back, drowsiness, coma, paralysis, convulsions, muscular incoordination, and psychoses.

Treatment *None* (handwritten)

There is no specific treatment for viral encephalitis. Analgesics for pain and other supportive therapy are used.

Prevention/Control

The following are ways to prevent and control viral encephalitis: control of mosquitoes by spraying and destruction of breeding places; use of screened living quarters and mosquito bed nets if necessary; avoidance of exposure to mosquitoes during times when they are known to bite; and use of repellants.

*West Nile * Crows * / Birds migrating South* (handwritten)
In N.C. — Bird Dead. (handwritten)
West Nile Virus (no treatment) /Death - 13% (handwritten)

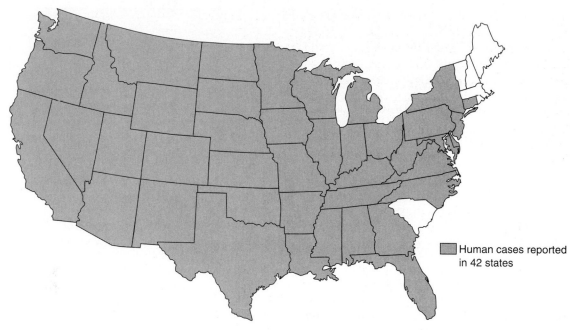

Average: 131 cases/year; 75/year excluding the epidemic of 1975

Human cases reported
in 42 states

Figure 9-9

Confirmed and probable St. Louis encephalitis cases in humans, by state, 1964–1997.

HERPES SIMPLEX

Herpes simplex is a recurrent, localized viral infection. Herpes simplex virus Type I generally infects the upper part of the body, usually the lips and face. Herpes simplex virus Type II generally infects the lower part of the body, most often the genital area. Infections from both types can occur in any part of the body depending on sexual practices and area exposed. (The incubation period for both types is two to twelve days. The viruses are found worldwide, and everyone is susceptible.) Both viruses can enter through a break in the skin or through the mucous membrane. Reactivation, which may or may not occur, can be due to a number of traumatic events, including stress or anything else that impairs the effectiveness of the immune system. Individuals with AIDS are especially vulnerable to reactivation, which can lead to a generalized infection and death. Once a person is infected with either type, he or she is infected for life.

Most adults (70% to 90%) have been exposed to HSV Type I (worldwide). Visible symptoms occur in only about ten percent of the cases. Once the virus enters the body it is there for life. In about sixty percent of those infected, the disease is reactivated in later life and may occur as sores around the mouth during periods of stress or lowered resistance. The virus has been found in saliva for as long as seven weeks after the lesion is healed. Genital herpes, most often caused by herpes virus Type II, is infective for about seven to twelve days. Asymptomatic shedding of virus is probably common for both types.

Transmission

Transmission is by contact with saliva of infected individuals or by sexual activities. Both kinds can be transmitted by oral-genital or oral-anal contact.

---

encephalitides   en-SEF-a-LI-ti-des

---

*not contageous - w/ no outbreak
may have internal outbreak*

CASE STUDY

Herpes Simplex Virus Type I

In July 1989, the Minnesota Department of Health (MDH) investigated an outbreak of herpes simplex virus Type I in participants at a Minnesota wrestling camp. The camp was held from July 2 through July 28 and attended by 175 male high school wrestlers from throughout the United States. The participants were divided into three groups according to weight (group 1, lightest; group 3, heaviest). During most practice sessions, wrestlers had contact only with others in the same group. The outbreak was detected during the final week of camp, and wrestling contact was subsequently discontinued for the final two days.

Clinical and questionnaire data were examined for 171 (98%) persons. Sixty (35%) persons met the case definition, including 21 (12%) who had HSV-I isolated from the skin or eye. All affected wrestlers had onset during the camp session or within one week after leaving camp. Two wrestlers had a probable recurrence of HSV, one oral and one cutaneous, during the first week of camp. Lesions were located on the head or the neck in 44 (73%) persons, the extremities in 25 (42%), and the trunk in 17 (28%). Herpetic conjunctivitis occurred in 5 persons; none developed keratitis. Associated signs and symptoms included lymphadenopathy (60%), fever and /or chills (25%), sore throat (40%), and headache (22%). Forty-four (73%) persons were treated with acyclovir.

Twenty-three percent of affected wrestlers continued to wrestle for at least two days after rash onset. Athletes who reported wrestling with a participant with a rash were more likely to have confirmed or probable HSV-I infection.

From *Morbidity and Mortality Weekly Report* 39:69, 1990.

Symptoms

Herpes may be asymptomatic or there may be varying degrees of typical prodromal symptoms. Itching and tingling precede the development of vesicular lesions around the mouth or in the genital or anal regions. The lesions are usually painful. There may also be fever, swollen glands, and painful urination. If lesions are internal, the symptoms may not be noticed. Figure 9-10 is an example of oral herpes. The fluid-filled vesicles break open and heal in one to three weeks during the primary infection; the interval is shorter in reactivated disease. Figure 9-11 is an example of genital herpes.

The virus can also cause conjunctivitis or a corneal ulcer, encephalitis, meningitis, or herpetic whitlow, an infection of the fingers that sometimes occurs in nurses, dentists, and others working with infected people.

Treatment

An analgesic antipyretic (pain and fever reducer) may be prescribed for a primary infection. If the mouth is affected, a mouthwash with a numbing agent may be used. Calamine or another drying lotion may be used to make the lesions on the lips and face less painful. Acyclovir, which comes in tablets or ointment form, has been found to reduce viral shedding, diminish pain, and speed up the healing for primary infections. It is also used prophylactically. Two other antiviral drugs are now available. Oral medications are more effective than ointments. As stated before, *there is no cure* for herpes infections at this time. Once a person is infected with the virus, it is with him or her for life.

Prevention/Control

Although personal hygiene is always a good practice to follow, the high rate of infection among adults makes it unlikely that oral herpes infection can be avoided. The use of condoms in sexual practices may reduce the risk of acquiring herpes in the genital or anal area. Close contact with anyone having apparent infection should be avoided.

Type 1 - almost all of us have it
10 % - have outbreaks

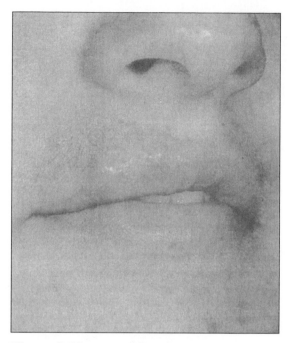

Figure 9-10
Herpes simplex on the lips and face.

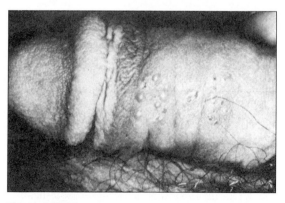

Figure 9-11
Genital herpes.

Individuals with herpetic lesions should be isolated from newborns, children, and immunosuppressed individuals. For pregnant women, a cesarean section is recommended before the membranes rupture, because a herpes infection can be fatal for the newborn child.

WARTS

Warts are caused by the human papilloma virus (HPV). There are a number of different kinds, including common warts, which usually appear on sites subject to injury, such as the hands (Figure 9-12), face, knees, or scalp, particularly in young children. They are firm, sharply defined, round or irregular, flesh-colored to brown growths. They may grow up to about one-quarter inch in diameter and often have a rough surface. Flat warts occur mainly on the wrists, the backs of hands, and the face. They are flesh colored and flat topped and may itch. Filiform warts appear more often in overweight, middle-aged people. They are long and slender and occur on the eyelids, armpits, or neck. Plantar warts appear as a hard, horny, rough-surfaced area on the sole of the foot. They may occur singly or in a cluster. Genital warts are pink and cauliflower-like (Figure 9-13). They are now the most common cause of STD and a proven factor in cancer of the cervix. The virus can be present without the warts. It is estimated that up to forty percent of the population have genital human papilloma virus.

The incubation period for warts is usually two to three months but may be as short as one or as long as twenty months. Warts wherever they occur are communicable, probably as long as the lesions are present. Young children generally have more common or flat warts, but genital warts are more prevalent in sexually active young adults. Plantar warts occur more often in school-age children and adolescents. Individuals whose immune system is depressed, such as those with HIV, are more susceptible to warts.

Transmission
Warts are usually transmitted by direct contact. Autoinoculation is also possible. Plantar warts may be acquired by walking barefoot on contaminated

herpetic whitlow   her-PET-ik HWIT-lo
antipyretic   an-ti-pi-RET-ik
acyclovir   a-SI-klo-vir
papilloma   pap-i-LO-ma

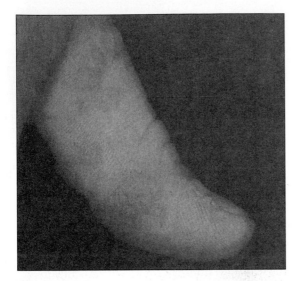

Figure 9-12
Common warts.

floors. Genital warts are usually transmitted by sexual contact.

Symptoms
Warts by themselves cause no pain or discomfort. If they become infected or if they are in a location such as plantar warts, where weight is placed upon them, or under a nail, they can be uncomfortable and painful.

Treatment
When the body builds up enough resistance, warts will disappear spontaneously. However, this can take months or years. If they are in a location that causes problems, such as plantar warts, there are procedures to help get rid of them. These may or may not be effective, and many times the warts return. Because the number of people infected with genital warts has increased dramatically, a variety of new methods of treatment are being investigated. Interferons are among the most promising.

Prevention/Control
To reduce the risk of getting warts, bath sandals should be worn on shower room floors or pool decks. Individuals should avoid direct contact with lesions on self or others. The chance of acquiring genital warts may be reduced by using condoms.

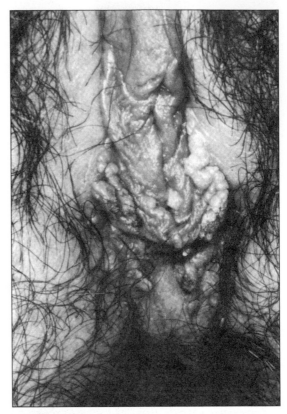

Figure 9-13
Genital warts.

ACQUIRED IMMUNE DEFICIENCY SYNDROME (AIDS, HIV INFECTION)

Rise in Opportunistic Disease

It wasn't a new group of symptoms that warned the CDC in 1981 that a strange, death-dealing virus was invading human bodies; it was an increase in reported cases of two rare diseases. *Pneumocystis carinii,* a type of pneumonia that had previously affected only those with suppressed immune systems, was infecting healthy homosexual men in Los Angeles; later on, cases of **Kaposi's** sarcoma, a rare skin tumor that previously affected only elderly men in the United States, was reported among young homosexual men. Soon it was evident that there was an increasing epidemic of opportunistic diseases, those that affect people with inefficient immune defenses. Opportunistic infections were also increasing in intravenous drug users and hemophiliacs, suggesting that the cause of the epidemic had something to do with transmission of blood as well as homosexual activity.

Identifying the Virus

In 1984, scientists in France and America identified the virus responsible for the new epidemic. The French named it lymphadenopathy-associated virus (LAV), whereas the Americans named it human T cell lymphotropic virus, strain III (HTLV III). In 1986, it was renamed human immunodeficiency virus (HIV).

The virus infects a cell known as a T-helper cell that is crucial in the immune system's defense of the body (see Chapter 2). Figure 9-14 is a highly magnified picture of HIV infecting T-helper cells. Figure 9-15 is a comparison of the reaction of the immune system to an invading organism under normal conditions and when AIDS is present.

Epidemiology

As of June 30, 1999, more than 665,000 cases of AIDS had been reported to the CDC. At least 385,000 of these persons have died. AIDS has infected people of every race, age, sex, and sexual persuasion (Tables 9-1 and 9-2). In less than ten years, it became the second leading cause of death in men twenty-five to forty-four years of age in the United States and rose to five on the list of leading causes of death among women in this age group (Figure 9-16). Figure 9-17 shows the cases reported among various groups by year of diagnosis. AIDS cases have also been reported in every state (Figure 9-18). Estimates suggest that 650,000 to 900,000 Americans are now living with HIV and at least 40,000 more are infected each year. Table 9-2 shows the total number of cases since the epidemic began by age group, exposure category, and sex.

Although AIDS incidence has remained highest among men who have sex with men, AIDS incidence from 1986 to 1996 increased the most among women, blacks, and people infected heterosexually.

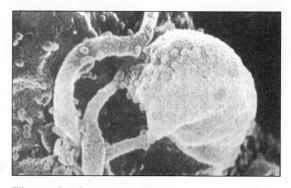

Figure 9-14

Human immunodeficiency virus released from infected T-helper cells (spherical particles) spread over adjacent T-helper cells, infecting them in turn. The individual AIDS particles are very tiny; over 200 million would fit on the period at the end of this sentence.

The incubation period is variable. It takes one to three months for antibodies to build up in the blood, and two to ten years or longer from the time of HIV infection to a diagnosis of AIDS. The period of communicability is uncertain, but is thought to start soon after infection with HIV and to last throughout life.

Global Epidemic

Although America has made some progress in preventing and controlling AIDS, it is imperative to recognize that most countries throughout the world also are dealing with epidemics of AIDS. By the end of 1999, it is estimated that 33.6 million people will be living with HIV (Figure 9-19a). The estimated number of new HIV infections in young people (Figure 9-19b) is a sober reminder that this epidemic could leave a large age gap among peoples of the world, especially in developing countries. In the *AIDS Epidemic Update*, it is stated that "More than ninety-five percent of all HIV-infected people now live in the developing

---

Pneumocystis carinii   NU-mo-SIS-tis ka-RI-ne-i
Kaposi   KAP-o-SE
lymphadenopathy   lim-FAD-e-NOP-a-the
lymphotropic   lim-FOT-ro-pic

Blood Transfusions were not screened
before 1985

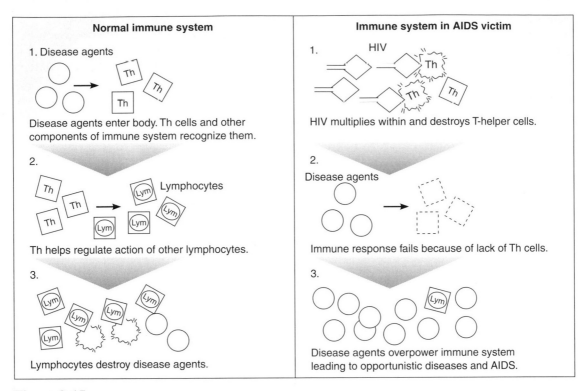

Figure 9-15

HIV and the immune system.

TABLE 9-1	Deaths in Persons with AIDS, by Race/Ethnicity, Age at Death, and Sex, Reported through June 1999, United States		
Race/Ethnicity and Age at Death[1]	**Males Cumulative Total**	**Females Cumulative Total**	**Both Sexes Cumulative Total**
WHITE, NOT HISPANIC			
Under 15	553	409	962
15–24	2,491	461	2,952
25–34	53,347	4,457	57,804
35–44	77,536	4,731	82,267
45–54	35,003	1,826	36,829
55 or older	14,747	1,648	16,395
All ages	183,839	13,555	197,394
BLACK, NOT HISPANIC			
Under 15	1,394	1,386	2,780
15–24	2,367	1,346	3,713
25–34	32,223	11,037	43,260

TABLE 9-1 *Continued*			
BLACK, NOT HISPANIC—CONT'D			
35–44	47,017	13,562	60,579
45–54	20,282	4,612	24,894
55 or older	8,598	2,048	10,646
All ages	111,985	34,025	146,010
HISPANIC			
Under 15	617	561	1,178
15–24	1,304	464	1,768
25–34	19,555	4,304	23,859
35–44	24,833	4,542	29,375
45–54	9,936	1,586	11,522
55 or older	4,076	765	4,841
All ages	60,371	12,233	72,604
ASIAN/PACIFIC ISLANDER			
Under 15	18	15	33
15–24	36	5	41
25–34	687	73	760
35–44	1,070	96	1,166
45–54	519	59	578
55 or older	232	44	276
All ages	2,564	294	2,858
AMERICAN INDIAN/ALASKA NATIVE			
Under 15	11	8	19
15–24	24	3	27
25–34	352	65	417
35–44	358	60	418
45–54	113	23	136
55 or older	39	8	47
All ages	900	167	1,067
ALL RACIAL/ETHNIC GROUPS			
Under 15	2,595	2,380	4,975
15–24	6,227	2,281	8,508
25–34	106,222	19,940	126,162
35–44	150,925	23,001	173,926
45–54	65,897	8,111	74,008
55 or older	27,713	4,516	32,229
All ages	359,902	60,299	420,201

[1]Data tabulated under "all ages" include 393 persons whose age at death is unknown. Data tabulated under "all racial/ethnic groups" include 268 persons whose race/ethnicity is unknown.

Center for Disease Control and Prevention. *HIV/AIDS Surveillance Report,* 1999; 11(No. 1)28.

TABLE 9-2	AIDS Cases by Age Group, Exposure Category, and Sex, Reported through June 1999, United States

	Males				Females				Totals[1]			
	July 1998–June 1999		Cumulative Total		July 1998–June 1999		Cumulative Total		July 1998–June 1999		Cumulative Total[2]	
Adult/Adolescent Exposure Category	No.	(%)	No.	(%)	No.	(%)	No.	(%)	No.	(%)	No.	(%)
Men who have sex with men	15,999	(45)	334,073	(57)	—	—	—	—	15,999	(34)	334,073	(48)
Injecting drug use	7,493	(21)	130,727	(22)	3,043	(28)	48,501	(42)	10,536	(23)	179,228	(25)
Men who have sex with men and inject drugs	1,940	(5)	45,266	(8)	—	—	—	—	1,940	(4)	45,266	(6)
Hemophilia/ coagulation disorder	150	(0)	4,741	(1)	21	(0)	269	(0)	171	(0)	5,010	(1)
Heterosexual contact:	2,754	(8)	24,984	(4)	4,296	(40)	45,597	(40)	7,051	(15)	70,582	(10)
Sex with injecting drug user	*604*		*8,370*		*1,208*		*18,895*		*1,812*		*27,265*	
Sex with bisexual male	*—*		*—*		*200*		*3,263*		*200*		*3,263*	
Sex with person with hemophilia	*7*		*49*		*27*		*396*		*34*		*445*	
Sex with transfusion recipient with HIV infection	*20*		*382*		*18*		*569*		*38*		*951*	
Sex with HIV-infected person, risk not specified	*2,123*		*16,183*		*2,843*		*22,474*		*4,967*		*38,658*	
Receipt of blood transfusion, blood components, or tissue[3]	146	(0)	4,811	(1)	120	(1)	3,619	(3)	266	(1)	8,430	(1)
Other/risk not reported or identified[4]	7,436	(21)	43,522	(7)	3,361	(31)	16,635	(15)	10,798	(23)	60,159	(9)
Adult/adolescent subtotal	35,918	(100)	588,124	(100)	10,841	(100)	114,621	(100)	46,761	(100)	702,748	(100)
Pediatric (<13 years old) Exposure Category												
Hemophilia/ coagulation disorder	1	(1)	226	(5)	—	—	7	(0)	1	(0)	233	(3)
Mother with/at risk for HIV infection:[4]	141	(90)	3,886	(88)	156	(94)	3,942	(95)	297	(92)	7,828	(91)
Injecting drug use	*38*		*1,552*		*37*		*1,532*		*75*		*3,084*	
Sex with an injecting drug user	*27*		*728*		*15*		*691*		*42*		*1,419*	
Sex with a bisexual male	*3*		*85*		*1*		*85*		*4*		*170*	
Sex with person with hemophlia	*—*		*17*		*—*		*12*		*—*		*29*	

TABLE 9-2 *Continued*												
	Males				**Females**				**Totals**[1]			
	July 1998–June 1999		Cumulative Total		July 1998–June 1999		Cumulative Total		July 1998–June 1999		Cumulative Total[2]	
Pediatric (<13 years old) Exposure Category	No.	(%)	No.	(%)	No.	(%)	No.	(%)	No.	(%)	No.	(%)
Sex with transfusion recipient with HIV infection	—		*11*		*1*		*14*		*1*		*25*	
Sex with HIV-infected person, risk not specified	28		*564*		*45*		*603*		*73*		*1,167*	
Receipt of blood transfusion, blood components, or tissue	*1*		*74*		*1*		*81*		*2*		*155*	
Has HIV infection, risk not specified	*44*		*855*		*56*		*924*		*100*		*1,779*	
Receipt of blood transfusion, blood components, or tissue[3]	—	—	236	(5)	—	—	140	(3)	—	—	376	(4)
Risk not reported or identified[4]	14	(9)	80	(2)	10	(6)	79	(2)	24	(7)	159	(2)
Pediatric subtotal	156	(100)	4,428	(100)	166	(100)	4,168	(100)	322	(100)	8,596	(100)
Total	**36,074**		**592,552**		**11,007**		**118,789**		**47,083**		**711,344**	

[1]Includes 3 persons whose sex is unknown.

[2]Includes 12 persons known to be infected with human immunodeficiency virus type 2 (HIV-2). See *MMWR* 1995; 44:603–06.

[3]Thirty-eight adults/adolescents and 2 children developed AIDS after receiving blood screened negative for HIV antibody. Thirteen additional adults developed AIDS after receiving tissue, organs, or artificial insemination from HIV-infected donors. Four of the 13 received tissue or organs from a donor who was negative for HIV antibody at the time of donation. See *N. Engl J Med* 1992; 326:726–32.

[4]See table 17 and figure 6 for a discussion of the "other" exposure category. "Other" also includes 124 persons who acquired HIV infection perinatally but were diagnosed with AIDS after age 13. These 124 persons are tabulated under the adult/adolescent, not pediatric, exposure category.

Centers for Disease Control and Prevention. *HIV/AIDS Surveillance Report,* 1999; 11(No. 1):12.

world which has likewise experienced ninety-five percent of all deaths to date from AIDS."*

The report goes on to estimate that eleven men, women, and children around the world were infected per minute in 1998—close to six million people, and one-tenth of the newly infected people were under fifteen years of age, bringing the number of HIV-infected children to 1.2 million. Table 9-3 is a global summary of a disease that, over fifteen years after it was identified in the United States, is still uncontrolled.

AIDS Epidemic Update 1999 (UNAIDS/WHO, December 1999).

Transmission

For a person to acquire AIDS, semen, vaginal secretions, or blood of an individual infected with HIV must be introduced into the bloodstream. This has occurred through sexual intercourse, sharing HIV-contaminated needles and syringes, and through transfusions of infected blood or its components. The AIDS virus has been detected in saliva, tears, urine, and bronchial secretions, but no cases have been reported that were the result of contact with these secretions. There has also been no evidence that AIDS has ever been transmitted by a mosquito or other biting insect. One of the

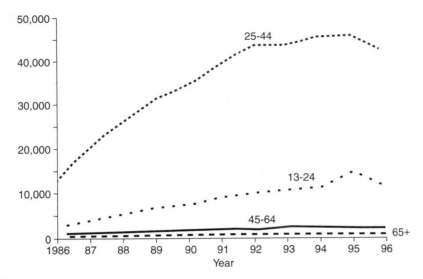

Figure 9-16a

Annual AIDS incidence by age group, United States, 1986–1996.

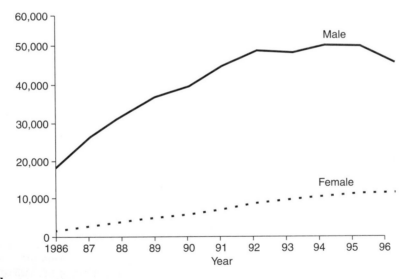

Figure 9-16b

AIDS incidence by gender, United States, 1986–1996.

greatest tragedies of the AIDS epidemic is the number of infants who are infected by HIV-infected mothers before, during, or shortly after birth. In America, guidelines for counseling pregnant women issued by the Public Health Service to health care workers across the country have caused perinatal AIDS incidence to drop dramatically.

Symptoms

A person may be infected with HIV and be asymptomatic (have no symptoms). Most people infected with HIV are asymptomatic. But some develop nonspecific symptoms from six days to six weeks after they are infected. These acute symptoms may include fever, headache, sore throat, muscle aches,

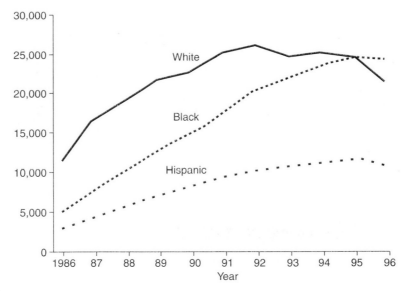

Figure 9-16c

AIDS incidence by race, United States, 1986–1996.

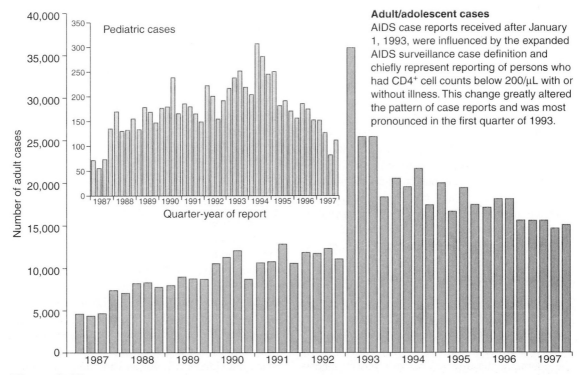

Figure 9-17

AIDS cases by quarter-year of report and age group, reported 1987 through 1997.

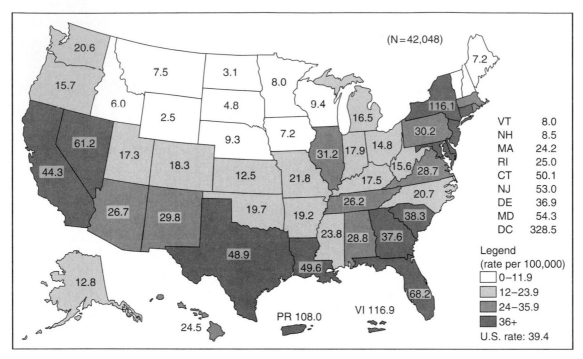

Figure 9-18a

Male adult/adolescent AIDS annual rates per 100,000 population, for cases reported July 1997 through June 1998, in the United States.

enlarged lymph nodes, generalized rash, and, rarely, moodiness, seizures and paralysis. If there are symptoms, they will resolve spontaneously, with no treatment and may be attributed to the "flu." With or without symptoms, the virus stays "quietly" in the body for up to ten years, but the disease advances in the person and can be transmitted to others. Antibodies can usually be detected in one to three months. The asymptomatic period generally ends with swollen lymph nodes and more flulike symptoms. A diagnosis of AIDS is now based on the appearance of certain opportunistic infections and T-cell count.

Treatment

A cure for AIDS has not been found. So far, **zidovudine** (formerly called azidothymidine [AZT]) and other drugs have only slowed down the course of the disease. No cure has ever been

discovered for any viral disease. It is possible to treat the opportunistic diseases, the most likely cause of AIDS fatalities, but there are slim chances for a cure.

Prevention

The only sure means of prevention are: sexual relations with uninfected individuals only, use of only sterilized needles for injections, and use of sterile gloves and equipment by all health care personnel. These seem like viable rules to follow, but unfortunately there are too many factors involved. Persons who use illicit drugs often do not care how they get their shots. People who drink too much will not care who their sex partners are. Even health care personnel are sometimes careless or, particularly in emergency situations, too rushed to take proper precautions. And many individuals will not take the time to find out

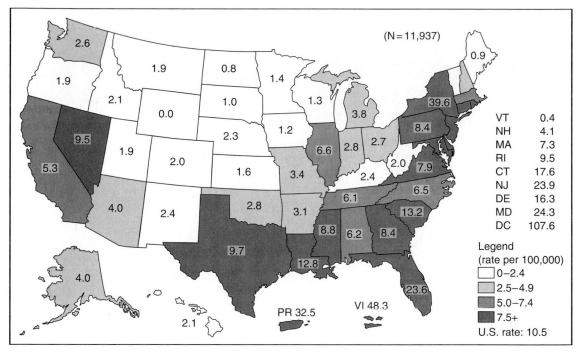

VT	0.4
NH	4.1
MA	7.3
RI	9.5
CT	17.6
NJ	23.9
DE	16.3
MD	24.3
DC	107.6

Legend
(rate per 100,000)
☐ 0–2.4
▢ 2.5–4.9
▨ 5.0–7.4
▮ 7.5+
U.S. rate: 10.5

Figure 9-18b

Female adult/adolescent AIDS annual rates per 100,000 population, for cases reported July 1997 through June 1998, in the United States.

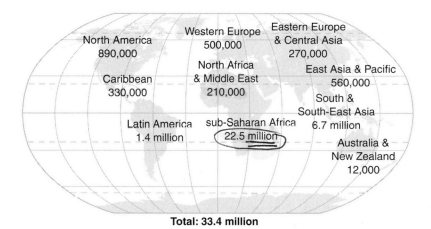

Total: 33.4 million

Figure 9-19a

Adults and children estimated to be living with HIV/AIDS as of end 1998.

zidovudine	zid-O-vu-DINE

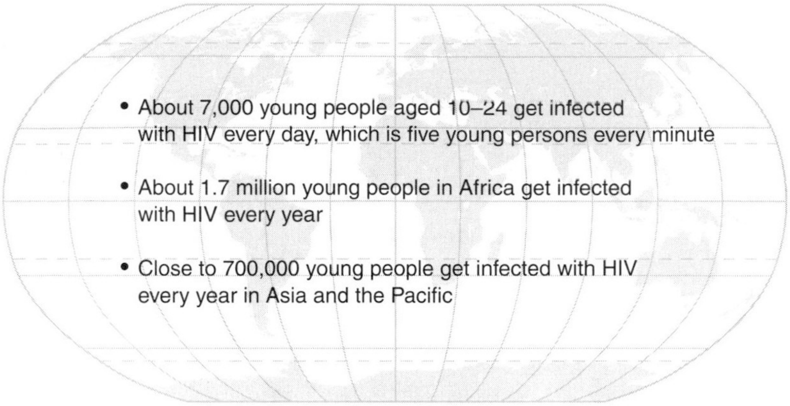

- About 7,000 young people aged 10–24 get infected with HIV every day, which is five young persons every minute

- About 1.7 million young people in Africa get infected with HIV every year

- Close to 700,000 young people get infected with HIV every year in Asia and the Pacific

Figure 9-19b

Estimated number of new HIV infections in young people.

TABLE 9-3	Global Summary of the HIV/AIDS Epidemic, December 1999		
People Newly Infected with HIV in 1999	**Total**		**5.6 million**
	Adults		5 million
	Women		*2.3 million*
	Children <15 years		570,000
Number of People Living with HIV/AIDS	**Total**		**33.6 million**
	Adults		32.4 million
	Women		*14.8 million*
	Children <15 years		1.2 million
Aids Deaths in 1999	**Total**		**2.6 million**
	Adults		2.1 million
	Women		*1.1 million*
	Children <15 years		470,000
Total Number of AIDS Deaths since the Beginning of the Epidemic	**Total**		**16.3 million**
	Adults		12.7 million
	Women		*6.2 million*
	Children <15 years		3.6 million

the sexual history of their sex partners. The use of condoms will decrease the risk of infection and is probably the best means of prevention at present.

Control

Because prevention of AIDS transmission is not a realistic expectation at present, the best hope for stopping the epidemic is a vaccine. At first it was thought that no vaccine was possible, but now researchers are more hopeful. The FDA has approved the first large-scale test of a vaccine to prevent HIV infection. Trials of the vaccine, named "AIDSVAX," will be conducted with 5000 volunteers at high risk for AIDS in the United States, Canada, and Thailand. Some in the scientific community are skeptical of its ability to protect people from anything but a few subtypes of HIV. This is to

be a three-year study, but as in any double-blind study, the ethical question of how long to keep giving the placebo to the control group if the vaccine is known to offer some protection to those in the experimental group before the three-year period is up may have to be answered. In the meantime, people need to realize that the only way this disease can be controlled is for everyone who is sexually active to have the facts. Sexual relations with someone who is not known well enough to rule out any possibility of having the virus (including a negative blood test if necessary) is an open invitation to infection with HIV. Communication between partners and with public health personnel to help with contact investigation, and developing monogamous long-term relationships will also help control this devastating disease.

SUMMARY

Table 9-4 summarizes relevant data on viral diseases acquired through the alimentary and other routes.

TABLE 9-4	**Viral Diseases Acquired through the Alimentary and Other Routes**			
Disease	**Special Characteristics**	**Transmission**	**Common Symptoms**	**Prevention/ Control**
Poliomyelitis	Once a dreaded disease, now rare because of vaccine. Post-polio syndrome sometimes occurs	Direct contact with respiratory secretions or oral-fecal route in areas of poor sanitation	90% asymptomatic; 5% typical prodromal symptoms; 1%–2% prodromal plus back pain and muscle spasms; 0.1%–2% have paralysis	Immunization in early childhood; contact investigation for possible treatment
Hepatitis A	Rare in U.S. but reported cases have begun to rise. Also called infectious hepatitis	Oral-fecal	Sudden onset of fever, malaise, anorexia, nausea, abdominal discomfort; jaundice	Good sanitation and personal hygiene; IgM prophylaxis for at-risk individuals

Continued

TABLE 9-4	Continued			
Disease	**Special Characteristics**	**Transmission**	**Common Symptoms**	**Prevention/ Control**
Hepatitis B	Also called serum hepatitis. Has a higher mortal- ity rate than A	Blood to blood or blood to mucous mem- brane contact	Insidious onset of anorexia, abdominal dis- comfort, nau- sea, and vomiting	Vaccination for those at high risk; proper disposal and sterilization of all needles and syringes
Hepatitis C	Formerly called non-A, non-B, 3.9 million Americans are infected	Bloodborne; mother to unborn child; through breast feeding	Fatigue, abdomi- nal pain, anorexia, nau- sea, vomiting, jaundice	Same as HBV
Rabies	Animal disease communicated to humans by a bite. Almost always fatal without treatment	Introduction of saliva of infected animal into bloodstream; no case of per- son-to-person transmission	Local or radiating pain or burning, sensation of cold, itching, and tingling at bite site; typical prodromal symptoms plus persistent loose cough; nervous- ness, anxiety, irritability, hyperesthesia, pupillary dila- tion, tachycar- dia, shallow respiration, excessive saliva, tears, perspiration; 2–10 days later, other CNS dis- orders, intense thirst, and hydrophobia	Registration, licensing, and vaccination of all dogs and cats; wild and stray animal control; vacci- nations for high-risk individuals
Encephalitis	Inflammation of the brain, can be sequela of other viral ill- ness. Occurs more in sum- mer and early fall	Bite of an infected mosquito	Sudden onset of fever, headache, and vomiting; pro- gresses to stiff neck and back, drowsiness, coma,	Mosquito control and elimination of breeding places; avoid- ance of mosquitoes during times

TABLE 9-4	*Continued*			
Disease	**Special Characteristics**	**Transmission**	**Common Symptoms**	**Prevention/ Control**
Encephalitis— Cont'd			paralysis, convulsions, muscular incoordination, psychoses	when they are known to bite; use of repellants
Herpes simplex Type I	Generally infects the lips and face. Once the virus enters the body it is there for life. Can be reactivated in 60% of those infected. Occurs mostly in children	By contact with saliva of infected individuals	May be asymptomatic or may have typical prodromal symptoms; vesicular lesions	Avoid close contact with infected individuals; isolate persons with lesions from newborns, children, and immuno-suppressed individuals
Herpes Simplex Type II	Usually located in the genital area or on the cervix in women. Occurs mostly in adults	By sexual contact	Lesions in first attack typically painful and vesicular; possible fever, swollen glands, painful urination	Cesarean section to protect newborn; condoms in sexual practices reduce risk
Warts	Various kinds include: common; flat; filiform; plantar; genital. Usually disappear without treatment in time. Most common cause of STDs	Direct contact or autoinoculation	None unless infected or in weight-bearing area	Avoid direct contact with lesions; use condoms to reduce risk of genital warts
Acquired immune deficiency syndrome (AIDS)	First reported in 1981 among male homosexuals in U.S. Now found in all kinds of people, male and female, young and old,	Introduction of blood, semen, or vaginal secretions of infected person into bloodstream; usually by sexual intercourse,	Typical prodromal symptoms; opportunistic diseases	Sexual relations with uninfected individuals only, use of sterilized needles only, use of sterile gloves and

Table 9-4	***Continued***			
Disease	**Special Characteristics**	**Transmission**	**Common Symptoms**	**Prevention/ Control**
Acquired immune deficiency syndrome (AIDS)— Cont'd	heterosexual and homosexual. It is a global epidemic. No recovered cases have been documented. Over 665,000 cases reported, over 385,000 of these have died	anal sex, unclean needles, or from mother to fetus		equipment by health care personnel at all times; use of condoms to decrease risk of infection; education of the public

There is no specific treatment for most viral diseases. At present, immunization is the main defense against them. Drugs including interferon and antibiotics have been developed that relieve symptoms or extend lives but there are no cures.

Questions for Review

1. What was the "iron lung"?
2. Among what people do outbreaks of polio still occur?
3. What are the four possible outcomes of poliomyelitis?
4. What five viruses are known to cause hepatitis?
5. Compare the means and results of infection with viral hepatitis A and viral hepatitis B.
6. Why is infection with hepatitis A a particular concern in day-care centers?
7. What determines the time from the bite of a rabid animal to symptoms in the victim?
8. Why is it necessary to determine whether an animal that has bitten someone without provocation is rabid?
9. What are the initial symptoms of rabies?
10. What is the treatment for a bite from an animal with rabies?
11. What is the cause of viral encephalitis?
12. What symptoms are specific for encephalitis?

13. What is the difference between infections caused by herpes simplex virus Type I and those caused by herpes simplex virus Type II?
14. For how long after the sores have healed can the herpes simplex virus Type I still be found in saliva?
15. Who is susceptible to herpetic whitlow?
16. How does acyclovir help a herpes infection?
17. What five kinds of wart were discussed in the text?
18. How are warts transmitted?
19. When might warts cause symptoms?
20. What opportunistic infections are most often connected with AIDS?
21. What is the difference between LAV, HTLV III, and HIV?
22. How does AIDS cause damage to the immune system?
23. How is AIDS transmitted?
24. What are the symptoms of AIDS?
25. How may AIDS be prevented or controlled?

FURTHER READING

Ahmed Aijaz, and Emmet B. Keeffe. 2000. Cost effective evaluation of acute viral hepatitis. *Western Journal of Medicine* 172:29.

All sites up and running on AIDS vaccine trials *AIDS Alert* 14:68, 1999.

Anderson, Rune, et al. 1999. Successful treatment of generalized primary herpes simplex type 2 infection during pregnancy. *Scandinavian Journal of Infectious Diseases* 31:201–2.

Apgar, Barbara. 1998. Treatment of recurrent genital herpes infections. *American Family Physician* 58:236.

Baer, George M. 1998. Defining the rabies problem *Public Health Reports* 113:245.

Bloom, Barry R. 1998. The highest attainable standard: Ethical issues in AIDS vaccine. *Science* 279:186.

Bradbury, Jane, and Michael McCarthy. 1998. Perinatal HIV transmission discussed in Geneva. *The Lancet* 351:39.

Cacciola, Irene, et al. 1999. Occult hepatitis B virus infection in patients with chronic hepatitis C liver disease. *New England Journal of Medicine* 341:22.

Centers for Disease Control and Prevention. [www.cdc.gov/nchstp/hiv_aids/pubs/rrfr]. "Draft guidelines for national HIV case surveillance, including monitoring for HIV infection and acquired immunodeficiency syndrome (AIDS)."

Centers for Disease Control and Prevention. [www.cdc.gov/ncidod/diseases/hepatitis/slidesct/httoc.htm]. "Epidemiology and prevention of viral hepatitis A to E: An overview."

Centers for Disease Control and Prevention, hepatitis branch. [www.cdc.gov/ncdod/diseases/hepatitis]. "Hepatitis can affect anyone."

Centers for Disease Control and Prevention. "Information on *Aedes albopictus*." [www.cdc.gov/ncidod/arbor/albopic-new.htm].

Centers for Disease Control and Prevention. "Manual for the surveillance of vaccine-preventable diseases." [www.cdc.gov/nip/manual/vpd].

Centers for Disease Control and Prevention. "Neato mosquito: An elementary curriculum guide." [www.cdc.gov/ncidod/dvbid/arbor].

Chintu, C., and Alwyn Mwinga. 1999. An African perspective on the threat of tuberculosis and HIV/AIDS can despair be turned to hope? *The Lancet* 353:997.

Cohen, Jon. 1999. The scientific challenge of hepatitis C. *Science* 285:5424.

Cohen, Jon. 1997. Exploiting the HIV-chemokine nexus. *Science* 275:1261.

Dandoy, Suzanne, and Frank Scanlon. 1999. Teaching kids about rabies. *American Journal of Public Health* 89:413.

Diaz-Mitoma, Francisco, R. Gary Sibbald, Stephen D. Shafran, et al. 1998. Oral famciclovir for the suppression of recurrent genital herpes. *Journal of the American Medical Association* 280:887.

Exotic diseases close to home. *The Lancet* 354:1221, 1999.

Friedrich, M. J. 1999. Third millennium challenge: hepatitis C. *Journal of the American Medical Association* 282:221.

Gacouin, A., et al. 1999. Human rabies despite postexposure vaccination. *European Journal of Clinical Microbiology and Infectious Diseases* 18:233.

Gillchrist, James A. 1999. Hepatitis viruses A, B, C, D, E, and G: implications for dental personnel. *Journal of the American Dental Association* 103:509.

Gorgoulis, V. G. 1999. Human papilloma virus is possibly involved in laryngeal but not in lung carcinogenesis. *Human Pathology* 30:274–83.

Haupt, W. 1999. Rabies—risk of exposure and current trends in prevention of human cases. *Vaccine* 17:1742.

"Herpes simplex virus-2 infection: An emerging Disease?" *Infectious Disease Clinics of North America,* March '98, 12(1):47.

An HIV vaccine: How long must we wait? *The Lancet* 1323, 1998.

Hoff, Rodney, and James McNamara. 1999. Therapeutic vaccines for preventing AIDS: their use with HAART. *The Lancet* 353:1723.

Hwang, Mi Young, Richard M. Glass, and Jeff Molter. 1998. Genital herpes. *Journal of the American Medical Association* 280:944.

International multicenter pooled analysis of postnatal mother to-child transmission of HIV-1 infection. *The Lancet* 352:597, 1998.

Kirchner, Jeffrey T. 1998. Risk of maternal-infant transmission of hepatitis C. *American Family Physician,* 57:1420.

Koff, Raymond S. 1999. Advances in the treatment of chronic viral hepatitis. *Journal of the American Medical Association* 282:511.

Koff, Raymond S. 1999. Advances in the treatment of chronic viral hepatitis. *Journal of the American Medical Association* 282:8907.

Kumar, Sanjay. 1999. When the threat to public health is in the shape of a dog. *The Lancet* 353:2219.

Lindberg, Claire E. 1999. Sexual behavior and condom use among urban women attending a family planning clinic in the United States. *Health Care of Women International* 20:303.

Logie, Alex W. 1999. African AIDS conference offers hope for the future. *The Lancet* 354:1104, 1999.

Luzuriaga, Katherine, and John L. Sullivan. 1998. Prevention and treatment of pediatric HIV infection. *Journal of the American Medical Association* 280:17.

Makulowich, Gail S. 1999. HIV and STD prevention update: perception of risk varies dramatically. *AIDS Patient Care and STDs* 13:445.

Manocha, A. P. 1999. Prevalence and predictors of severe acute pancreatitis in patients with acquired immune deficiency syndrome. *American Journal of Gastroenterology* 94:784–9.

Marton, Betty. 1998. Haunted by polio: Decades later, many survivors relive devastating symptoms. *AHA News* 34:7.

Marx, James F. 1998. Understanding the varieties of viral hepatitis. *Nursing* 28:43.

Making sense of hepatitis C. *The Lancet* 352:1485, 1998.

Mayo Clinic. "Genital warts. What you should know." [www.mayohealth.org/mayo].

Minuk, G. Y. 1999. The influence of host factors on the natural history of chronic hepatitis C

viral infections. *Journal of Viral Hepatitis* 6:271–6.

New drug therapies shown to delay development of AIDS. *Science News Update.* [www.wmw-assn.org/sci-pubs/sci-news/1998].

Page, W. John. 1999. Risk for rabies transmission from encounters with bats, Colorado 1977–1996. *Emerging Infectious Diseases* 5:433.

Pianko, Stephen, and John McHutchison. 1999. Chronic hepatitis B: new therapies on the horizon? *The Lancet* 354:1662.

Progress toward global eradication of poliomyelitis, 1997. *Morbidity and Mortality Weekly Report* 47:414, 1998.

Progress toward poliomyelitis eradication—Europe and central Asian republics, 1997–May 1998. *Morbidity and Mortality Weekly Report* 47:504, 1998.

Recommendations for prevention and control of hepatitis C virus (HCV) infection and HCV-related chronic disease. *Morbidity and Mortality Weekly Report* 47:1, 1998.

Robinson, D., et al. 1999. Human rabies—Virgina, 1998. *Journal of American Medical Association* 281:891.

Rose, Verna L. 1999. CDC issues new recommendations for the prevention and control of hepatitis C virus infection. *American Family Physician* 59:1321.

Rose, Verna L. 1999. CDC issues revised guidelines for the prevention of human rabies. *American Family Physician* 59:2007.

Rose, Verna L. 1999. New home test for hepatitis C virus. *American Family Physician* 60:320.

Sadovsky, Richard. Hepatitis C virus infection: Diagnosis and treatment. *American Family Physician* 58:962, 1998.

Sidley, Pat. 1999. Doctors demand AIDS drug for women who have been raped. *British Medical Journal* 318:1507.

Smith, Scott R., and Duane M. Kirking. 1999. Access and use of medications in HIV disease. *Health Services Research* 34:123.

Stephenson, Joan. 1998. AIDS vaccine moves into stage 3 trials. *Journal of the American Medical Association* 280:7.

Update: West Nile-like viral encephalitis—New York. *Journal of the American Medical Association* 282:1714, 1999.

White, P. J., and G. P. Garnett. 1999. Use of antiviral treatment and prophylaxis is unlikely to have a major impact on the prevalence of herpes simplex virus type 2. *Sexual Transmitted Infectious Diseases* 75:49–54.

Women and HIV: closing the treatment gap. *Patient Care* 33:187, 1999.

Wyatt, Jeffrey D., et al. 1999. Human rabies postexposure prophylaxis during a raccoon rabies epizootic in New York, 1993 and 1994. *Emerging Infectious Diseases* 5:415.

Zoulim, F., and C. Trepo. 1999. New antiviral agents for the therapy of chronic hepatitis B virus infection. *Intervirology* 42:125–44.

10

DISEASES CAUSED BY FUNGI

OBJECTIVES

1. *Compare coccidioidomycosis and histoplasmosis.*

2. *Identify factors that predispose an individual to candidiasis.*

3. *State the location for the various forms of tinea.*

4. *Explain why fungal diseases have become more common.*

5. *State symptoms, treatment, prevention, and control for the diseases in this chapter.*

INTRODUCTION

Fungal infections have become a serious problem for the immuno-compromised individual. In less than a decade, some fungi that were once rare and "inconvenient" have become stronger and, in the case of high-risk individuals, life-threatening. As can be seen by the list of conditions and therapies listed in Box 10-1, the technologic advances that have lengthened and saved lives are now a target for opportunistic fungi that can shorten and take lives.

The first group of fungal diseases in this chapter, including coccidioidomycosis, histoplasmosis, candidiasis, and dermatophytoses have been and are common in the United States although some are limited to certain geographic areas. These are treated in more detail than the five listed in Table 10-1 that represent fungi that are still comparatively weak in the general population but a great risk to those with the conditions and/or therapies appearing in Box 10-1.

Conditions and Therapies Predisposing to Invasive Fungal Infections*

CONDITIONS

Granulocytopenia (low white blood cell count)
Advanced HIV infection
Bone marrow and solid organ transplant
Very low birth weight
Diabetes mellitus
Fibrotic and cavitary lung disease
Severe burns or trauma
Intravenous drug use

THERAPIES

Intravenous hyperalimentation (intravenous feeding)
Broad-spectrum antibiotics
Indwelling catheters and devices
Prosthetic devices
Corticosteroid treatment
Hemodialysis and peritoneal dialysis
Intravascular implants (cardiac valves, shunts)

*Dixon, Dennis M., Michael M. McNeil, Mitchell L. Cohen, et al. "Fungal infections: a growing threat," *Public Health Reports* 111:3.

TABLE 10-1   Opportunistic Fungi

	Characteristics	Transmission	Symptoms
Aspergillus (Aspergillosis)	Can infest many parts of the body: bronchi, lungs, ear canal, skin, eye, nose, urethra, lungs, kidney, and other organs. Found in fermenting compost piles, damp hay	Inhalation of airborne spores	Dependent on location; if in lung, may be none or mimic tuberculosis
Pneumocystis carinii (pneumonia) PCP	Most humans infected early in life. Thought until recently to be a protozoan, but DNA more like fungi	Uncertain, may be airborne; reservoir unknown	Shortness of breath, nonproductive cough; may be followed by anorexia and weight loss
Cryptococcus (Crypto-coccosis)	Common in the environment. Occurs more in AIDS patients and those over 60. Lungs are primary site but may disseminate and cause infection of the meninges, kidneys, prostate, and bones	Inhalation of airborne spores	Primary infection may be asymptomatic; usually identified by central nervous system symptoms
Blastomyces (Blastomycosis)	Endemic to Mississippi River valley. Primarily infects lungs and skin. Pulmonary infection may be acute or chronic	Inhalation of airborne spores	Low-grade fever, cough, dyspnea, hemoptisis, pleuritic chest pain, weight loss, and fatigue
Sporothrix (Sporotrichosis)	Usually infects the skin. Can be cutaneous, pulmonary, or disseminated. Occupational disease for farmers, gardeners, and horticulturists. Found in soil, wood, moss, and decaying vegetation	Contact with contaminated plant life; bales of hay implicated in some outbreaks; pulmonary assumed to be inhaled	Skin—subcutaneous nodules; pulmonary—productive cough; disseminated—many lesions that spread from skin or lungs; weight loss, anorexia, other lesions, arthritis, or osteomyelitis

COCCIDIOIDOMYCOSIS (VALLEY FEVER)

The incidence of **coccidioidomycosis** has increased sharply since the early 90s. In Kern County, California, the case number has grown from 250 a year to 8200 cases that occurred between September 1991 and January 1995. In Arizona, the number of cases increased 144 percent during 1990 to 1995. Weather and increasing population are thought to be the reason for the resurgence of this fungus. The disease is found mainly in the southwestern United States and Central and South America (Figure 10-1). It is found in two forms, primary coccidioidomycosis, which is an acute respiratory disease, and progressive coccidioidomycosis, a progressive, chronic, frequently fatal disease. The progressive form occurs more frequently in dark-skinned men, pregnant women, and individuals whose immune systems are suppressed. The reser-

voir for the fungus, ***Coccidioides immitis,*** is in the soil. In the United States it is found from California to southern Texas. Incubation is one to four weeks for primary infection and variable for progressive coccidioidomycosis. The disease is not communicable. Susceptibility is general, but one attack confers lifelong immunity.

Transmission

Transmission is generally by inhalation of the spores found in the soil in endemic areas. Dry weather coupled with sparse foliage and high winds provides the ideal conditions for the spores to be airborne.

Symptoms

The primary illness may be asymptomatic or resemble a flulike illness with cough, fever, sore throat, chills, malaise, headache, and in some cases an itchy rash. About five percent of infected individuals develop tender red nodules on their

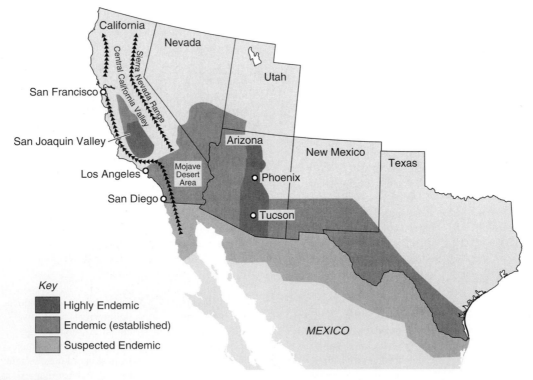

Figure 10-1

Geographic distribution of coccidioidomycosis.

D.I.C. = Body's clotting fails
Bleeding Out

legs, especially the shins, with joint pain in the knees and ankles. The primary disease generally heals spontaneously within a few weeks. In rare cases (1 in 1000) the disease disseminates throughout the body, causing fever and abscesses. Disseminated coccidioidomycosis is frequently fatal (up to sixty percent of cases).

Treatment

The primary form usually requires only bed rest and relief of symptoms. Various antifungal agents are effective in treating more severe primary cases and the disseminated form.

Prevention/Control

Dust control measures should be used in endemic areas. Individuals from nonendemic areas need to be careful about selecting occupations in which they will be exposed to dust. Skin testing can be done to determine exposure. Individuals who have to work in risky locations should wear dust masks.

HISTOPLASMOSIS (SPELUNKER'S DISEASE)

Raising chickens would not seem to be a very dangerous occupation, but in certain parts of the United States, chickens can provide the source of an infection that in its most severe form can be fatal. The organism that causes this fungal infection, **Histoplasma capsulatum,** is found in the feces of bats and birds. It grows in soil with a high nitrogen content and has been endemic in the Midwest for many years but is now spreading to other parts of the country (Figure 10-2). An estimated 500,000 cases occur in the United States

coccidioidomycosis   kok-SID-i-oyd-o-mi-KO-sis
Coccidioides immitis   kok-SID-I-oyd-IS imi-TY-tis
Histoplasma capsulatum   HIS-to-PLAZ-ma kap-siu-LA-tum

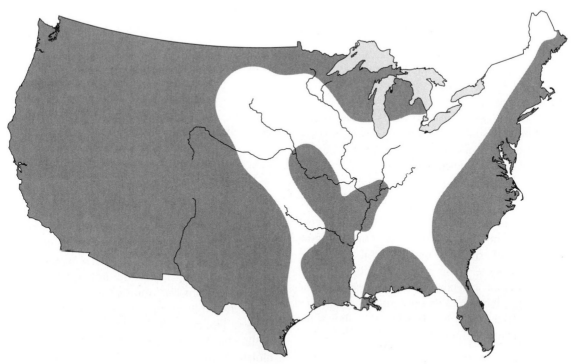

Figure 10-2

Endemic areas (white) of histoplasmosis in North America.

CASE STUDY

Histoplasmosis

On June 27, 1995, a crew of five workers began partial demolition of an abandoned city hall building in a community in Kentucky. At the time of demolition, a colony of bats had been observed in the vicinity of the building, and an approximately two-foot-deep pile of debris covered with bat guano had accumulated in the building. During the demolition, none of the workers wore personal protective equipment (PPE) (i.e., respirators, eye protection, gloves, or protective clothing). Within three weeks, all five workers required treatment for acute respiratory illnesses, and three had been hospitalized. Tests suggested the presence of *H. capsulatum* (histoplasmosis).

From the demolition crew, local physicians, medical records, personnel from local hospitals and clinics, and community members, Kentucky Department of Human Services investigators gathered information about per-sons who possibly had been exposed to *H. capsulatum* during the demolition. A total of fifty-five persons (including the demolition crew) were identified who had worked in or near the building or lived in the area during the demolition. Each was questioned about a history of symptoms (including fever greater than or equal to 101°F, chills, night sweats, cough, headache, fatigue, and myalgia) during July 1 to August 3.

Overall, nineteen of the fifty-five persons tested positive. Of these, twelve persons had participated in the demolition: five had worked as the crew, one truck driver had hauled the debris to the dump site, four workers from the city workshop had helped the truck driver haul and dump the debris, and two had washed the building. Three persons had visited the building during the demolition, and four others had lived or worked within 500 yards of the building.

From *Morbidity and Mortality Weekly Report* 44(38):701–703, 1995.

each year. Areas of infection are also found in South and Central America, Africa, Europe, eastern Asia, and Australia. When the soil of chicken houses or bat caves is stirred up by raking, windy conditions, or some other means, the spores rise into the air and may be inhaled by anyone in the area. The incubation period is five to eighteen days. Susceptibility is general, and inapparent infections are common, leading to increased resistance.

Transmission

There is no person-to-person transmission. Inhalation of spores from the soil that have become airborne is the main means of transmission. A person can also become infected if the spores are rubbed into an open sore, but this type of transmission is rare. Figure 10-3 shows the common sources of infection with histoplasmosis.

Symptoms

The primary lesion for histoplasmosis is in the lungs. Most often, the individual is asympto-matic. There are four cases in which symptoms appear: (1) primary acute, with flulike symptoms such as fever, malaise, headache, myalgia, anorexia, cough, and chest pain; there may also be small scattered nodules in the lung, lymph nodes, and spleen; (2) acute disseminated, with enlarged liver and spleen, swollen lymph nodes, fever, and prostration; can be fatal without treatment; (3) chronic disseminated, with variable symptoms, which may include fever, anemia, hepatitis, endocarditis, meningitis, ulcers of mouth, larynx, stomach, or bowel, and infection of the adrenal glands; this, too, is usually fatal unless treated; (4) chronic pulmonary, which mimics tuberculosis and causes a productive cough, difficult breathing, and sometimes bloody sputum. Eventually there is weight loss, extreme weakness, breathlessness, and cyanosis (dark bluish or purplish skin). Periods of remission may occur, and often there is spontaneous cure of this type.

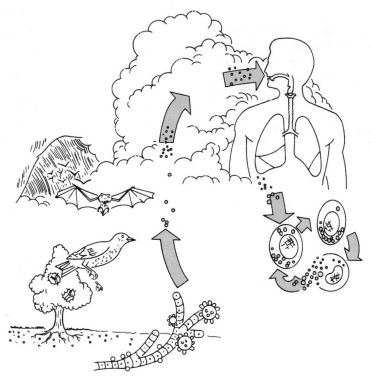

Figure 10-3
Possible sources of histoplasmosis.

Treatment

Primary acute histoplasmosis requires no treatment. For the other two kinds, antifungal therapy is effective, either amphotericin B or Ketoconazol, depending on the condition of the patient. This is generally a long-term treatment of about ten weeks.

Prevention

Protective masks should be used when working in areas that may be contaminated, such as chicken coops and their surrounding soil, bat-infested caves, and starling nesting places. Dusty, contaminated areas should be sprayed with water or oil to reduce dust.

Control

In case of an outbreak, there should be investigation of contacts to determine whether there is an environmental source of infection that can be eliminated.

[handwritten: Thrush = white in babies mouth or vaginal area]
[handwritten: Diaper Rash]
[handwritten: Fungus - enhabited in body]

CANDIDIASIS (MONILIASIS, THRUSH)

Candidiasis is an opportunistic yeastlike fungal infection of the skin or mucous membranes. It is generally caused by ***Candida albicans.*** It often occurs in babies (diaper rash), in the mouth (thrush), or in the vulvovaginal area (**moniliasis**). The infection occurs worldwide, and the fungus is a natural inhabitant of the human body. The incubation period for candidiasis is variable. Thrush, in infants, has an incubation period of two to five days. Candidiasis is communicable as long as the lesions are present.

candidiasis	KAN-di-DI-a-sis
Candida albicans	KAN-di-da AL-bi-kans
moniliasis	MO-ni-LI-a-sis

If you are on medicine antibiotics = kill bad bacteria & good bacteria = can get yeast inf.

Transmission

Candidiasis can be transmitted by secretions or excretions of infected individuals or carriers. A baby can get thrush while passing through the birth canal of a mother with the infection; candidiasis can be transmitted through sexual intercourse, and endogenous infections occur whenever resistance is lowered. *old / young / aids*

Symptoms

Symptoms for candidiasis depend upon the site of the infection. When on the skin, there is a scaly, red, papular rash, often appearing in creases of skin, such as under the breasts or in the vaginal area. In diaper rash, there are papules at the edges of the rash.

Candidiasis in the mouth is called "thrush" and causes cream-colored or bluish white patches on the tongue, mouth, or pharynx. There may be only a burning sensation in the mouths and throats of adults, but in infants they can swell and cause difficulty in breathing.

When candidiasis occurs in the vagina, there is a white or yellow "cheesy" discharge that is extremely itchy. There are white or gray raised patches on the vaginal wall, and intercourse may be painful. Different symptoms occur when the infection is in the kidneys, lungs, brain, endocardium, esophagus, nails, or eye, all of which are susceptible to infection by the fungus. The infection may also be systemic and cause chills, high fever, low blood pressure, prostration, and sometimes a rash.

Treatment

The first aim of treatment is to control the underlying condition that allowed this opportunistic infection to occur. There are many antifungal drugs that are effective in treating candidiasis, and some, particularly those effective for vaginal infection, are now sold over the counter.

Prevention/Control

Treatment of vaginal candidiasis in pregnant women can prevent thrush in the newborn. Partner treatment is necessary, because the infection can be transmitted through sexual intercourse. The effectiveness of the immune system can be improved by maintaining a healthful lifestyle.

DERMATOPHYTOSES (TINEA) *= worm*

These common fungal infections may occur anywhere on the skin and under and around the nails. They are caused by dermatophytes (fungi). The word *tinea,* followed by the Latin term for the part of the body infected, is often used. The terms are *tinea capitis* (head), *tinea barbae* (beard), *tinea corporis* (body), *tinea cruris* (inguinal), *tinea pedis* (foot), *tinea manuum* (hand), and *tinea unguium* (nail).

Tinea barbae or Tinea capitis *ringworm*

Tinea barbae infects the beard area of men and is often accompanied by bacterial folliculitis and inflammation secondary to ingrown hairs. *Tinea capitis* is sometimes called "ringworm of the scalp" and primarily affects school-aged children. It is more common in large cities and overcrowded conditions. The reservoir for most of the organisms is people, although some have animal hosts. Incubation is ten to fourteen days, and the fungi are communicable through contaminated materials as long as the lesions are present.

Transmission

The infection is transmitted by direct or indirect contact. The backs of theater seats, barber clippers, toilet articles, combs, hairbrushes, or clothing and hats that have been contaminated with hair or beard of an infected person are common fomites. Animals also can transmit the infection and sometimes are carriers.

Symptoms

Tinea capitis and *tinea barbae* begin as small papules and spread across the head or bearded areas. Figure 10-4 shows a patch of scaly baldness left on the back of a boy's head by the fungal infection. The hairs that are in the area of infection become brittle and break off easily. One variety of *tinea capitis* is characterized by a mousy odor. In this kind, there are small, yellowish, cuplike crusts that appear stuck on the scalp. The hair does not break off but becomes gray and lusterless and eventually falls out. The baldness caused by this infection may be permanent.

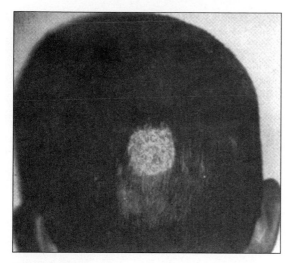

Figure 10-4
Tinea capitis.

Treatment

There are several antifungal drugs that are taken by mouth for at least four weeks. There are also over-the-counter remedies that may be effective if the infection is mild. If there is a secondary bacterial infection, antibiotics may be used.

Prevention

The public needs to be educated to the danger of acquiring the infections from infected children and animals. If there is an epidemic, for most fungal species involved, ultraviolet light (Wood's lamp) can detect lesions on the head; this can be used before children enter school. Children with unkempt hair should be examined for lesions.

Control

If the cases are mild, daily washing of the hair will remove loose hairs. In severe cases, hair should be washed daily and covered with a cap. Household contacts, pets, and farm animals should be examined and treated if infected.

Tinea corporis and Tinea cruris

These fungal infections occur worldwide, and males are more often infected than females. *Tinea cruris* infects the skin in the pubic area and almost always occurs in males. It is commonly called "jock itch." The reservoir for the organisms that cause *tinea corporis* is in humans, animals, and soil. For *tinea cruris,* it is usually in men. The incubation period is four to ten days, and the infection is communicable as long as lesions are present or as long as infective fungus is on contaminated materials. Friction and excessive perspiration in the armpits or inguinal area will predispose to fungal infection.

Transmission

Fungal infections are transmitted by direct or indirect contact with skin of an infected person or lesions of infected animals. Floors, shower stalls, benches, and similar locations can also be a source of infection.

Symptoms

This fungus disease of the body begins with red, slightly elevated scaly patches that contain minute vesicles or papules. The lesions are ring-shaped, and new patches arise on the periphery while the central area clears up, leading to the "ringworm" appearance (Figure 10-5). The periphery may be dry and scaly or moist and crusted. Often there is considerable itching.

Treatment

The individual must bathe thoroughly and frequently with soap and water. Scabs and crusts are removed, and a fungicide ointment applied. An oral fungicide is also effective.

Prevention

Towels and clothing used for workouts should be laundered with hot water and/or a fungicidal agent; showers and gymnasiums should be kept antiseptic with frequent washing of benches and floors with a fungicidal agent. Showers and dressing rooms should be hosed, with allowance for rapid draining, at regular intervals.

---

tinea   TE-ne-a
tinea capitis   Te-ne-a KAP-i-tis
tinea barbae   TE-ne-a BA-be
tinea corporis   TE-ne-a KOR-po-ris
cruris tinea   KROO-ris TE-ne-a
tinea manuum   TE-ne-a MAN-u-um
tinea pedis   TE-ne-a PE-dis
tinea unguium   TE-ne-a un-gwim

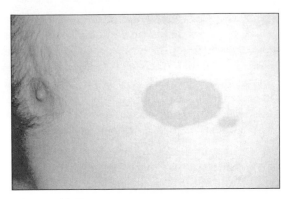

Figure 10-5
Tinea corporis.

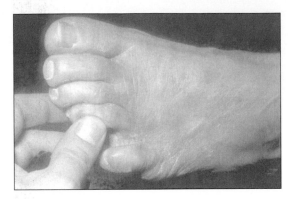

Figure 10-6
Tinea pedis.

Control

Individuals who are being treated for a tinea infection should be excluded from swimming pools and activities likely to lead to exposure of others. Clothing of infected individuals should be laundered frequently with a fungicidal agent. School and household contacts and pets should be examined for identification and treatment of a possible source.

Tinea pedis

This fungus infection of the foot, especially between the toes, is commonly called "athlete's foot." It is the most common of all the fungal skin diseases. The fungus infects adults more often than children, males more than females. The infections occur more often and are more severe in hot weather. Warm, moist conditions (such as exist between sweaty toes) predispose to the infection. The reservoir of infection is people. The incubation period is unknown, but the infection is communicable as long as lesions are present or infective spores are on contaminated materials. Some people seem more susceptible than others, and inapparent infections occur. Those who are susceptible may have repeated attacks.

Transmission

Means of transmission are the same as for tinea corporis.

Symptoms

There is scaling or cracking between the toes and watery blisters (Figure 10-6). In severe cases, lesions may appear on other parts of the body, particularly the hands, but this is an allergic reaction to the fungus products and not infective. Itching can be severe, and cracking can become extremely painful.

Treatment

Fungicide in salve or powder form should be applied after every bath or shower. Feet should be kept dry and exposed to the air as much as possible.

Prevention Wear Shower Shoes

Prevention is the same as for tinea corporis, except that special attention to drying between toes after bathing and regular use of a fungicidal powder will reduce chances of infection.

Public and private pools used to have a foot bath for swimmers to walk through as they went from the dressing rooms to the pool. It is now known that unless someone changes these foot baths every ten to fifteen minutes, the solution no longer is effective and will eventually support the growth of tinea, thus spreading the infection.

Open (from the top) dressing facilities that can be kept comparatively dry by the sun and scrubbed nightly with disinfectant (fungicide) are best. A fungicide should be applied to the pool decks and dressing rooms and office area at night to reduce the risk of spreading tinea pedis. These measures should also be applied to locker and shower rooms in schools and sports facilities.

Control

In some cases, tinea pedis is very difficult to eradicate. If this is the case, socks and shoes of infected individuals need to be boiled if possible or replaced if not. Inspection of individuals before entering locker rooms or shower facilities should be done regularly, and those who have lesions on their feet should be restricted from usage of public areas.

Tinea manuum

Fungal infection of the hands is less common than tinea pedis. There is some itchiness and lesions that eventually scale off. When the hands are infected, often the feet are also. Prevention, control, and treatment of tinea pedis will normally lead to elimination of tinea manuum. (Treatment is the same.)

Tinea unguium

Tinea can also infect the fingernails or toenails. It more commonly affects the toenails. It may infect one or more nails and is a fairly common occur-

rence. The reservoir of infection is people, sometimes animals or soil. The incubation period is unknown; infection is communicable as long as the lesion is present. If a nail is injured, it is more susceptible to infection, and reinfection often occurs.

Transmission

There is a low rate of transmission, and it is thought to spread mainly by direct contact with infected skin or nails.

Symptoms

The infected nail gradually thickens and becomes discolored, and cheesy-looking material collects under the nail. In some cases, the nail becomes chalky and disintegrates.

Treatment

The treatment of choice is griseofulvin by mouth. It is given until the nails grow out. There are other topical applications that can be purchased over the counter, but they are not generally effective.

Prevention

Preventive measures are the same as for tinea pedis.

Control

There are no specific control measures, because the infection is not often transmitted, even to family members.

SUMMARY

Table 10-2 summarizes significant data concerning diseases caused by fungi.

TABLE 10-2 Diseases Caused by Fungi

Disease	Special Characteristics	Transmission	Common Symptoms	Prevention/ Control
Coccidioido-mycosis	Occurs mainly in southwestern United States. Common name is valley fever.	Inhalation of spores from soil; most favorable conditions—	May be asymptomatic or may have flulike symptoms and an itchy rash.	Dust control measures; masks when working in high-risk areas; tests for *Continued*

	Special		**Common**	**Prevention/**
Disease	**Characteristics**	**Transmission**	**Symptoms**	**Control**
Coccidioido-mycosis—Cont'd	May be acute or chronic. Sharp increase in incidence. Fungus spores found in soil from California to southern Texas	summer dust and windstorms	Rarely disseminates but if so, may be fatal. May have lesions in lung similar to TB. May also be systemic abscesses	susceptibility; strong immunity after recovery
Histoplasmosis	Endemic in midwest and East, spreading to other parts of country. Bats and birds carry disease agent in feces. Spore form of fungus found in soil around bat-infested caves, chicken houses, etc. Estimated 500,000 cases a year	Inhalation of spores from soil; no person-to-person transmission	Primary lesion is in lungs. May be asymptomatic or may be flulike illness, acute disseminated, chronic disseminated, or chronic pulmonary. Last three may be fatal if untreated but spontaneous remissions occur also	Protective masks in high risk areas; dusty contaminated areas sprayed with water or oil; in outbreak, contact investigation for environmental source
Candidiasis	Opportunistic yeastlike fungus is natural inhabitant of human body. Different locations show different forms, i.e., thrush, moniliasis, diaper rash. Resistance lowered by chemotherapy, antibiotics, AIDS, diabetes, and other diseases	Endogenous infection or contact with excretions or secretions of infected individuals	Depend on site of infection, i.e., scaly, red, papular rash in creases of skin. Cream-colored or bluish white patches in mouth or pharynx can cause breathing difficulty. Cheesy discharge from vaginal area, extreme pruritis. Systemic infection causes chills, high	Treat pregnant women with infection, treat sexual partners, improve immune system

TABLE 10-2 *Continued*

TABLE 10-2	*Continued*			
Disease	**Special Characteristics**	**Transmission**	**Common Symptoms**	**Prevention/ Control**
Candidiasis— Cont'd			fever, LBP, prostration, rash. Cause of diaper rash	
Dermatophytoses Tinea capitis	Occurs mainly in children (ringworm of the scalp)	Direct or indirect contact with hair or articles used by infected person or sometimes animals	Begins as a small papule and spreads across head or bearded areas. Hairs become brittle and break easily	Education of parents and children; daily washing of hair and wearing of cap in severe cases; examination and treatment of contacts and pets
Tinea corporis and tinea cruris	Ringworm of the body and pubic area (jock itch). More common in men. Friction and excessive perspiration are factors	Same as above	Red, slightly elevated scaly patches that contain tiny vesicles or papules. Periphery may be dry and scaly or moist and crusted. Causes considerable itching	Launder towels and clothing used for workouts in hot water; antiseptic measures used in gymnasiums, showers, dressing rooms; exclude infected persons from swimming pools and other activities at high risk for exposing others; examine school and household contacts and pets for possible source
Tinea pedis	"Athletes foot," most common fungal infection. Fungus thrives in warm, moist	Same as tinea corporis	Symptoms include scaling or cracking between toes, watery blisters. Severe itching	Feet kept dry, fungicidal salve or powder application after bath or shower;

TABLE 10-2	*Continued*			
Disease	**Special Characteristics**	**Transmission**	**Common Symptoms**	**Prevention/ Control**
Tinea pedis— Cont'd	conditions, especially interdigital areas		and pain possible	contaminated socks and shoes disinfected
Tinea unguium	Infection of toe-nails and sometimes fin-gernails	Direct contact with infected skin or nails	Nail thickens, becomes dis-colored, cheesy-looking material collects under nails	Same as tinea corporis

QUESTIONS FOR REVIEW

1. In what part(s) of the country is coccidioidomycosis found?
2. How is coccidioidomycosis transmitted?
3. When is coccidioidomycosis fatal?
4. In what part of the country is histoplasmosis found?
5. What are the common sources of infection for histoplasmosis?
6. In what five ways may infection with histoplasmosis affect the individual?
7. How can coccidioidomycosis and histoplasmosis be avoided?
8. What are the common sites for infection with candida?
9. What symptoms occur at each site of candidiasis?
10. What factors predispose an individual to candidiasis?
11. Why is treatment of pregnant women with candidiasis important?
12. What are the most common sites of tinea infections?
13. What treatments are effective for tinea infections?
14. How are the symptoms for the various kinds of tinea infection alike and how do they differ?
15. How can each kind of tinea discussed in the chapter be prevented and controlled?

FURTHER READING

Busick, Natisha P., Peter C. Fretz, Jeffrey R. Galvin, et al. "Histoplasmosis." Virtual Hospital: Lung cancer and related topics. [http://vh.radiology.uiowa.edu].

Chenoweth, C. E. 1999. In consultation. Diagnosing massive candidiasis with blood cultures. *Journal of Critical Illness* 14:183–4.

Clancy, R., et al., 1999. Recurrent vulvovaginal candidiasis—allergy or immune deficiency? *International Archives of Allergy and Immunology* 118:349.

Cummins, Rebecca E., and Rowena C. Romero. 1998. Disseminated North American blastomycosis in an adolescent male: A delay in diagnosis. *Pediatrics* 102:977.

Dennerstein, G. 1998. Pathogenesis and treatment of genital candidiasis. *Australian Family Physician* 27:363.

Disseminated candidiasis. *Consultant* 1999. 39:3177.

Elewski, B. E., et al. 1999. Treatment of *tinea pedis* when bacterial presence is suspected: a review of the literature. *Journal of New Developments in Clinical Medicine* 17:159.

Faul, J. L. 1999. Constrictive pericarditis due to coccidioidomycosis. *Annual Thoracic Surgery* 68:4.

Fichtenbaum, Carl J., and Judith A. Aberg. Candidiasis. The AIDS Knowledge Base. [http://hivinsite.ucsf.edu].

Fidels, P. L., Jr. 1999. Host defense against oropharyngeal and vaginal candidiasis: site-specific differences. *Revista Iberoamericana De Micologia* 16:8.

Flaitz, M., and M. J. Hicks. 1999. Oral candidiasis in children with immune suppression: clinical appearance and therapeutic considerations. *ASDC Journal of Dentistry for Children* 66:161–6.

Fluconazole: most cost effective vaginal candidiasis treatment, modeling study finds. *Formulary* 34:278, 1999.

Forrest, L. A., and H. Weed. 1998. Candida laryngitis appearing as leukoplakia and GERD. *Journal of Voice* 12:91.

Galgiani, John N. 1999. Coccidioidomycosis: a regional disease of national importance. *Annual of Internal Medicine* 130:293.

Glaser, Dee Anna, and Anne T. Riordan. 1998. Tinea barbae: Man and beast. *The New England Journal of Medicine* 338:735.

Goldman, M. 1999. Fungal pneumonias: the endemic mycoses. *Emerging Infectious Diseases* 5:672.

Guttman, Cheryl. 1999. Clinicians taking fresh approach to management of fungal infections. *Dermatology Times* 20:43.

Guttman, Cheryl. "Valley fever epidemic leads to description of a new manifestation." *Dermatology Times,* Apr. '98, Supplement 2, 19(4):16–7.

Hay, J. R. 1999. The management of superficial candidiasis. *Journal of the American Academy of Dermatology* 40:2.

Hubbard, Thomas W. 1999. The predictive value of symptoms in diagnosing childhood *tinea capitis. Archives of Pediatric & Adolescent Medicine* 153:51.

Jenkin, G. A., M. Choo, P. Hosking, et al. 1998. Candidal epididymoorchitis. *Clinical Infectious Diseases* 26:942.

Jensen, J. L., and P. Barkvoll. 1998. Clinical implications of the dry mouth. Oral mucosal diseases. *Annual New York Academy of Science* 842:156.

Jones, Timothy F., and Gary L. Swinger. 1999. Acute pulmonary histoplasmosis in bridge workers: a persistent problem. *American Journal of Medicine* 106:480.

Kirchner, Jeffrey T. 1999. Treatment options for *tinea capitis. Family Physician* 60:2387.

Koehler, A. P., A. F. Cheng, K. C. Chu, et al. 1998. Successful treatment of disseminated coccidioidomycosis with amphotericin B lipid complex. *Journal of Infection* 36:113.

Lawrence, M. A. 1999. Coccidiomycosis prostatistis associated with prostate cancer. *AADE ED Journal* 84:3.

Linsangan, L. C. 1999. Coccidioides immitis infection of the neonate: two routes of infection. *Pediatric Infectious Disease Journal* 18:2.

Lipman, Jeffrey, and Roger Saadia. "Fungal infections in critically ill patients: rates are rising but diagnosis and treatment remain difficult." *British Medical Journal,* Aug. 2, '97, 315(7103):266–7.

Liu, J. W., et al. 1999. Acute disseminated histoplasmosis complicated with hypercalcaemia. *Journal of Infection* 39:88.

Lortholary, O., et al. 1999. Review. endemic mycoses: a treatment update. *Journal of Antimicrobial Chemotherapy* 43:321–331.

Masur, Henry, Jonathan Kaplan, Holmes, et al. 1998. 1997 USPHS/IDSA report on the prevention of opportunistic infections in persons infected with human immunodeficiency virus. *Pediatrics* 102:1063.

Medical mycology research center. The University of Texas Medical Branch at Galveston, Texas, USA. [http://fungus.utmb.edu/f-atlas/cocci.htm].

Meszaros, Liz. 1999. Current therapies fight mycotic infections in adolescents. *Dermatology Times* 20:50.

Meszaros, Liz. 1999. Triple therapy approach aids children with *tinea capitis. Dermatology Times* 20:30.

Mikamo, H., K. Kawazoe, Y. Sato, et al. 1998. Comparative study on the effectiveness of antifungal agents in different regimens against vaginal candidiasis. *Chemotherapy* 44:364.

Minamoto, G. Y., and A. S. Rosenberg. Fungal infections in patients with acquired immunodeficiency syndrome. *Medical Clinic of North America,* Mar. '97, 81(2): 381–409.

Moraes, P. S. 1998. Recurrent vaginal candidiasis and allergic rhinitis: A common association. *Annual Allergy and Asthma Immunology* 81:165.

Moser, S. A. 1999. Laboratory diagnosis of histoplasmosis. *Clinical Microbiology Newsletter* 21:95.

Noble, Sara L., Robert C. Forbes, and Pamela L. Stamm. 1998. Diagnosis and management of common tinea infections. *American Family Physician* 58:163.

Nogueira, S. A., M. J. Caiuby, V. Vasconcelos, et al. 1998. Paracoccidioidomycosis and tuberculosis in AIDS patients. *International Journal of Infectious Diseases* 2:168.

O'Dell, Michael L. 1998. Skin and wound infections: An overview. *American Family Physician* 57:2424.

Oldfield the 3rd, E. C.; W. D. Bone; C. R. Martin; et al. "Prediction of relapse after treatment of coccidioidomycosis." *Clin Infect Dis (A47),* Nov. '97, 25(5):1205–10.

Olivere, J. W. 1999. Coccidioidomycosis—the airborne assault continues: an unusual presentation with a review of the history, epidemiology, and military relevance. *Aviation, Space and Environmental Medicine* 70:790–6.

"*Pneumocystis carinii* infection." Clinical care options for HIV Care Series. [www.healthcg.com/hiv/hsv].

Pomeranz, Albert, J. Svapna, and S. Sabnis. 1999. Asymptomatic dermatophyte carriers in the households of children with tinea capitis. *Archives of Pediatric & Adolescent Medicine* 153:483.

Rodgers, C., and F. Young. 1999. Look out for the symptoms of Candidiasis. *Practice Nurse* 17:536, 538, 540.

Rodgers, C. A., and A. J. Beardall. 1999. Recurrent vulvovaginal candidiasis: why does it occur? *International Journal of STD & AIDS* 10:435.

Sarkar, Soumitra, Michael P. Dube, Brenda E. Jones, et al. Pneumocystis carinii pneumonia masquerading as tuberculosis. *Archives of Internal Medicine*, Feb. 10. '97, 157(3):351–6.

Schneider, Eileen, Rana A. Hajjeh, Richard A. Spiegel, et al. A coccidioidomycosis outbreak following the Northbridge, Calif, earthquake. *Jama: The Journal of the American Medical Association*, Mar. 19, '97, 277(11):904–5.

Shahi, S. K., et al. 1999. Broad-spectrum antimycotic drug for the control of fungal infection in human begins. *Current Science* 76:836.

Silachamroom, U., and S. Shuangshoti. 1998. Massive pulmonary cryptococcosis in an immunocompetent patient. *Southeast Asian Journal of Tropical, Medical, and Public Health* 29:105.

Spinelli, Nancy A., and Amy Goldstein. 1999. Pruritic rash on the left palm. *Patient Care* 33:246.

Thompson, Craig, and Robert McEachern. 1998. Blastomycosis as an etiology of acute lung injury. *Southern Medical Journal* 91:861.

Vaz, A., M. Pineda-Roman, A. R. Thomas, et al. 1998. Coccidioidomycosis: An update. *Hospital Practices* 33:105.

Vincent, J. L., E. Anaissie, H. Bruining, et al. 1998. Epidemiology, diagnosis and treatment of systematic candida infection in surgical patients under intensive care. *Intensive Care Medicine* 24:206.

Walling, Anne D. 1999. A cost-effective strategy for diagnosing vaginal candidiasis. *American Family Physician* 59:1308.

Wheat, J. Histoplasmosis. Experience during outbreaks in Indianapolis and review of the literature. *Medicine (Baltimore) (MNY),* Sept. '97, 76(5):339–54.

Diseases Caused by Protozoa and Metazoa

Objectives

1. *State means of avoiding giardiasis and amebiasis.*

2. *Describe precautions that should be taken to prevent toxoplasmosis.*

3. *Explain why malaria is still a problem in the world.*

4. *Describe the sequence that produces the periodic chills and other symptoms in malaria.*

5. *Distinguish among pinworm, roundworm, hookworm, and tapeworm.*

6. *Discuss the source of trichinosis.*

7. *Distinguish among the three kinds of parasitic lice that cause pediculosis.*

8. *Identify symptoms, treatment, prevention, and control for the diseases discussed in this chapter.*

Introduction

In addition to the protozoan and metazoan infestations to be covered in this chapter, others have received increased attention in the past few years. Four of these are identified briefly in Table 11-1.

Many parasites can be present in the body without any outward signs or symptoms, or such mild symptoms they aren't identified. What may be a nuisance or minor illness for the average person can become deadly for the immunocompromised. For a number of reasons (see Box 10-1), the numbers of people with little resistance to pathogenic agents in our society are increasing rapidly.

Most parasitic infections are more of a problem in other countries than they are in the United States, but with increasing immigration, more immunocompromised individuals, and more global travel, predictions of a "coming plague" should not be taken lightly.

CASE STUDY

Cryptosporidiosis

On July 10, 1997, the Minnesota Department of Health (MDH) was notified by a parent about four cases of gastroenteritis among a group of ten children whose only common exposure was a birthday party at the Minnesota zoo on June 29. The zoo provided MDH with a list of registered groups that had visited the zoo during June 28–30; group members were contacted and interviewed about illness and zoo exposures. All of the children diagnosed with gastroenteritis had played in a water sprinkler fountain in the zoo, compared with 7 (6%) of 109 controls. Cryptosporidium oocysts were identified in nine of ten stool specimens of case-patients tested at MDH.

The fountain was closed on July 11, and MDH issued a public statement advising persons who had visited the zoo and subsequently developed diarrheal illness to contact their physician and MDH. The public statement also stated that children who developed diarrhea after exposure to the fountain should not visit swimming beaches, swimming and wading pools, and other recreational water facilities until at least two weeks after recovery from diarrheal symptoms.

A standard questionnaire was used to document illness history and zoo exposures in persons responding to the public statement.

The source of contamination of the fountain was not established, but contamination by a child wearing a diaper and playing in the fountain was suspected. Animals (including ruminants) in a petting zoo approximately fifty yards from the fountain tested negative for *Cryptosporidium* before being placed in the petting zoo area and again during the outbreak investigation.

From *Morbidity and Mortality Weekly Report* 47:856, 1998.

TABLE 11-1	Emerging Protozoan and Metazoan Diseases		
	Characteristics	**Transmission**	**Symptoms**
Cryptosporidiosis	Among the most common causes of diarrhea in patients with AIDS and other impairments of the immune system; 1993 Milwaukee outbreak involved 400,000; 2.2% of AIDS cases reported to CDC are infected	Fecal-oral, person-to-person, waterborne, and foodborne	Asymptomatic or profuse and watery diarrhea; children may vomit before diarrhea
Schistosomiasis (snail fever)	Second most prevalent tropical disease after malaria; over 200 million infected worldwide, 400,000 now live in U.S.; severe form leads to 200,000 deaths a year	Immature organism lives in fresh water, penetrates the skin of waders, bathers, and swimmers	First, itchy rash, then fever, malaise, diarrhea, cough, and enlarged liver and spleen
Strongyloidiasis (threadworm)	Infection of the duodenum and jejunum; found in	Infective larvae found in feces, penetrate the skin,	Varied as they pass through the body, then include

TABLE 11-1	*Continued*		
	Characteristics	**Transmission**	**Symptoms**
Strongyloidiasis (threadworm)— Cont'd	tropical and temperate areas including southeastern U.S.; estimated 400,000 cases in southeastern U.S. and Puerto Rico	enter circulation and are carried to the lungs, penetrate capillary walls, enter alveoli, ascend the trachea to the epiglottis, descend into digestive tract and reach the upper part of the small intestine where development of the female is completed	abdominal pain, diarrhea, rash, nausea, weight loss, vomiting, and constipation
Trichuriasis (whipworm)	Worldwide, 350 million infected; only lives in humans; most common in the tropics	Person-to-person through exposure to human feces or dirt containing eggs; enters digestive tract through mouth	May be asymptomatic if light infection; heavy infections cause abdominal pain, diarrhea, internal bleeding, bowel obstruction, loss of muscle tone

GIARDIASIS

Giardiasis is an infection of the small intestine caused by a protozoan, *Giardia lamblia*. The disease occurs worldwide but is most common in developing countries and other areas where sanitation and hygiene are poor. In the United States, it is found more often in children. The rapid increase of day-care centers has put more children at risk. Giardiasis is more common in people who have returned from countries where it is endemic and in campers who drink water from contaminated streams without purifying it. The incubation period is three to twenty-five days or longer. The disease is communicable as long as the person has the infection. Many people are asymptomatic carriers.

Transmission

Giardiasis is acquired by ingesting the cysts in fecally contaminated water or by the fecal-oral transfer of cysts, person-to-person or less often, by contaminated food. Figure 11-1 shows how giardiasis is spread. Many victims are asymptomatic and transmission is more likely to be by those without symptoms. Individuals who are symptomatic are restricted in socialization and activities, to a greater or lesser extent, depending on the severity of the symptoms. Chlorine used in water treatment does not destroy the cysts.

Symptoms

When there are symptoms from giardiasis, they are gastrointestinal. They include abdominal cramps, pale, loose, greasy stools, and nausea. With chronic giardiasis, there may be fatigue and weight loss.

Treatment

The drug of choice for giardiasis is **metronidazole.** There are other drugs that can be used alternatively, and **furazolidone** is used in suspension for very young children. Severe diarrhea may necessitate fluid replacement.

---

giardiasis   JI-ar-DI-a-sis
metronidazole   ME-tro-ni-da-ZOL
furazolidone   fure-AZ-ola-DON

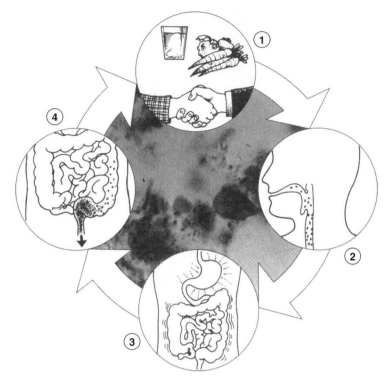

Figure 11-1
Cycle of giardiasis.

Prevention

The best means of prevention is education of the public in personal hygiene and the need for hand washing before eating and after toilet use. Protection of public water supplies from contamination with human or animal feces and sanitary disposal of feces are also mandatory. Campers need to boil or filter any water not connected to a city purification system.

Control

If there is an outbreak, contacts should be examined for signs of infection, and there should be a search for environmental sources that can be eliminated.

AMEBIASIS (AMEBIC DYSENTERY)

This acute or chronic disease is caused by a tiny parasitic protozoan named ***Entamoeba histolytica.*** The infection may or may not be symptomatic. **Amebiasis** occurs worldwide but is found more often in areas where sanitation is poor. Incidence

in the United States averages from one percent to three percent but is higher in mental institutions and among homosexual males who have many sexual partners. The incubation period is commonly two to four weeks, and the disease is communicable as long as an infected individual is passing cysts. Most persons who harbor the organism do not develop disease.

Transmission

Transmission occurs principally through ingesting feces-contaminated food and water. It may also occur sexually through oral-anal contact. The cycle by which amebiasis is spread is shown in Figure 11-2.

Symptoms

Symptoms of the acute form of amebic dysentery include sudden high fever, chills, abdominal cramping, profuse, bloody diarrhea with **tenesmus,** and abdominal pain. Chronic amebic dysentery lasts one to four years, with periods of bloody, mucoid diarrhea, mild fever, and abdominal

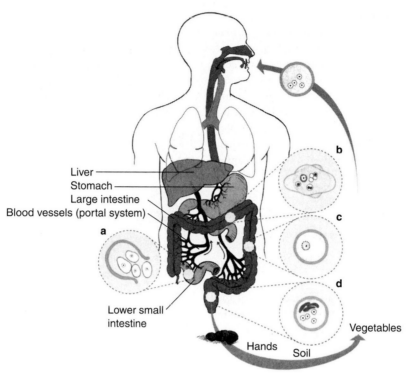

Figure 11-2
Cycle of amebiasis.

cramps. Complications may lead to more serious illness including abscess of the liver.

Treatment
A number of different drugs are used in treatment, depending upon the severity and nature of the disease.

Prevention
As with any disease that is passed through feces, the emphasis in prevention is on education of the public in sanitary disposal of feces and thorough hand washing after defecation. Fruits and vegetables need to be cleaned and cooked correctly, and water that may be contaminated needs to be boiled if other purification methods are not available. High-risk individuals need to be warned of the dangers of oral-fecal transmission.

Control
Infected individuals should be excluded from food handling and working with patients in health care institutions. Contacts should be investigated for infection and a search conducted for a possible source.

TOXOPLASMOSIS

One of the most common infectious diseases, **toxoplasmosis,** usually produces no ill effects except when transmitted by a woman to her unborn child or in people with immunodeficiency. The protozoan *Toxoplasma gondii* causes the infection. The most common method for people to get it is through eating undercooked lamb or pork. About

entamoeba histolytica   EN-ta-ME-ba his-TO-lit-ika
amebiasis   AM-e-BI-a-sis
tenesmus   te-NEZ-mus
toxoplasmosis   toks-o-plas-MO-sis
Toxoplasma gondii   TOKS-o-PLAS-ma GOND-i

twenty-five percent of the pork and ten percent of the lamb eaten by humans contains the *Toxoplasma* organisms. These organisms also multiply in the intestines of cats, and about one percent of cats excrete cysts containing *Toxoplasma* eggs in their feces. The infection occurs worldwide in mammals and birds. Cats acquire the infection from eating infected birds and mammals (particularly rodents) and are the main host, although other animals act as intermediate hosts. Incubation is five to twenty-three days depending on the source.

Transmission

Toxoplasmosis is transmitted from the host to humans in the cysts, which can live outside the host. As has been stated, the most common means of infection is through eating undercooked meat. It can also be transmitted by contaminated water supplies. Because the cysts are in the feces of the host, cat litter boxes and unprotected sandboxes may also contain them. Children who play in these areas may become infected. One of the most serious forms of infection occurs when a pregnant woman has a primary infection and it is transmitted through the placenta to the unborn child. Figure 11-3 shows the different means by which toxoplasmosis may be transmitted.

Symptoms

If toxoplasmosis is acquired in the first trimester of pregnancy, it often results in stillbirth. Infants who survive have congenital toxoplasmosis. Many problems may arise because of this infection, such as hydrocephalus and **hepatosplenomegaly.** Some defects do not become evident for months or years. The symptoms for the acute form of toxoplasmosis are similar to those for mononucleosis. Immunodeficient patients may have a generalized infection with encephalitis, fever, headache, vomiting, delirium, convulsions, and a rash. Complications of the generalized infection include myocarditis, pneumonitis, and hepatitis.

Treatment

Treatment is not necessary unless the infection is during early pregnancy or there are complications. Immunocompromised individuals including AIDS

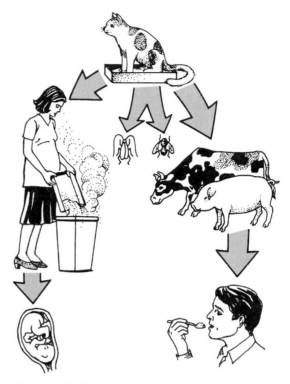

Figure 11-3
Transmission of toxoplasmosis.

patients need to have prophylactic treatment throughout life. Several drugs are effective and used for these cases.

Prevention

All meats should be cooked thoroughly. If cats are kept inside and fed only commercially prepared cat food, then they should not become infected. Litter boxes should be cleaned frequently and children not allowed near them. Pregnant women should not be involved with cleaning litter boxes or have contact with strange cats. Sandboxes should be protected from stray cats. The public and, especially, pregnant women should be educated as to the dangers and means of acquiring toxoplasmosis.

Control

If infection with toxoplasmosis occurs, contacts should be examined and the source of the infection identified.

MALARIA

Malaria is the single most important disease hazard for Americans traveling to foreign countries. Malaria is no longer endemic in most Western countries but is brought into the United States by travelers who have been in Asia, Africa, or Latin America, where it is most prevalent. Figure 11-4 shows reported cases and some of the reasons for the variation in number of cases from 1967 to 1997 in the United States. Malaria is a disease caused by four species of plasmodium, *Plasmodium vivax, Plasmodium malariae, Plasmodium **falciparum,*** and *Plasmodium **ovale.*** The incubation period varies from twelve days to ten months or longer, depending on the infecting strain. Untreated or insufficiently treated patients may be a source of mosquito infection for one to more than three years. There is a fatality rate of ten percent for untreated cases. Individuals with certain genetic traits seem to have some natural immunity, and adults in endemic areas have built up tolerance to the infection. Otherwise, susceptibility is universal. The WHO has been trying to eliminate malaria in developing nations, but little progress has been made in the last twenty years because the mosquitoes have developed resistance to insecticides, and the plasmodia have developed resistance to drugs.

Transmission

Malaria is most often transmitted by the bite of an infected female ***Anopheles*** mosquito. It can also be transmitted by injection or transfusion of the blood of infected persons or by contaminated needles. Congenital infection is rare. When an infected mosquito bites, it injects the plasmodia into the bloodstream of the victim. The infective microorganisms move through the circulation to the liver, where they

hepatosplenomegaly	HEP-a-to-SPLE-no-MEG-a le
falciparum	FAL-si-PA-room
ovale	OV-a-l
Anopheles	a-NOF-e-lez

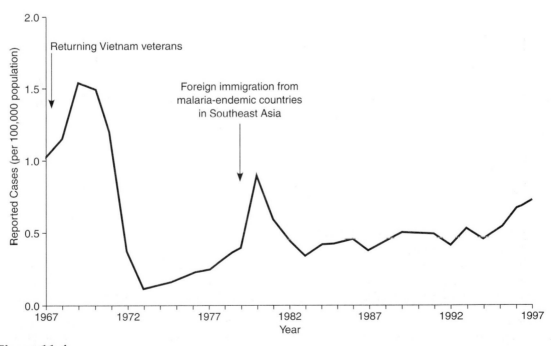

Figure 11-4
Malaria, by year, United States, 1967–1997.

form cystlike cells. When the cysts rupture, they invade erythrocytes (red blood cells) and feed on the hemoglobin (iron-containing pigment). Eventually, the erythrocytes rupture, releasing the contents into the bloodstream to infect other erythrocytes. At this point, the person becomes a reservoir for malaria and infects any mosquito that feeds on him or her. When the infected mosquito bites a person, the cycle continues as shown in Figure 11-5.

Symptoms

The classic symptoms of malaria are chills, fever, myalgia, and headache, interspersed with periods of well-being. Acute attacks occur when the erythrocytes rupture, releasing their contents into the bloodstream. These attacks have three stages: (1) cold stage—chills and shaking that last one to two hours; (2) hot stage—high fever up to 107°F, which lasts three to four hours; (3) wet stage—profuse sweating that lasts two to four hours. Other more serious symptoms may occur and vary with the form of the disease. The cycles of wellness and malarial attacks may continue for as long as fifty years.

Treatment

For all but *P. falciparum,* treatment with **chloroquine** is effective, and the victim usually recovers in three to four days. Quinine and other drugs, used together, are effective against *P. falciparum,* which has become resistant to chloroquine, but ten days of treatment are necessary.

Prevention

Because a mosquito is the means by which malaria is transmitted, one of the most important preventive measures is elimination of any breeding places. In endemic areas, screens need to be used in living and sleeping areas, and bed nets impregnated with an insecticide can also reduce the risk of acquiring the disease. Insecticides are also helpful when applied to the skin of people who may be exposed to the *Anopheles* mosquito. Blood donors

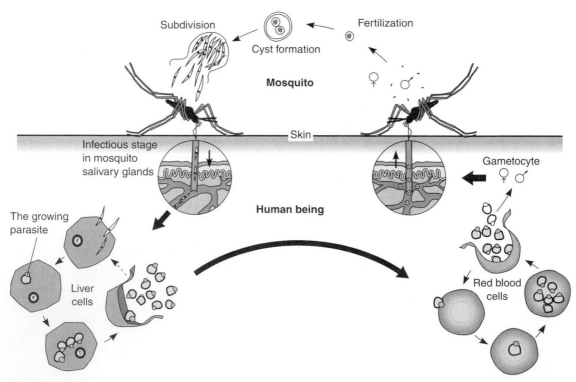

Figure 11-5
Cycle of malaria.

need to be questioned about possible infection with malaria. Finally, drugs should be used prophylactically for those traveling to an endemic area.

Control

If someone is diagnosed with malaria, an investigation should be made to determine the source. If it is a case of needle sharing, all participants must be treated.

ENTEROBIASIS (PINWORM INFECTION)

Enterobiasis is the most prevalent infection with worms in the United States. Children are the main victims, with as many as one-fifth of all children in the United States infected at one time. The infection occurs worldwide and among all socioeconomic classes. Humans are the reservoir of infection. There is no evidence of an animal reservoir for these **helminths.** The life cycle (incubation period) of the worm is two to six weeks. The disease is communicable as long as the eggs are being discharged, usually about two weeks. Everyone is susceptible to pinworm infestation.

Transmission

Pinworms live in the human intestine. Female worms are white and usually about a third of an inch long. They migrate to the **perianal** (around the anus) area at night to lay their eggs. Direct transmission occurs when a person's hands transfer the eggs from the anus to the mouth. Indirect transmission occurs by contact with clothing, bedding, food, or other articles that have been contaminated with the eggs. In households where there is heavy contamination, dust-borne infection may occur. Figure 11-6 shows how pinworm infestation may occur.

helminths	hel-MINTHS
perianal	PER-e-A-nal

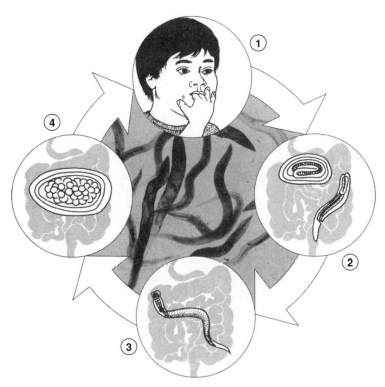

Figure 11-6
Cycle of enterobiasis.

Symptoms

In some cases, there are no symptoms, but for most, tickling and intense itching at night are present. The itching disturbs sleep, and scratching may lead to a secondary infection. Rarely, complications may occur, such as appendicitis and vaginitis.

Treatment

When pinworm infestation is suspected, a physician will apply cellophane tape to the anal area and examine it under the microscope for signs of the eggs. Drugs can destroy the worms, but everyone in the family needs to be treated to avoid reinfection.

Prevention

Education of children in personal hygiene is the best means of prevention. Emphasis should be placed on keeping the hands away from the mouth (discourage fingernail biting), daily bathing (preferably showers), the need for hand washing after defecation and before handling food, and changing underwear daily.

Control

All members of the family should be examined, and the source of the infection identified. Families should adhere to cleanliness as far as bed linens, underclothing, and other articles that might be contaminated.

ASCARIASIS (ROUNDWORM INFECTION)

Infection with roundworms (**ascariasis**) occurs worldwide in approximately one billion people. In the United States, about four million are infected. It is more prevalent in the South, particularly among children four to twelve years of age. Up to ninety percent of the population may be infected in poorer countries, whereas only about one percent have a light infestation in the United States and other developed countries. Although the disease is largely asymptomatic, the worms compete for food with the host and in children can retard growth because of malnutrition. It takes approximately sixty days for eggs to appear in the feces after their ingestion (incubation period). The reservoir is in humans or the soil. The disease is communicable as long as female worms live in the intestine. Infective eggs can also live in the soil for years. Everyone is susceptible to infestation with these worms.

Transmission

Ascariasis is acquired by humans through ingestion of soil contaminated with human feces that harbor the eggs. This process can occur directly by eating contaminated soil or indirectly by eating raw vegetables grown in contaminated soil and not well washed. After the eggs are eaten, they hatch and release larvae, which penetrate the intestinal wall and reach the lungs through the bloodstream. The larvae grow in the lungs, pass into the alveoli, ascend the trachea, and are then swallowed, thus entering the gastrointestinal tract. Here they grow to maturity, mate, and the female lays her eggs, which pass out with the feces, beginning the cycle anew. Figure 11-7 shows the cycle for ascariasis.

Symptoms

Often, the first sign of a roundworm infection may be a live worm noticed in the stools or one that passes out of the mouth or nose. There may be mild stomach discomfort, and if the infection is severe, stomach pain, vomiting, restlessness, disturbed sleep, and, in extreme cases, intestinal obstruction.

Treatment

Antiworm medications are effective in temporarily paralyzing the worms so that they can be expelled by peristaltic movements of the intestines.

Prevention

Proper sanitation methods to keep soil from being polluted with feces, and training children to wash hands before eating and handling food, are the best methods of prevention.

Control

The source of infection should be identified and any environmental sources eliminated. Family members should be checked and treated if necessary.

TRICHINOSIS

Infection with the worm responsible for **trichinosis** occurs when meat containing the cyst is ingested. These cysts are found primarily in pork and are infective when the pork is not cooked thor-

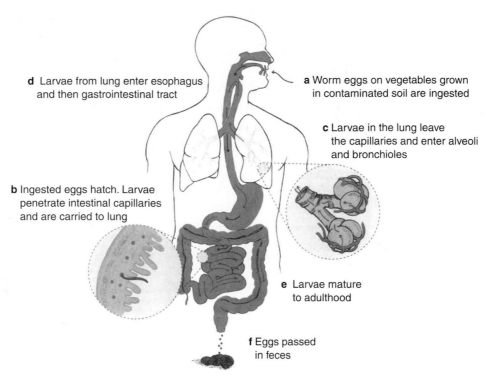

d Larvae from lung enter esophagus and then gastrointestinal tract

a Worm eggs on vegetables grown in contaminated soil are ingested

c Larvae in the lung leave the capillaries and enter alveoli and bronchioles

b Ingested eggs hatch. Larvae penetrate intestinal capillaries and are carried to lung

e Larvae mature to adulthood

f Eggs passed in feces

Figure 11-7

Cycle of ascariasis.

oughly. The reservoir for the organism is in swine, dogs, cats, rats, and many wild animals, including fox, wolf, and bear. Gastrointestinal symptoms may appear within a few days of eating the meat; systemic symptoms usually appear in eight to fifteen days, but this varies from five to forty-five days, depending upon the number of worms ingested. There is no person-to-person communicability, but animal hosts remain infective for months. Figure 11-8 shows reported cases in the United States from 1967 to 1997. Although there has been a steady decline, outbreaks still occur. Everyone is susceptible to trichinosis, and an initial infection results in partial immunity.

Transmission

Humans acquire the disease by eating raw or insufficiently cooked meat containing the encysted larvae. Although beef is not a source, hamburger is sometimes purposely or inadvertently mixed with pork and, if undercooked, can also contain infec-

tive cysts. Figure 11-9 shows how infection with trichinosis may occur.

Symptoms

Ingesting just a few worms usually causes no symptoms. A heavy amount of worms may cause diarrhea and vomiting within a day or two of eating the meat. A week later, more symptoms may occur as the larvae spread through the body. These symptoms include fever, swelling around the eyelids, and severe muscle pains. In most people, the symptoms gradually disappear, but in rare cases, the person may become seriously ill and die.

Treatment

Different drugs are used during the intestinal stage and the muscular stage. Corticosteroids may be used in severe cases.

ascariasis	AS-ka-RI-a-sis
trichinosis	TRIK-in-O-sis

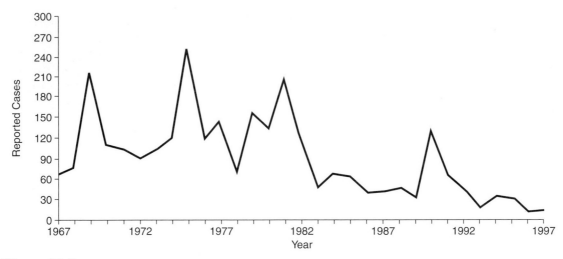

Figure 11-8
Trichinosis, by year, United States, 1967–1997.

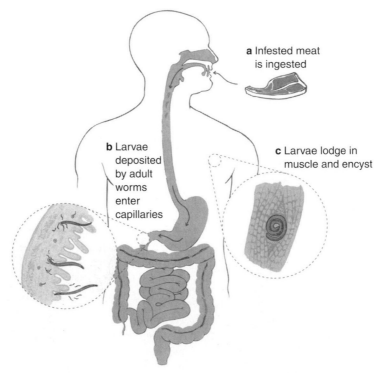

Figure 11-9
Cycle of trichinosis.

Prevention

The disease can be prevented by thorough cooking of all pork, pork products, and any meats that may be mixed with pork or contain the worms, such as bear meat.

Control

The source of infection should be identified, and any remaining infected meat confiscated. Other family members and persons who have eaten suspected meat should be examined for infection.

HOOKWORM DISEASE

Sandy soil, high humidity, a warm climate, and failure to wear shoes provide the conditions for acquiring hookworm disease. It occurs mostly in tropical and subtropical countries where poor sanitation allows human feces to get into the soil. In the United States, the disease is most common in the Southeast. Incubation may be from a few weeks to several months, depending upon degree of infection and condition of the host. The disease is not communicated from person to person, but infected individuals can contaminate the soil for several years. If conditions are favorable, the larvae will remain infective in the soil for several weeks. Everyone is susceptible to the hookworm. Some immunity is thought to develop after the first infection.

Transmission

Humans are infected when infective larvae penetrate the skin, usually of the foot. The larvae pass through the circulatory system to the lungs, enter the alveoli, migrate up the windpipe, and are swallowed, entering the gastrointestinal tract. Here they mature, mate, and the female deposits eggs, which are excreted in the feces to begin the cycle again. Figure 11-10 shows the life cycle of the hookworm.

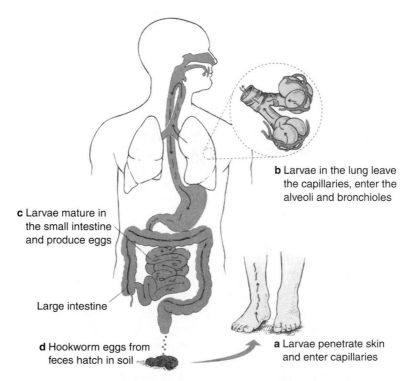

b Larvae in the lung leave the capillaries, enter the alveoli and bronchioles

c Larvae mature in the small intestine and produce eggs

Large intestine

d Hookworm eggs from feces hatch in soil

a Larvae penetrate skin and enter capillaries

Figure 11-10
Cycle of hookworm disease.

Symptoms

A red, intensely itchy rash may develop at the point of entry, usually on the feet. This is called *ground itch* and may last several days. If the infestation is light, there may be no symptoms. In heavier infestations, after the ground itch, the migration of the larvae through the lungs may produce a cough and pneumonia. When the adult worms form in the intestines, there may be abdominal discomfort. The most serious result of hookworm disease is the loss of blood, which can lead to anemia, enlarged heart (from increased oxygen demand), and heart failure.

Treatment

Administration of drugs to destroy the worms and correction of any iron deficiency through diet or iron supplements are the usual treatment.

Prevention

Hookworm disease can be prevented by the sanitary disposal of human feces and the wearing of shoes in endemic areas.

Control

The source of the infection should be identified and eliminated.

TAENIASIS (TAPEWORM DISEASE)

People may become infected with various species of tapeworm that are sometimes present in beef, pork, or fish. These worms can grow to be twenty or thirty feet long and lodge in the intestines. The occurrence of **taeniasis** is worldwide, particularly where beef and pork are eaten raw and where sanitary conditions allow swine and cattle to have access to human feces. It is rare in the United States but is frequently found in immigrants from other countries. From the time of ingestion, it takes eight to fourteen weeks for the eggs to appear in the stools. Pork tapeworm is communicable person to person, but the others are not. The eggs of beef and pork tapeworm may be released into the environment for as long as they are in the intestines, sometimes as long as thirty years. The eggs may remain infective in the environment for months. Everyone is susceptible to tapeworm infection.

Transmission

Humans acquire tapeworms by ingesting undercooked or raw meat or fish or by hand-to-mouth contact in some cases. Figure 11-11 shows the life cycle of a fish tapeworm.

Symptoms

Although these worms become very large, there may be no symptoms besides mild abdominal discomfort and diarrhea. In the case of the tapeworm found in pork, a more serious effect occurs when the embryos escape from the egg shells, penetrate the intestinal wall, move into the circulation, and are carried to various tissues where they develop into cysts that may lead to dangerous systemic and central nervous system symptoms.

Treatment

Drugs are available that are effective in the treatment of tapeworm.

Prevention

Means of prevention include education of the public regarding proper cooking of meats and sanitary disposal of human feces. If beef or pork are frozen to −5° Celsius (23° Fahrenheit) for more than four days, the infecting organism will be destroyed.

Control

Rigid sanitation measures should be taken and the source of the infection identified and eliminated.

SCABIES

Scabies results from infestation with mites that burrow under the skin and lay eggs. Figure 11-12 is an enlarged view of *Sarcoptes scabiei,* the scabies mite. Scabies infestation can occur anywhere, and although it was once thought to be a sign of poverty or poor sanitation, recent outbreaks in the United States and Europe have developed in all socioeconomic groups. The incubation period is two to six weeks before itching begins in persons who are newly infected. For those who have been exposed before, it is one to four days after re-exposure. Scabies is highly communicable until mites and eggs are destroyed. Some individuals seem to be more resistant than others to the infection, and those who have had one infestation are not infected as easily as before.

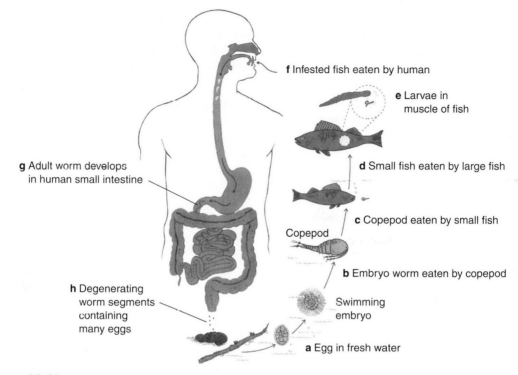

f Infested fish eaten by human

e Larvae in muscle of fish

g Adult worm develops in human small intestine

d Small fish eaten by large fish

c Copepod eaten by small fish

Copepod

b Embryo worm eaten by copepod

Swimming embryo

h Degenerating worm segments containing many eggs

a Egg in fresh water

Figure 11-11

Life cycle of fish tapeworm.

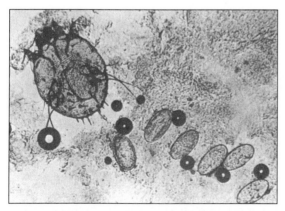

Figure 11-12

Scabies mite.

Transmission

The scabies mite is usually acquired by skin-to-skin contact. Sexual relations are often a means of transmission.

Symptoms

The major symptom is itching that is greater at night. Evidence of the presence of the mites is visible as papules, vesicles, or tiny burrow lines. They generally appear between fingers, on anterior surfaces of wrists and elbows, in the armpit, at the waistline, on nipples in females, and genitalia in males. In infants, the burrows may appear on the head and neck. Scratching of the lesions can lead to secondary bacterial infections.

Treatment

Topical application of an insecticide, lindane, is the treatment for scabies, immediately preceded and followed the next day by a soap-and-water bath. Itching often persists for one to two weeks, even after the treatment has eliminated the mites.

taeniasis   te-NI-a-sis

Prevention

The best prevention for scabies is education of the public on the means of transmission and the need for early diagnosis and treatment of infested individuals and their contacts.

Control

Contacts need to be examined to determine the source of infection and administer treatment.

PEDICULOSIS

Three kinds of parasitic lice feed on human blood and cause **pediculosis**: *Pediculus capitis,* the head louse; *Pediculus corporis,* the body louse (Figure 11-13); and *Phthirus pubis,* the crab louse. *P. capitis* is the most common species and feeds on the scalp and, rarely, in the eyebrows, eyelashes, and beard. It occurs where there are overcrowded conditions and poor personal hygiene and generally affects children. *P. corporis* stays in the seams of clothing, close to the skin, and lives only to feed on blood. Prolonged wearing of the same clothing, overcrowding, and poor personal hygiene are factors in this infestation. *P. pubis* is usually found in the pubic area but may also be in other hairy parts of the body. Infestation with lice may occur in any part of the world, and outbreaks of head lice are common among school children and in institutions.

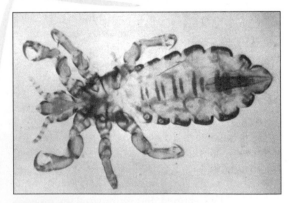

Figure 11-13
Body louse.

The eggs of the lice hatch in about a week, and the lice reach sexual maturity in eight to ten days, when mating takes place and more eggs are laid. Everyone is susceptible to louse infestation if suitable conditions are present.

Transmission

The means of transmission for head and body lice is direct contact with an infested person or indirect contact with their belongings. Pubic or crab lice are acquired through sexual intercourse or use of infested bedding. When an individual develops a fever, lice leave them, and thus crowding and illness with fever increase transmission from person to person.

Symptoms

For head lice, there is severe itching; matted, foul-smelling, lusterless hair (severe cases); swollen lymph nodes; and a rash on the body. The adult lice crawl down the hair shafts and deposit oval, gray-white nits (eggs) on the hair shafts. When body lice are present, there are usually small red papules on the shoulders, trunk, or buttocks, which change to hives from scratching. If the infestation is not treated, the skin becomes dry, discolored, thickly encrusted, and scaly, and there may be a bacterial infection and scarring. Pubic lice cause skin irritation from scratching, which is usually more obvious than the bites. Small gray-blue spots may appear on the thighs and upper body.

Treatment

Treatment for head lice is a lindane cream rubbed into the scalp at night, then rinsed out in the morning with lindane shampoo. This treatment is repeated the following night. A fine-tooth comb dipped in vinegar is used to remove nits from the hair. Washing the hair with ordinary shampoo will remove crustations. Body lice may be removed by bathing with soap and water. In severe cases, lindane may have to be used. The lice can be removed from clothes by washing, ironing, or dry cleaning. Pubic lice are treated with lindane cream or lotion that is left on for twenty-four hours, or by shampooing with lindane shampoo. Treatment is

Head lice = Current Epidemic

repeated in one week, and clothes and bed sheets must be laundered to prevent reinfestation. There are other preparations that can be used in treating pediculosis if lindane is not effective.

Prevention

All primary schoolchildren should be inspected regularly for head lice. If conditions are present that favor body lice, then children should be inspected for these also. The public should be educated on the value of laundering clothing and bedding in hot water or dry cleaning to destroy the nits and lice. Children should be cautioned against borrowing combs or other cosmetic supplies or clothing capable of transmitting the lice. Contact with infested individuals and their belongings should be avoided.

Control

Infested individuals should be isolated from contact with others until twenty-four hours after treatment with lindane or other effective insecticide. Along with treatment of infested individuals, clothing, bedding, and other possible vehicles of transmission must be disinfected. Household and other close contacts should be examined and treated when necessary.

pediculosis   pe-DIK-u-LO-sis
Pediculus capitis   pe-DIK-u-lus ka-pi-TI-tis
Pediculus corporis   pe-DIK-u-lus cor-POR-is
Phthirus pubis   THIR-us pu-BIS

SUMMARY

Table 11-2 summarizes relevant data on diseases caused by protozoa and metazoa.

TABLE 11-2	**Diseases Caused by Protozoa and Metazoa**				
Disease	**Special Characteristics**	**Transmission**	**Common Symptoms**	**Prevention/ Control**	**Treatment**
Giardiasis	Found more in children in U.S.; common in travelers from endemic areas and campers drinking impure water	Ingestion of cysts in contaminated water or by fecal-oral route, person to person	Often none; when present, abdominal cramps, pale, loose, greasy stools, nausea	Sanitary disposal of feces, thorough hand washing after defecation, well-cleaned raw fruits and vegetables; exclusion of infected individuals from food preparation; protection of water supplies.	Metronidazole is the drug of choice in the United States. Other drugs can be used alternatively. Furazolidone is available in pediatric suspension for children and infants.

Continued

TABLE 11-2	*Continued*				
Disease	**Special Characteristics**	**Transmission**	**Common Symptoms**	**Prevention/ Control**	**Treatment**
Amebiasis (amebic dysentary)	Acute or chronic; parasitic protozoan, *E. Histolytica;* 1% to 3% incidence in U.S., higher in mental institutions and among male homosexuals; communicable as long as an infected individual carries cysts	Through ingestion of feces-contaminated food and water and oral-anal sex	Sudden high fever, chills, stomach cramps, bloody diarrhea with tenesmus; may last 1–4 years	Sanitary disposal of feces, hand washing after defecation; fruits and vegetables cleaned, contaminated water boiled; infected individuals excluded from food-handling; contact investigation	Can be treated by a number of different drugs
Toxoplasmosis	Dangerous for unborn child if mother is infected and for immunodeficient individuals; if early in pregnancy, more serious infection in child	Most common: ingestion of undercooked lamb or pork; also by contact with feces of cats and some other animals	Acute form similar to mononucleosis; generalized form in immunodeficient patients: encephalitis, fever, headache, vomiting, delirium, convulsions, rash	Thorough cooking of lamb and pork; keep cats inside and feed only commercially prepared cat food; clean litter boxes frequently, do not allow children to play in them nor pregnant women to clean them; cover sand boxes when not in use to keep cats out.	Treatment for toxoplasmosis is usually not necessary but in the case of immunocompromised individuals, it is essential. A number of drugs are available
Malaria	Single most important disease hazard for travel-	By the bite of an infected female *Anopheles*	Chills, fever, myalgia, headache	Elimination of breeding places for mosquitoes;	Chloroquine is used for all forms of malaria

TABLE 11-2	*Continued*				
Disease	**Special Characteristics**	**Transmission**	**Common Symptoms**	**Prevention/ Control**	**Treatment**
Malaria— Cont'd	ers to Asia, Africa, Latin America; WHO efforts to eliminate malaria hampered by insecticide-resistant mosquitoes and drug-resistant plasmodia; 10% fatality rate if untreated; humans are only important reservoir; life cycle of mosquito in two hosts	mosquito; also by injection or transfusion of blood from an infected person or with contaminated needles; mosquito is infective for life, sporozoites develop in her glands; mosquito is unaffected by the disease		screened living and sleeping areas; insecticides; there is no vaccine; drugs used prophylactically	except *P. falciparum,* for which quinine and other drugs are used concurrently
Enterobiasis (pinworm)	Most prevalent infection with worms in U.S.; mostly in children	Direct from anal area to mouth; indirect on contaminated articles; rarely by inhalation in dust	Tickling and intense itching at night in anal area	Emphasis on good personal hygiene for children, particularly hand washing after defecation; daily change of underwear and cleanliness of bed linens	A number of drugs are available that destroy pinworms
Ascariasis (roundworm)	More prevalent in southern U.S. and among children 4–12 years of age	Ingestion of contaminated soil or unwashed contaminated raw vegetables or fruit	Mild stomach discomfort; stomach pain, vomiting, restlessness, disturbed sleep, in severe cases	Good sanitation and training of children in personal hygiene	Paralyzing drugs are used to treat roundworms so they are expelled by peristaltic movements of the intestines

TABLE 11-2	Continued				
Disease	**Special Characteristics**	**Transmission**	**Common Symptoms**	**Prevention/ Control**	**Treatment**
Trichinosis	Cysts found primarily in pork; beef can be accidentally or purposely mixed with pork	Ingestion of raw or insufficiently cooked meat containing encysted larvae	At first, diarrhea and vomiting; later, fever, swelling around eyelids, severe muscle pains caused by movement of larvae in muscles	Thorough cooking of pork and pork products (150°F. Or until meat is grey)	The worms or trichinae are destroyed by drugs and iron deficiency may need to be corrected
Hookworm	Most common in southeastern U.S.; worm usually enters through foot; may be cause of mental and physical retardation in children; eggs in feces confirm diagnosis	Penetration of skin, usually of the foot, by infective larvae; eggs are produced in intestines and excreted in feces	Red, intensely itchy rash at point of entry; abdominal discomfort; cough, pneumonia, anemia, and complications possible; symptoms may not show for months; occur during lung migration phase	Sanitary disposal of human feces, wearing of shoes	A number of effective drugs are available to treat hookworm
Taeniasis (tapeworm)	Can grow to be 20 or 30 feet long in intestines; occurs where beef or pork are eaten raw or where pigs and cattle have access to human feces	Usually by ingesting undercooked or raw meat or fish	Mild abdominal discomfort, diarrhea; pork tapeworm may produce serious systemic effects	Thorough cooking of all meats and sanitary disposal of human feces	A number of drugs are available to treat tapeworm
Scabies (mites)	Mites burrow under the	Skin to skin contact	Itching that increases at	Education of the public on	Topical application of an

TABLE 11-2	*Continued*				
Disease	**Special Characteristics**	**Transmission**	**Common Symptoms**	**Prevention/ Control**	**Treatment**
Scabies (mites)— Cont'd	skin		night; papules, vesicles, or tiny burrow lines	means of transmission; early diagnosis and treatment	insecticide is used to treat scabies
Pediculosis (lice)	Head louse, body louse, and pubic louse (crabs); body louse is vector for typhus and other diseases	Direct contact with an infested person, bedding, or other articles used or worn by infested person	Head lice: severe itching, foul-smelling, lusterless hair, swollen lymph nodes, rash Body lice: small, red papules on shoulders, trunk, or buttocks, hives; skin becomes dry, discolored, encrusted and scaly without treatment Pubic lice: itching, skin irritation from scratching; small gray-blue spots on thighs and upper body	Inspection of all primary school-children for head lice; inspection for body lice also when infestation likely; avoidance of physical contact with infested individuals; public education on laundering and cleaning procedures to destroy nits and lice; infested individuals should be isolated until 24 hours after treatment	Lindane cream or lotion is used for all kinds of lice infestations. For head lice, a fine-toothed comb dipped in vinegar is also used. Bedding and clothing worn by the victims need to be laundered in hot water and all members of the household should be treated

QUESTIONS FOR REVIEW

1. What groups of people are more likely to acquire giardiasis?
2. What precautions can be taken to prevent giardiasis?
3. What similarities are there between amebiasis and giardiasis?
4. For what people is toxoplasmosis most dangerous? Why?
5. What is the most common method for acquiring toxoplasmosis?
6. What precautions can be taken to prevent transmission of toxoplasmosis by cats?
7. Why have efforts by WHO to control and eliminate malaria failed in recent years?
8. How is malaria transmitted?

9. When persons with malaria have an acute attack of chills and other symptoms, what has taken place in their bodies?

10. Describe the three stages of an acute attack of malaria.

11. What means of prevention are recommended for malaria?

12. Why are children more likely to have pinworms?

13. What causes the nocturnal itching of pinworms?

14. What methods are recommended for prevention of pinworms?

15. Where in the United States is roundworm most prevalent?

16. How are roundworms transmitted?

17. What method is used to expel roundworms?

18. What meat is usually the source of trichinosis?

19. How can trichinosis be prevented?

20. How do humans become infected with hookworm?

21. What is the most serious result of hookworm disease?

22. In which meats can tapeworms be found?

23. To what dangerous results can infection with pork tapeworm lead? How?

24. How is scabies transmitted?

25. Describe the infestation and results caused by the three kinds of parasitic lice discussed in the text.

26. What means of treatment, prevention, and control are used for lice?

FURTHER READING

Apgar, Barbara. 2000. Efficacy and safety of therapy for human scabies infestation. *American Family Physician* 61:513.

Balter, Michael. 1999. Gene sequencers target malaria mosquito. *Science* 285:508.

Bonn, Dorothy. 1998. Susceptibility to malaria during pregnancy explained. *The Lancet* 352:1447.

Brainerd, Elaine. 1998. From eradication to resistance: Five continuing concerns about pediculosis. *Journal of School Health* 68:146.

Brody, Jane E. 1999. Sly parasite menaces pets and their owners. *New York Times* 149:F7.

Campbell, Lee Ann, Cho-Chou Kuo, and J. Thomas Grayston. 1998. Chlamydia pneumoniae and cardiovascular disease. *Emerging Infectious Diseases* 4:4.

Coleman-Jones, Emma. 1999. Ronal Ross and the great malaria problem: Historical reference in the biological sciences. *Journal of Biological Education* 33:181.

Dawes, M., et al. 1999. Treatment of head lice. *British Medical Journal* 318:385.

Deneen, V. C., P. A. Belle-Isle, C. M. Taylor, et al. 1998. Outbreak of cryptosporidiosis. *Morbidity and Mortality Weekly Report,* 47:856–61.

Dunn, David, et al. 1999. Mother-to-child transmission of toxoplasmosis: risk estimates for clinical counseling. *The Lancet* 353:1829.

E. B. 1998. FDA approves of irradiation of food products to control infection. *Medical Update* 21:4.

Ectoparasitic infections. *Morbidity and Mortality Weekly Report* 47:105, 1998.

Fedarko, Kevin. 1998. A lousy, nit-picking epidemic. *Time* 151:73.

Fleming, Alan F., and Leonard B. Lerer. 1999. Cost-effectiveness of malaria control in sub-Saharan Africa. *The Lancet* 354:1123.

Frost, Floyd, Gunther F. Craun, and Rebecca L. Calderon. 1998. Increasing hospitalization and death possibly due to clostridium difficile diarrheal disease. *Emerging Infectious Diseases.*

Furlow, Bryant. 1999. The body snatchers. *New Scientist* 163:42.

Henderson, C. W. 2000. Invasive amoebiasis is an emerging parasitic disease. *AIDS Weekly* p. 12.

Jelinek, T., et al. 1999. Self-use of rapid tests for malaria diagnosis by tourists. *The Lancet* 354:1609.

Kirchner, Jeffrey T. 1998. Diagnosis, treatment and prevention of giardiasis. *American Family Physician* 57:802.

Kitchen, Lynn W. 1999. Case studies in international travelers. *American Family Physician* 60:471.

Lazarevic, Aleksandar M., and Aleksandar N. Neskovic. 1999. Low incidence of cardiac abnormalities in treated trichinosis: a prospective study of 62 patients. *American Journal of Medicine* 107:18.

Levy, Deborah A., Michelle S. Bens, Gunther F. Craun, et al. 1998. Surveillance for waterborne-disease outbreaks—United States, 1995–1996. *Morbidity and Mortality Weekly Report,* 47:1.

Lousy news: pesticide resistance. *Science News* 156:207, 1999.

MacKenzie, Debora. 1999. Tropical killer flies north. *New Scientist* 163:14.

MacKenzie, Debora. 1999. The comeback killer. *New Scientist* 163:13.

Malakooti, M. A., K. Biomndo, and G. D. Shanks. 1998. Re-emergence of epidemic malaria in the highlands of Western Kenya. *Emerging Infectious Diseases.*

Marsh, Kevin. 1998. Malaria disaster in Africa. *The Lancet* 352:924.

McClure, Jane Blaum, and Emily F. Omura. 1998. Cutaneous larva migrans. *The New England Journal of Medicine* 338:1733.

McQuiston, John T. 1999. Two Suffolk county boys contract malaria at local scout camp. *New York Times* 148:B2.

"Parasitic roundworm diseases," National Institute of Allergy and Infectious Diseases, [www.niaid.nih.gov/factsheets].

Pneumonia and severe haemoptysis. *The Lancet* 352:198, 1998.

Price, James H., et al. 1999. School nurses' perceptions of and experiences with head lice. *Journal of School Health* 69:153.

Rampaging malaria. *Geographical Magazine* 71:64, 1999.

Rivera, Rachel. 1998. Killer mosquitoes. *Science World* 54:14.

Shandera, Wayne X., and Padma Bollam. 1998. Hepatic amebiasis among patients in a public teaching hospital. *Southern Medical Journal* 91:829.

Stanley Jr., Samuel L. 1998. Malaria vaccines: Are seven antigens better than one? *The Lancet* 352:1163.

Summertime blues: It's Giardia season. *Journal of Environmental Health* 61:51, 1998.

The virus and the hookworm. *British Medical Journal* 7199:1693, 1999.

Walling, Anne D. 1999. Toxoplasmosis in pregnancy. *American Family Physician* 59:685.

Wallon, Martine, et al. 1999. Congenital toxoplasmosis: systematic review of evidence of efficacy of treatment in pregnancy. *British Medical Journal* 318:1511.

Watts, Jonathan. 1999. Japan and WHO join forces to develop new antimalarial drugs. *The Lancet* 354:1624.

Woo, P. C. Y., et al. 1999. A woman with ascites and abdominal masses. *The Lancet* 355:546.

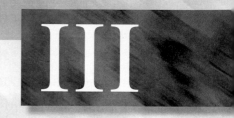

Chronic Disease and Disorders

With the use of vaccinations and antibiotics, many infectious diseases that have besieged humans for centuries have been brought under control. Scientists, physicians, and health personnel everywhere foresaw a world free of infectious disease as vaccines for more diseases and more "wonder drugs" became available. But this vision was not to be. Microorganisms able to change and resist the new drugs and new and more virile pathogens have required researchers to continue seeking the elusive victory over infectious disease. While men and women of science have been involved in a life or death struggle with infectious disease, noninfectious diseases have been increasing steadily, taking a growing number of lives and claiming the top positions on the charts for disease morbidity and mortality.

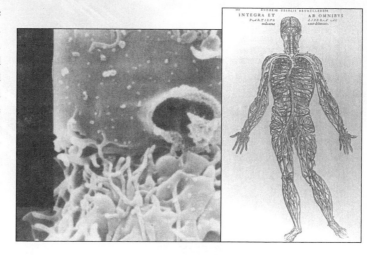

(right) Vena cava from Vesalius's *De humani corporis fabrica* (1543).

(left) Electron micrograph of natural killer cell attacking cancer cell.

Cardiovascular disease is the number one killer in the United States today. In 1995, nearly one million people in the United States died of cardiovascular disease. This is almost as many as died from cancer, accidents, pneumonia, influenza, and all other causes of death combined (excluding AIDS). According to 1995 estimates by the American Heart Association (AHA), 58,200,000 Americans have some form of cardiovascular disease. Headway has been made against some chronic diseases but it is obvious that a chance to celebrate the conquest of disease is a long way off.

In addition to the chronic diseases that have made the list of the ten leading causes of death, there arc others such as arthritis and ulcers which, although not often fatal, cause unending pain, crippling, and suffering. It is estimated that forty percent of the American population have one or more chronic conditions.

CARDIOVASCULAR AND CEREBROVASCULAR DISEASE

OBJECTIVES

1. *Describe the disease process in atherosclerosis.*

2. *Distinguish among major risk factors for atherosclerosis that can be and cannot be altered.*

3. *Identify five risk factors that may be related to the development of atherosclerosis.*

4. *Distinguish among essential, secondary, and malignant hypertension.*

5. *Explain the significance of angina pectoris.*

6. *Explain possible causes of congenital heart defects.*

7. *Describe the cardiovascular diseases in this chapter, including predisposing factors, symptoms, prevention, and treatment.*

8. *Identify the signs of a cerebrovascular accident (stroke).*

PHYSIOLOGY OF THE CARDIOVASCULAR SYSTEM

The cardiovascular system is composed of the heart (Figure 12-1), blood vessels (Figure 12-2), and lymphatics (Figure 12-3). The heart is a muscular pump that consists of four chambers: two atria or upper chambers and two ventricles or lower chambers. Figure 12-4 shows the direction of blood flow through the chambers, valves, and blood vessels. Although the following description of blood flow discusses one side at a time, it is important to remember that both atria contract at the same time and both ventricles contract at the same time.

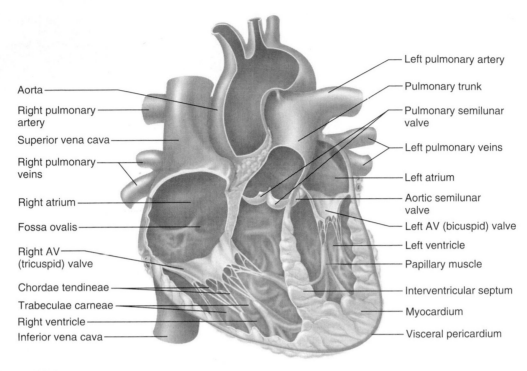

Aorta

Right pulmonary artery

Superior vena cava

Right pulmonary veins

Right atrium

Fossa ovalis

Right AV (tricuspid) valve

Chordae tendineae

Trabeculae carneae

Right ventricle

Inferior vena cava

Left pulmonary artery

Pulmonary trunk

Pulmonary semilunar valve

Left pulmonary veins

Left atrium

Aortic semilunar valve

Left AV (bicuspid) valve

Left ventricle

Papillary muscle

Interventricular septum

Myocardium

Visceral pericardium

Figure 12-1
The human heart.

Blood returns to the heart from the upper and lower body by the superior (upper) and inferior (lower) venae cavae, into the right atrium (see Figure 12-4). The blood passes from the atrium through the tricuspid valve into the right ventricle. Approximately eighty percent of the blood flows from the atrium to the ventricle by gravity. When the right atrium contracts, the rest of the blood is pushed into the ventricle. When the right ventricle contracts, the tricuspid valve is closed by the pressure of the blood, and the pulmonary semilunar valve opens, allowing blood to pass into the pulmonary arteries, which carry the blood to the lungs for oxygenation. The oxygenated blood returns to the left atrium through the pulmonary veins and passes into the left ventricle, which is completely filled after left atrial contraction. Contraction of the ventricle then pushes the blood against the bicuspid valve, closing it, and against the aortic semilunar valve, causing it to open. The blood flows through the aorta and is distributed to the rest of the body,

including the heart muscle itself, which has its own supply of veins and arteries. These are the coronary (from the Latin for *crown*) arteries and veins and are shown in Figure 12-9.

CONDUCTION SYSTEM

The heart has specialized conducting tissue that allows electrical impulses to regulate the heartbeat. These structures are cardiac muscle like the rest of the heart but modified enough to specialize in initiating and conducting the heartbeat. The **sinoatrial** node, **atrioventricular** node, atrioventricular bundle, or bundle of His, and **Purkinje** fibers can be seen in Figure 12-5.

The *sinoatrial node* is the part of the heart called the pacemaker and initiates electrical contraction in the heart. The impulse generated at the sinoatrial node travels quickly through the muscle fibers of both atria to the atrioventricular node (AV node).

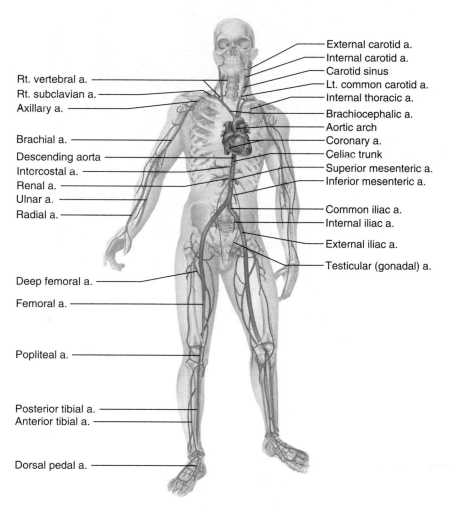

Rt. vertebral a.
Rt. subclavian a.
Axillary a.

Brachial a.
Descending aorta
Intercostal a.
Renal a.
Ulnar a.
Radial a.

Deep femoral a.

Femoral a.

Popliteal a.

Posterior tibial a.
Anterior tibial a.

Dorsal pedal a.

External carotid a.
Internal carotid a.
Carotid sinus
Lt. common carotid a.
Internal thoracic a.
Brachiocephalic a.
Aortic arch
Coronary a.
Celiac trunk
Superior mesenteric a.
Inferior mesenteric a.

Common iliac a.
Internal iliac a.

External iliac a.

Testicular (gonadal) a.

Figure 12-2a
The arteries of the body.

At this point the conduction pauses to allow for contraction of the atrium. When the impulse passes from the atrioventricular node, it picks up speed and is relayed through the *atrioventricular bundle* and to the *Purkinje fibers,* which together stimulate the ventricles to contract.

This conduction system of the heart works with no noticeable flaws for many years for most people. But abnormal rhythms, referred to as *cardiac* **arrhythmias** or *cardiac* **dysrhythmias** can be caused by a number of disorders. These dysrhythmias vary in severity from those that are mild, occur infrequently, and are accompanied by no other symptoms, to those that are life threatening, such as *ventricular fibrillation.* In any case, cardiac dysrhythmias involve a disturbance of the heart's electrical conduction and the amount of

sinoatrial   sin-o-A-tre-al
atrioventricular   a-tre-o-ven-TRIK-u-lar
purkinje   pur-KIN-je
arrhythmias   a-RITH-me-as
dysrhythmias   dis-RITH-me-as
ventricular fibrillation   ven-TRIK-u-lar fi-bril-A-shun

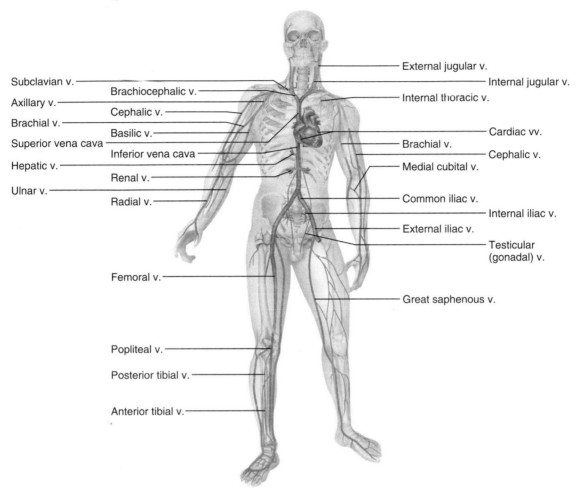

Figure 12-2b
The veins of the body.

blood being pumped from the heart. If the ability of the heart to pump blood to the body is impaired enough, it can lead to sudden death. It should be understood that an occasional irregular beat may happen to anyone and is not indicative of any problem. However, if irregular beats occur in a pattern over time, a physician should be consulted. When the electrical conduction from the atria to the ventricles is slowed or blocked, a temporary or permanent pacemaker can be placed into or on the heart to maintain the contraction of the ventricles.

PREVENTION OF CARDIOVASCULAR DISEASES

As was discussed in Chapter 2, heredity, environment, and lifestyle all play a part in determining whether an individual will develop a chronic disease. Although research is going on today that may make it possible to alter genes and thus affect the heredity factor, it will be years before this can be done. There are risk factors that we cannot change, including age, heredity, and gender, but

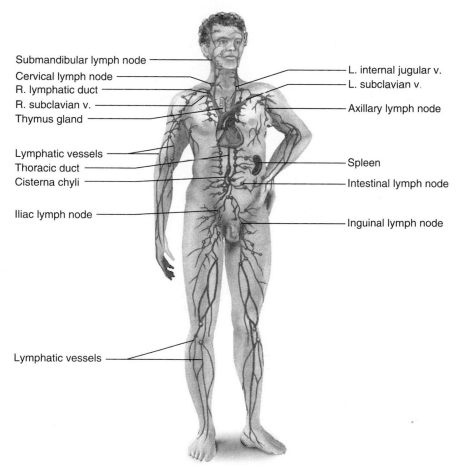

Figure 12-3

The lymphatic system.

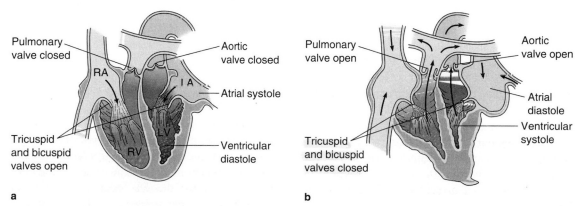

a   b

Figure 12-4

Path of blood through the heart during contraction of atria (a) and ventricles (b). RA: right atrium; LA: left atrium; RV: right ventricle; LV: left ventricle; AO: aorta; PA: pulmonary artery (see Figure 12-1 also).

Valves prevent back flow of Blood.

PQRST (EKG waves)

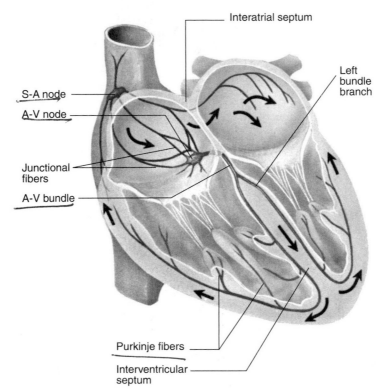

S-A node

A-V node

Junctional
fibers

A-V bundle

Interatrial septum

Left
bundle
branch

Purkinje fibers

Interventricular
septum

Figure 12-5
The conduction system of the heart.

there are many we can change. Certainly we can make changes in the way we eat, sleep, work, and play. For those who make the effort, it can mean not only added years of life but added quality of life for the years they live.

Often cardiovascular disease is far advanced when diagnosed. According to studies and research, the onset of the disease can be as early as childhood. Educational and preventive measures need to begin in childhood and continue throughout life. Proper nutritional habits, abstention from smoking, regular activity, weight control, and stress management can greatly reduce the risk for atherosclerosis and hypertension. Atherosclerosis and hypertension are present in many cardiovascular diseases.

TYPES OF CARDIOVASCULAR DISEASE

Atherosclerosis

Atherosclerosis is discussed first because of its involvement in many forms of cardiovascular disease. Information in this section will be referred to as other diseases of the heart and blood vessels are discussed.

The term *atherosclerosis* (AS) is from the Greek *athero* (gruel) plus *sclerosis* (hardening). Figure 12-6 shows deposits of plaque on the endothelium (inner lining) of an artery. These fatty deposits resemble the fat observed on a fresh chicken. The terms *arteriosclerosis* and *athero-*

normal heartbeat = 60-100 Bpm (beats per min.)

> ### CASE STUDY
>
> ## Heart Disease
>
> A forty-seven year-old married white male school teacher was a two pack per day smoker with a history of diabetes mellitus, hyperlipidemia and obesity, and a family history of coronary artery disease. He was awakened from his sleep at three a.m. with crushing substernal chest pain that radiated to his left arm and was accompanied by shortness of breath. When paramedics arrived, they found the patient cool, clammy, bradycardic, and hypotensive. Intravenous
>
> fluids and atropine were given and he was transported to a suburban hospital.
>
> On arrival in the emergency department at the hospital, the patient was in considerable distress. The patient was treated with morphine, atropine, and aspirin, but he remained bradycardic and hypotensive. Other measures to keep him alive were tried, but the evolving clinical data made it clear that his prognosis was extremely grim. He was given comfort measures and he died peacefully.

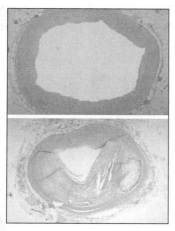

Figure 12-6

Buildup of atheromatous plaque reduces the lumen (opening) within the artery.

sclerosis are often used interchangeably although technically, AS is a form of arteriosclerosis. Arteriosclerosis refers to hardening and thickening of the arteries and loss of elasticity of the vessel walls. There are several disease processes that cause this. Most of these are rare, but AS has become epidemic in economically developed societies, and in the Western world it is now the disease that most often leads to illness and death.

Because all nations do not have the high incidence of AS found in the Western world, it seems

reasonable to believe that the disease is not inevitable. Studies have shown that when natives of Japan, which has a relatively low rate of AS, immigrate to the United States, they soon develop the same rates of illness and death from AS as persons born in the United States. Some factor or factors in our society or in our lifestyles must contribute significantly to the incidence of death from this cardiovascular disease.

Although atheromas can develop in any artery, the most common sites are the aorta and the coronary and cerebral arteries. As a result, **myocardial infarcts** (MIs), or heart attack, and **cerebrovascular** accidents (CVAs), or stroke, are the major results of AS. AS also affects other parts of the body, including the legs, where it can result in peripheral vascular disease, and gangrene (death of tissue, usually because of an inadequate supply of oxygen to the area).

A number of theories of **atherogenesis** (the formation of atheromas) have developed. Figure 12-7 shows successive stages in the formation of an atherosclerotic plaque according to the

atherosclerosis	ath-er-o-skle-RO-sis
myocardial	mi-o-KAR-de-al
cerebrovascular	ser-e-bro-VAS-ku-lar
atherogenesis	ath-er-o-JEN-e-sis

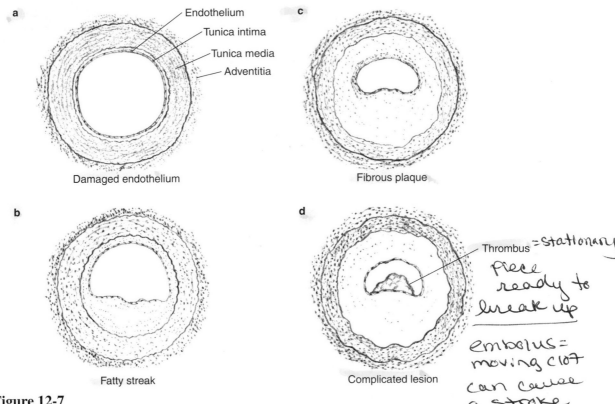

Figure 12-7

Progression of atherosclerosis from normal artery (a) to complicated lesion with thrombus (d).

[handwritten annotations on figure: Thrombus = stationary piece ready to break up; embolus = moving clot can cause a stroke]

reaction to injury theory. This theory, which seems to be the most popular, states that (1) the endothelium is somehow injured, perhaps by bacteria, nicotine, **hyperlipidemia** (too much fat), or high blood pressure. When any injury occurs in the body, our natural defenses are activated (see Chapter 3), and blood cells are able to attach to the endothelium; (2) cholesterol, foamy (containing lipids) **macrophages,** smooth muscle cells (which multiply), and other cellular debris are added to the lesion; and (3) it eventually becomes a fibrous plaque; (4) finally, a thrombus is formed, calcification may occur, and more lipids accumulate; it is then referred to as a "complicated lesion." Treatment for AS in any of these stages may reverse the process.

The components of a plaque—cholesterol, foamy macrophages, smooth muscle cells, and cellular debris—are present in each plaque in varying amounts, resulting in differences between the lesions. It should also be remembered that this process occurs over many years of a person's lifetime (the beginning of atherosclerotic plaques has been found in young children), and there are no apparent signs until the disease is far advanced.

As the plaques increase in size, the lumen (opening) of the arteries becomes smaller (see Figure 12-7). With progression of the disease, the flow of blood through the artery is restricted, leading to insufficient blood flow to tissue in the area. If the plaque is in a coronary artery or the aorta, and a thrombus (stationary clot) develops or an embolus (moving clot) occludes the artery, a myocardial infarct, or heart attack, may occur. If the plaque is in an artery supplying the brain and the above events occur, a cerebrovascular accident, or stroke, may be the result.

[handwritten notes at bottom of page: chest pain = heart not getting enough blood (O₂); blockages in corony arteries; cigarettes, stress constrict arteries]

Predisposing Factors

It is known that AS increases with age. As the passageways for blood through the arteries become narrower because of atheromas, ischemic heart disease (IHD), or insufficient blood supply to the heart, occurs. The formation of atheromas is probably not a natural result of age, but at present death from ischemic heart disease as a result of AS increases as people get older.

Gender is another risk factor that cannot be changed. Before sixty years of age, AS is more prevalent in men than in women. After menopause, the difference decreases, and recent studies indicate that women are more at risk for cardiovascular disease than was expected by the scientific community. This is because almost all studies on heart disease in the past were done using men as the subjects and the results were applied to women as well.

Some families suffer a higher death rate from IHD than others. The term *familial hyperlipoproteinemias* is used to describe a group of inborn abnormalities in lipid metabolism. Individuals who have inherited one of these disorders tend to develop AS, usually before the age of fifty, if not treated. There might also be a tendency toward *hypercholesterolemia* in some families because of dietary and other habits supported by the social customs of the family.

It is not possible to choose not to age or to choose our sex or parents, or to choose to be born in a part of the world where the risk for AS is low, but there are many ways by which all individuals can reduce their risk for AS and IHD. The following risk factors for AS can be reduced or eliminated.

Hyperlipidemia

Cholesterol is contained in the food we eat and is also manufactured in the liver. It is a major component of atheromatous plaques. A higher than normal amount of cholesterol and/or other fats in the blood is defined as "hyperlipidemia." There are a number of connections between cholesterol and AS that have been verified by such studies as the well-publicized Framingham Study and the

Multiple Risk Factor Intervention Trials (MR FIT), both of which have been ongoing for many years. Among those connections are the following:

1. Laboratory animals develop AD when fed diets that raise the level of cholesterol in their blood.
2. Genetic disorders that produce high levels of cholesterol in the blood lead to AS and increased risk of IHD.
3. Most populations with relatively high levels of cholesterol in their blood have more deaths caused by IHD.
4. Many different studies have shown that when patients with high cholesterol are treated by diet, regular exercise, and cholesterol-lowering drugs, cardiovascular mortality is reduced.

The damaging effects of a high cholesterol level received so much press when first recognized that the fact that other lipids (fats) in the blood also played a part in cardiovascular disease was largely ignored by advertisers eager to sell their products. Efforts to educate the public, as well as guidelines on advertising, are helping people make wiser choices when trying to reduce their risk of cardiovascular disease.

Lipoproteins

Lipids can be divided into five types according to their properties. All lipids in the plasma circulate attached to protein, thus the term *lipoprotein*. The lipids attached to the protein in varying amounts are phospholipids, cholesterol, and triglycerides. One type of lipoprotein, **chylomicron,** is composed primarily of triglycerides (80% to 95%) from dietary fats and is present only after a meal. The other four types are very-low-density lipoprotein (VLDL), intermediate-density lipoprotein

hyperlipidemia	hy-per-lip-i-DEE-mi-a
macrophages	MAK-ro-faj
ischemic	is-KE-mick
hypercholesterolemia	hi-per-ko-les-ter-ol-E-me-a
chylomicron	ki-lo-MI-kron

258   UNIT III   Chronic Disease and Disorders

Artherosclerosis

(IDL), low-density lipoprotein (LDL), and high-density lipoprotein (HDL).

Of these five lipids, LDL is the lipid most strongly correlated with AS and has the most cholesterol. It is sometimes referred to as the "bad" cholesterol. On the other hand, there is an inverse relationship between HDL and AS. HDL removes cholesterol from the blood and sends it to the liver to be processed and excreted and may even remove it from atheromatous plaques. HDL has been called "good" cholesterol. Chylomicron and IDL are normally removed from the plasma very quickly or converted to LDL and do not accumulate. It is not yet known how atherogenic VLDL is. It is only certain that LDLs are atherogenic and HDLs are not. In fact, higher levels of HDLs lower the risk for heart disease.

Because HDLs lower the risk for heart disease, the level of LDL in the plasma does not always identify those at risk for AS. It is possible to have low LDL and still be at risk because the HDL is also low. Conversely, LDL may be very high, but it is not considered a risk if the HDL is also high. The important measure for anyone is the ratio of total cholesterol to HDL. For men, a ratio of 4:1 is considered low risk, and for women a ratio of 3.8:1 is low risk (Table 12-1).

Hypertension, or High Blood Pressure

There is no doubt that untreated hypertension accelerates atherogenesis and the incidence of heart disease. The Framingham Study has shown that there is a higher rate of IHD in individuals with diastolic pressures greater than 105 mm Hg (millimeters of mercury) than in individuals whose diastolic pressure is less than 85 mm Hg, and that after forty-five years of age high blood pressure is a greater risk factor than high cholesterol levels. Recent studies have found that, by fifty-five years of age, women have the same incidence of hypertension as men. According to the data, hypertension is present in more than half of all women older than fifty-five years and in two-thirds of women over sixty-five years of age. Hypertension will be discussed in more detail later in the chapter.

TABLE 12-1	Ratio of Total Cholesterol to HDL Cholesterol	
Risk	Male	Female
Very low (1/2 average)	Under 3.4	Under 3.3
Low risk	4.0	3.8
Average risk	5.0	4.5
Moderate risk (2 × average)	9.5	7.0
High risk (3 × average)	Over 23	Over 11

Smoking

The association between smoking and heart disease is well documented. Included in the findings are the following: when autopsies are performed, there is a greater degree of aortic and coronary AS in smokers than in nonsmokers; when a smoker gives up smoking, his (most studies to date have been done on males) risk of dying of IHD decreases with each year that he is smoke-free; if a person smokes, there is a far greater risk of dying of a heart attack; since women have begun to smoke, their risk of coronary heart disease has been increasing; and finally, the death rate from IHD is 70 percent to 200 percent higher in men who smoke one or more packs of cigarettes a day than in those who don't smoke.

Diabetes Mellitus

Diabetes seems to make people susceptible to AS. It is estimated that about seventy-five percent of diabetics under forty years of age have moderate to severe AS in comparison to five percent of nondiabetics. Although research is still going on to find a definitive relationship, several factors are thought to increase the incidence of AS in diabetics. *Hyperlipidemia* occurs in one-third to one-half of diabetics. Type II diabetics have *lower levels of HDL,* making them more susceptible to AS. Diabetics also have *increased platelet adhesiveness,* which can affect atherogenesis. Finally, many Type II diabetics are *obese* and have *hypertension,* both of which can contribute to the formation of atherosclerotic plaques.

Miscellaneous Factors

There are other factors that may be related to the development of AS. Although the relationship has not yet been verified by research, evidence of their connection is gradually accumulating. These include (1) competitive, stressful lifestyle with type A behavior; (2) **hyperuricemia** (excess uric acid in the blood); (3) obesity; (4) lack of regular exercise; (5) high intake of carbohydrates; and (6) use of oral contraceptives, particularly combined with smoking (this applies more to those who have used oral contraceptives in the past; oral contraceptives are thought to be safer today).

Symptoms

Symptoms of AS do not appear until the disease is far advanced. They occur when the lumen of the artery has become so small that the blood supply to a body part is restricted. If this happens to be in a coronary artery, then the decrease in oxygen to the heart causes angina pectoris, a severe pain and/or feeling of pressure in the region of the heart that usually radiates to the left shoulder and down the left arm. Other symptoms may occur, depending upon the severity of the attack. If the blood flow is restricted to the muscles of the legs, there is pain in the legs during walking that is relieved by rest. A decrease of blood flow in the arteries supplying the brain may cause transient ischemic attacks (TIAs), which produce symptoms and signs of a stroke (see Cerebrovascular Accident, page 268) but last less than twenty-four hours, and/or episodes of dizziness. Rarely, a person might have no pain but instead, severe nausea, weakness, and sudden perspiration. Also, the pain can be referred to other sites as shown in Figure 12-8.

hyperuricemia	hi-per-u-ris-E-me-a

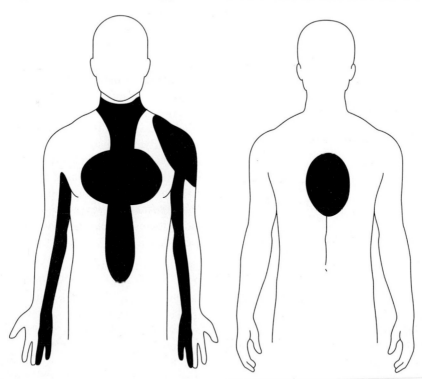

Figure 12-8

Some sites of pain and pressure for angina (left) and heart attack (right). Any severe pain in these areas should be reported to a physician.

Prevention

Prevention depends upon controlling or eliminating risk factors (which are discussed under Predisposing Factors) as much as possible with medical care and a healthful lifestyle (see Chapter 2).

Treatment

The severity and location of the diseased arteries have to be considered to prescribe treatment. In studies conducted by the Stanford Center for Research in Disease Prevention, it has been shown that HDL levels are increased by the right diet and regular exercise alone. This beneficial effect has occurred in all groups tested (by the Stanford Center as well as other institutions), including people with coronary heart disease, the elderly, men, women, and children. And according to the National Institutes of Health (NIH), for most people, "quitting smoking and paying rigorous attention to diet, weight control, and exercise are all that's needed" to optimize lipid levels and reduce the risk of coronary heart disease (resulting from AS). Drugs to decrease lipidemia are only used if dietary and lifestyle modifications do not succeed in lowering the LDL or increasing HDL or if lipid levels are dangerously high.

Hypertension

Hypertension is another condition that is a strong risk factor for heart disease (see Atherosclerosis). Blood pressure is measured by use of a stethoscope and cuff called a **sphygmomanometer.** When a reading is taken, the systolic pressure is heard first, and the diastolic second. The systolic reading is the amount of pressure placed against the walls of the arteries when the ventricles are contracting. The diastolic reading is the amount of pressure placed against the walls of the arteries when the heart is at rest.

There is controversy among clinicians as to when to start treatment for hypertension. Normal blood pressure in most young adults is 120/80 (120 systolic and 80 diastolic). Blood pressure of highly trained athletes could be much lower. Borderline hypertension, according to the NIH, is 140/90 to 160/95, with a diastolic pressure of 90 to

104 indicating a need for treatment. Generally, readings need to be done more than once on individuals before they can be diagnosed as hypertensive, because there are fluctuations that occur naturally during the day. Because the diastolic reading indicates how much rest the heart is getting, there is more concern over a high diastolic reading than a high systolic reading. For some people, the trip to the doctor's office is enough to raise their blood pressure. Other factors, including emotional and physical stress, can cause the systolic pressure to rise temporarily. This is the reason that at least two readings are taken before a diagnosis of hypertension is given.

There are two types of hypertension, *essential* and *secondary.* Another term used when speaking of high blood pressure is *malignant hypertension,* a severe form in which the blood pressure rises rapidly, resulting in the possibility of injury to the arterioles. It may be present in either kind of hypertension.

Essential Hypertension

Also referred to as primary or idiopathic hypertension, essential hypertension is the most common form. It is estimated by the AHA that fifty million Americans (approximately one-fourth) have high blood pressure. Although risk factors are known, an underlying cause has not been identified. The term *essential hypertension* may be confusing when the common meaning of *essential* is used; in referring to diseases, however, the words *essential, idiopathic,* and *primary* are used to indicate a condition that is present for which no cause has been identified.

Predisposing Factors

Risk factors for essential hypertension include family history, race, stress, obesity, high dietary intake of saturated fats or sodium, use of tobacco, use of oral contraceptives, and insufficient physical activity.

Some people are exposed to one or more of these factors and never develop hypertension. But people who do develop hypertension generally have one or more of these factors in their lives. Family history, race, and aging cannot be con-

most
High BP pills — are Potassium depleters / Diuretics — urinate out potassium

trolled, but the rest can, and if they are, then essential hypertension can be reduced to normal and kept there.

Symptoms

Most people with hypertension have no symptoms until the disease causes changes in the blood vessels. Severely elevated blood pressure damages the inner walls of the arteries, causing fibrin accumulation, swelling, and, possibly, blood clots. The symptoms of advanced disease vary, depending on the location of the damaged vessels. If they are in the area of the brain, a cerebrovascular accident (CVA), or stroke, may occur; in the retina, blindness; in the heart, myocardial infarction; and in the kidneys, **proteinuria,** edema, and eventually, renal failure.

Prevention

To prevent hypertension, any risk factors that can be changed should be. Persons with family histories of hypertension, stroke, or heart attack should have their blood pressure checked at least once a year. An annual checkup is wise for all young people and adults; anyone who has undergone a prolonged period of stress or who is obese should be checked more frequently.

Treatment

Exercise has proved to be just as effective as drugs in lowering blood pressure. A low-fat diet, salt restriction, and weight control can also help. If exercise, decreasing dietary fat and salt, and attaining the best body weight do not help, there are many drugs that can be used. The main categories are diuretics, beta blockers, calcium channel blockers, and ACE inhibitors that block a hormone known as angiotensin. Angiotensin has a strong influence on blood pressure. Some doctors will initiate drug therapy at a higher level of pressure than others, feeling that the side effects of the drugs may do more harm than a moderately raised pressure.

With proper treatment, most people are able to lower their pressure enough to avoid serious damage to the blood vessels. Unfortunately, it is difficult to get people to stay on a regular schedule of drugs and/or lifestyle changes, because symp-

toms are normally not present or are so mild as to be unnoticed.

Secondary Hypertension — caused b/c of some other disease

Secondary hypertension results from renal disease or other identifiable causes, including endocrine, vascular, and neurogenic disorders. Some of these will be discussed in Chapter 16.

Coronary Artery Disease (CAD)

The heart has its own blood supply (Figure 12-9). When the supply of blood to the heart is insufficient, it is usually a result of coronary artery disease (CAD). This disease is more prevalent in white people, the middle-aged, and the elderly. Before menopause, women have less heart disease than men, but after menopause, their chances of a heart attack gradually increase. White males under forty-five years of age in the United States have a six times greater risk than women of the same age. In males forty-five to fifty-four years of age there is a four- to fivefold difference, and by the eighth decade, there is only a twofold difference. The difference between men and women in susceptibility to CAD is not completely understood. It was thought that the female hormone estrogen had a protective effect, but when estrogen supplements were given to men in scientific studies, there was no difference in CAD mortality. It is possible that male hormones, including testosterone, are correlated with increased risk for CAD. As was stated earlier, researchers have just begun to use female subjects for cardiovascular research. This should result in more verifiable information.

Predisposing Factors

AS is the usual cause of CAD. When the atheromas, made of cholesterol, other fats, and cellular debris, build up on the walls of the coronary arteries, the blood flow to the heart muscle is reduced. This condition is referred to as cardiac ischemia.

---

sphygmomanometer   sfig-mo-man-OM-et-er
idiopathic   id-e-o-PATH-ik
proteinuria   pro-te-in-U-re-a

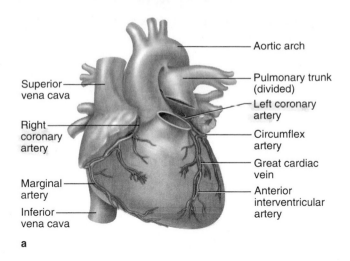

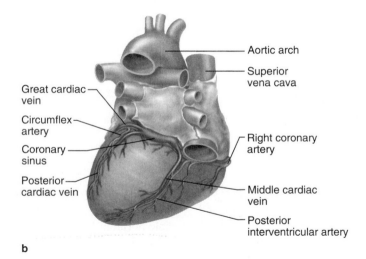

Figure 12-9

The coronary blood vessels (a) anterior aspect of the heart. (b) Posterior aspect of the heart.

Narrowing of a vessel lumen results in slowing the movement of blood, and a thrombus may form. If the thrombus occludes the lumen or an embolus moves to the site, the blood flow may be shut off completely, leading to a myocardial infarction, to be discussed next. The predisposing factors for AS were discussed earlier in the chapter.

Symptoms

Angina pectoris (generally shortened to angina) is the classic symptom of CAD. It is usually described as a squeezing or crushing tightness in the chest. The tightness may radiate to the left arm, neck, jaw, or shoulder blade, and sometimes is felt as a dull pain or burning (see

Figure 12-8). The pain or tightness may also be accompanied by nausea, vomiting, fainting, sweating, and cold hands and feet. These attacks often follow physical exertion, large meals, or stressful experiences.

Prevention

Prevention measures are the same as for AS.

Treatment

In addition to changes in lifestyle, drugs may be used to reduce oxygen consumption by the heart or to increase oxygen supply to the heart. Those now in use include nitrates, beta blockers, and calcium channel blockers, all of which (by different actions) increase oxygen supply to the heart and reduce myocardial demand for oxygen. Also, because excess platelets have been found to decrease the flow of blood to the heart, antiplatelet agents may be used.

Angioplasty, a procedure in which a balloon is inserted into the artery and then inflated, is sometimes used to treat CAD. This procedure helps to widen the lumen and establish an increased flow of blood to the heart (Figure 12-10).

Coronary artery bypass grafts are used to treat the condition surgically if the angina is severe, ventricular function is good, and the coronary arteries are in good condition. The techniques for this surgery have improved steadily, and one of the newest methods involves using an artery from the breast rather than a vein from the leg. These techniques are **palliative** rather than curative, because the atherosclerotic process will continue unless changes in diet, exercise, and other habits that are known to increase the risk of AS occur.

Myocardial Infarct (Heart Attack)

A heart attack, or myocardial infarct (MI), occurs when the blood flow is reduced, by AS or a clot, through one or more of the coronary arteries, causing ischemia and necrosis (death of tissue, or infarct). Death often results from the cardiac damage or complications, particularly when treatment is delayed. Almost half of sudden deaths caused

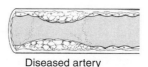
Diseased artery

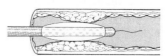
Balloon catheter positioned in stenotic area

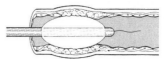
Inflated balloon presses plaque against arterial wall

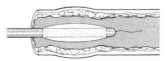
Balloon is deflated and blood flow is reestablished

Figure 12-10
Balloon angioplasty.

by MI occur within one hour of the onset of symptoms, before the individual is hospitalized. Death occurs in four to six minutes if the heart stops beating, but if cardiopulmonary resuscitation (CPR) is begun immediately, the chances of survival are greatly increased. As was discussed earlier, females have lower mortality rates from MI than males, especially before menopause.

Predisposing Factors

The causes of MI are the same as for coronary artery disease, because the latter leads to MI. A family history of MI, hypertension, smoking, elevated serum triglyceride and cholesterol levels, diabetes mellitus, obesity, sedentary lifestyle, and inability to control stress are all considered to be predisposing factors.

---

angioplasty AN-je-o-plas-te
palliative PAL-e-a-tiv

Symptoms

A persistent crushing pain in the chest area beneath the sternum (breastbone) is the most common symptom. This pain may radiate to the left arm, jaw, neck, or shoulder blades. It is often described as crushing, squeezing, or heavy and may be accompanied by vomiting, sweating, and difficulty in breathing. In some cases, the pain may not occur at all; indigestion is often the only sign. Angina of increasing frequency may indicate that an MI is imminent. Sometimes victims have a feeling of impending doom. They may also feel fatigued and experience vomiting and a feeling of suffocation.

Prevention

Preventive measures are the same as for AS.

Treatment

Immediate administration of CPR when the heart has stopped and emergency medical treatment can be lifesaving. Various drugs may be administered to relieve chest pain, stabilize heart rhythm, and reduce the load on the heart. Among these are antiarrhythmics, diuretics, nitroglycerin, and morphine.

RHEUMATIC HEART DISEASE

Rheumatic heart disease is a result of a systemic inflammatory disease of childhood (see Chapter 4, Rheumatic Fever) that generally follows a streptococcal infection. Inflammation of the heart (pancarditis, which includes endocarditis [Chapter 6], myocarditis, and pericarditis) can lead to heart damage, particularly to the valves. Eventually the valvular problem may lead to congestive heart failure. The incidence of rheumatic fever and its sequelae, including rheumatic heart disease, has decreased in the United States over the years since antibiotic treatment became available. For the period from 1985 to 1995, the death rate for rheumatic fever and rheumatic heart disease fell 36.8 percent according to the AHA.

Predisposing Factors

The predisposing factor for rheumatic heart disease is rheumatic fever.

Symptoms

About fifty percent of those who develop rheumatic fever go on to develop pancarditis and/or damaged heart valves. The symptoms of acute rheumatic fever are very similar to those of other disorders (see Rheumatic Fever in Chapter 4), and because they do not occur for one to five weeks after the streptococcal infection, they may not be recognized as symptoms of rheumatic fever. The earliest sign of rheumatic heart disease may be a murmur, caused by valve dysfunction, that has gone undetected for many years. There may also be other symptoms, including chest pain, extra heart sounds, heart block, and atrial fibrillation. However, once the acute stage of rheumatic fever is passed, there may be an undetected residual effect on the heart valves that is not diagnosed and only discovered years later when the individual is subjected to heart surgery (perhaps for another reason).

Prevention

Because rheumatic heart disease is always a result of rheumatic fever, which follows a streptococcal infection, prevention of rheumatic heart disease depends on early treatment of streptococcal infections and continued treatment and management of rheumatic fever should it develop.

Treatment

If there is severe valve dysfunction of the heart, then corrective valvular surgery can be performed. This seldom occurs before adolescence and, as was mentioned earlier, in the absence of apparent symptoms, may not be identified for many years.

CONGESTIVE HEART FAILURE (CHF)

Although the heart is a single organ, heart failure may begin on the right or left side but will eventually affect the whole heart.

Congestive heart failure (CHF) occurs when the heart cannot keep up its work load of pumping blood to the lungs and the rest of the body. This inability generally occurs because the left ventricle has been damaged, but it may also result if the right ventricle is damaged. In either case, failure of one side of the heart will gradually affect the whole heart. It may be acute, as a direct result of MI, but it is generally a chronic disorder resulting in decreased pumping of blood from the heart and associated with retention of salt and water, which leads to swelling in the legs and ankles.

⚒ Right-sided heart failure is most often a result of right ventricular strain caused by disease of the lungs or pulmonary arteries and is referred to as **cor pulmonale.**

Predisposing Factors

CHF can be caused by a number of factors. Included in these are MI, hypertension, **mitral stenosis** (narrowing of the mitral valve opening) secondary to rheumatic heart disease, and aortic stenosis (Figure 12-11).

Symptoms

Fatigue, **dyspnea** (shortness of breath), enlarged neck veins when the victim is in an upright posi-tion, nocturia (excessive urination at night), and enlargement of the liver are among the signs of CHF. Patients sometimes have coldlike symptoms with a dry cough and confuse the condition with an allergic reaction.

Prevention

Preventive measures are the same as for AS.

Treatment

Bed rest with diuretics to reduce blood volume, digitalis to strengthen myocardial contractility, and **vasodilators** to increase cardiac output are among the therapies used to treat CHF.

cor pulmonale	cor PUL-mon-al
mitral stenosis	MI-tral sten-O-sis
dyspnea	disp-NE-a, DISP-ne-a
vasodilators	vas-o-di-LA-tors

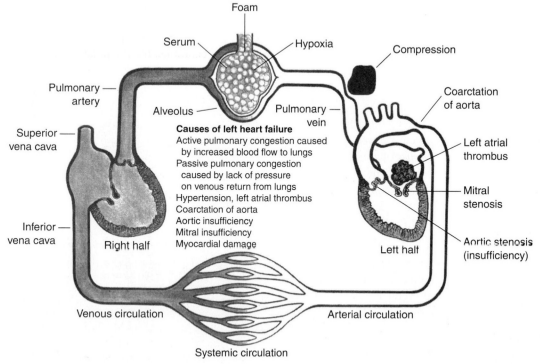

Figure 12-11

Conditions leading to congestive heart failure.

Thrombophlebitis

Inflammation of a vein accompanied by formation of a **thrombus** is called **thrombophlebitis.** The disease usually occurs in an extremity, and most often a leg. If it is in a superficial vein, it is not as serious and is less likely to lead to an **embolism.** In the deep veins, the condition has to be monitored carefully, because the thrombus can become an embolus and travel to the lungs, resulting in pulmonary embolism, which can be fatal.

Predisposing Factors

There are a number of factors involved in the formation of thrombi. Anything that causes an alteration of the epithelial lining of the vein can lead to a thrombus. The process may occur as a result of surgery or trauma. Cardiovascular disorders, obesity, heredity, increasing age, an excess of platelets and overproduction of fibrinogen, use of oral contraceptives, and prolonged bed rest are also among the identified causes. Intravenous drug abuse and extensive use of the intravenous route for medication and diagnostic tests may cause superficial thrombophlebitis.

Symptoms

As the thrombus grows, chemicals are released, resulting in heat, pain, swelling, redness, tenderness, and hardness along the length of the affected vein in superficial thrombophlebitis. There may be no symptoms for deep-vein thrombophlebitis, or the patient may experience pain, fever, chills, malaise, and possibly swelling and cyanosis (blueness caused by reduced oxygen in the general circulation) of the affected arm or leg.

Prevention

Although some predisposing factors cannot be changed, reducing the risk factors for AS, which have already been discussed, and making any other changes possible to reduce other risk factors will help to prevent thrombophlebitis.

Treatment

The main goal of treatment is to prevent the thrombus from becoming an embolus and traveling to the lungs. Pain relief is provided by administration of analgesics. Bed rest with elevation of the affected arm or leg, moist soaks, anticoagulants for deep-vein thrombophlebitis, and antiembolism stockings (after it is safe to walk) are used in treatment.

Varicose Veins

Varicose veins are dilated and twisted veins, usually superficial, in which blood tends to accumulate and stagnate because of defective valves. Because they are near the surface, the pressure of the excess blood produces a bluish raised area along the line of the vein. Nodules can be seen pushing the skin in front of them (Figure 12-12). Most often varicose veins occur in the legs but may also appear in the rectal area as hemorrhoids.

Predisposing Factors

Factors that may contribute to the development of varicose veins are obesity, hormonal changes during pregnancy or at menopause, pressure on the pelvic veins during pregnancy, and standing for long periods.

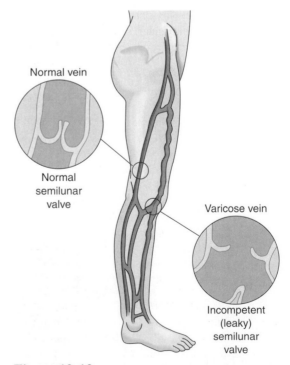

Normal vein

Normal semilunar valve

Varicose vein

Incompetent (leaky) semilunar valve

Figure 12-12
Varicose veins.

Symptoms

There may be no symptoms or mild to severe symptoms, including cramps at night, dull aching, fatigability, and pain in feet and ankles.

Prevention

Avoiding obesity and long periods of standing can reduce the risk. If weight gain during pregnancy does not go beyond the optimal level, this may also reduce the risk for women.

Treatment

Surgery is possible but not advised unless the problem becomes severe. Antiembolism stockings, prescribed exercise (to improve blood flow), rest, and elevation of the extremity are the usual treatment.

CONGENITAL HEART DEFECTS

An abnormality of the heart that is present from birth, congenital heart defect occurs in six to eight babies per 1000 born. Some defects are not apparent at birth and may not become evident until adolescence or adulthood. The most common heart deformities are ventricular septal defect (VSD), **patent ductus arteriosus** (PDA), atrial septal defect (ASD), pulmonic stenosis, coarctation of the aorta, and **tetralogy of Fallot** (Figure 12-13).

Symptoms

Defects in the structures of the heart lead to insufficient or excessive circulation of the blood to the lungs or to the body. In some cases, deoxygenated blood might be pumped to the body instead of to the lungs, or oxygenated blood might be pumped to the lungs instead of to the body. These conditions will cause cyanosis, difficulty in breathing, or both. Children with heart defects may tire rapidly with activity. As has been mentioned before, symptoms may not occur until adulthood.

Predisposing Factors

In most cases (over 90%) the cause is unknown. However, both environmental and genetic risk factors are thought to be involved. Environmental factors include conditions affecting the mother, such as rubella, smoking, and alcoholism and other drug use. There is well documented evidence

of the defects that can occur as a consequence of maternal rubella in the first trimester of pregnancy.

The age of the mother at time of pregnancy is a factor also because more defects tend to occur in babies as the mother's age increases, particularly over forty years of age. Hereditary factors do not seem to play a significant role. Because a couple has one child with a birth defect does not mean that a second child will be affected.

Prevention

Women need to abstain from alcohol if there is a chance that they could be pregnant, because some researchers believe that just one drink could cause a defect if it is taken early in the development of the fetus. If a woman is pregnant, she needs to stay away from anyone with rubella, and girls should not be vaccinated against rubella after puberty. Women over forty years of age should be aware of the possibility of congenital defects in the baby should they decide to have a child. During pregnancy, no drugs should be taken by the mother unless approved by the doctor.

Treatment

Rest, oxygen, and various drugs may be used initially and offer temporary or indefinite relief. Some defects present at birth may get smaller or disappear as the child gets older. However, if the condition of the child (or adult in some cases) worsens, then surgery may be considered.

Surgical correction of heart disease caused by congenital defects is an area of medicine in which there has been good progress, resulting in improved techniques. Corrective surgery is now available for most heart defects. Narrowed heart valves can be treated by balloon **valvuloplasty,** in which a catheter is introduced into the heart to widen the affected valve. In some cases, open

---

thrombus   THROM-bus
thrombophlebitis   throm-bo-fle-BI-tis
embolism   EM-bo-lizm
patent ductus arteriosus (PDA)   PAT-ent DUK-tus
tetralogy of Fallot   tet-RAL-o-gy of FAL-lut
valvuloplasty   VAL-vu-lo-plas-te

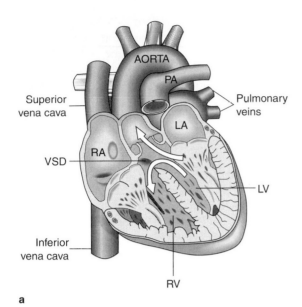

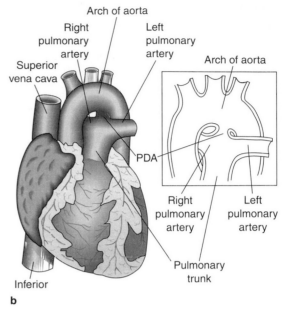

Figure 12-13

Three common congenital heart defects: (a), ventricular septal defect; (b), patent ductus arteriosus; (c), atrial septal defect.

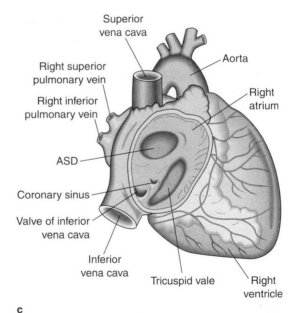

heart surgery is necessary, and some conditions can be treated only by a heart transplant.

Children who have successful heart surgery gradually have a near-normal life span. However, they are more susceptible to endocarditis, and preventive antibiotics may be prescribed.

CEREBROVASCULAR DISEASE

Cerebrovascular Accident (Stroke)

Although cerebrovascular accidents affect the brain, they are caused by disorders of or in the blood vessels.

A cerebrovascular accident (CVA), or stroke, is caused by a sudden impairment of cerebral circulation in one or more of the blood vessels supplying the brain. This impairment may be due to a thrombus, embolus, or hemorrhage. In older people, thrombosis is the most common cause. It tends to occur while the person is asleep or shortly after awakening. It can also occur during surgery or after a heart attack. An embolism, the second most common cause, may occur at any age but is more likely among people who have a history of some types of heart disease or after open-heart surgery. Hemorrhage may also occur at any age and results from chronic hypertension or aneurysms that cause sudden rupture of a cerebral artery.

The interruption or insufficiency of oxygen supply can lead to serious damage and death of

WARNING SIGNS OF STROKE

Although many stroke victims have little advance warning of an impending crisis, there are some warning signals of stroke that should be recognized. The American Heart Association encourages everyone to be aware of the following signs:

- Sudden, temporary weakness or numbness of the face, arm, and leg on one side of the body
- Temporary loss of speech or trouble in speaking or understanding speech
- Temporary dimness or loss of vision, particularly in one eye
- Unexplained dizziness, unsteadiness, or sudden falls
- Many major strokes are preceded by "little strokes," warning signals like the above, experienced days, weeks, or months before the more severe event

   Prompt medical or surgical attention to these symptoms may prevent a fatal or disabling stroke from occurring.

cells in brain tissue. About half of the people who survive a CVA remain permanently disabled and experience another stroke within weeks, months, or years. CVA is the third most common cause of death in the United States today and the most common cause of neurologic (brain and spinal cord) disability.

Predisposing Factors

All the risk factors for ischemic heart disease resulting from AS also apply to CVA; in addition, a history of transient ischemic attacks, gout, and postural hypotension (blood pressure below normal on standing) have been found to increase the risk.

Symptoms

Strokes are classified according to their course of progression. A transient ischemic attack (TIA) lasts only a few seconds to hours and is referred to as a "little stroke." A progressive stroke or stroke in evolution, begins with slight neurologic impairment that gradually worsens within a day or two. In a completed stroke, the damage is maximal in the beginning. The symptoms for the completed stroke generally occur suddenly, with unconsciousness and heavy breathing caused by paralysis of a portion of the soft palate. The pupils are sometimes unequal, with the larger one being on the side of the hemorrhage or occlusion. Paralysis usually involves one side of the body, skin is sweaty, and speech disturbances are present. If caused by a thrombosis, onset may be more gradual, with generalized symptoms such as headache, vomiting, mental impairment, convulsions, fever, and disorientation.

Prevention

Primary prevention involves elimination or reduction of any predisposing factors possible. For secondary prevention, the box above gives the warning signs for a stroke published by the AHA. These should be learned, and if any signs are present in anyone, medical help should be sought immediately.

Treatment

Following the stroke, anticonvulsants may be used to prevent seizures; stool softeners to avoid straining, which increases intracranial pressure; corticosteroids to minimize swelling; and analgesics to relieve headache, but not aspirin if hemorrhagic CVA has occurred. Surgery may be performed to improve cerebral circulation for patients with thrombotic or embolic CVA.

SUMMARY

Table 12-2 summarizes relevant data on cardiovascular and cerebrovascular diseases.

TABLE 12-2	Cardiovascular Disease				
Disease	**Special Characteristics**	**Predisposing Factors**	**Some Common Symptoms**	**Prevention/ Control**	**Treatment**
Atherosclerosis (AS) (A form of arterio-sclerosis)	Atheromas form on lining of arteries, most commonly in aorta, coronary, and cerebral arteries. Progressive narrowing of lumen causes decrease in blood flow to tissue in area. Clot may block the vessel completely and result in an MI, a CVA, or other tissue damage depending on location. One theory of cause is reaction to injury	Age, sex, family predisposition, hyperlipidermia, hypertension, smoking, and diabetes mellitus definite; stressful lifestyle, aggressive personality, obesity, lack of exercise and use of oral contraceptives possible; cholesterol is a major component of atheromatic plaque; LDL strongly related to AS; HDL disposes of cholesterol	Angina pectoris (severe, constricting pain in chest, often radiating to left shoulder and down the arm), TIAs, and other symptoms depending on location of plaques	Prevention depends upon controlling or eliminating risk factors as much as possible with medical care and a healthy lifestyle. The condition can be reversed with diet and exercise	HDL levels can be improved by the right diet and regular exercise if the disease is not too far advanced. For most cases, quitting smoking, a healthful diet, weight control, and exercise can optimize lipid levels and reduce the risk of AS. Nitroglycerine is often prescribed for angina
Hypertension (HBP or HT)	Essential HBP is most common, cause is unknown. Secondary HBP results from another identifiable cause. Malignant HBP can occur in either form—BP rises quickly, causing dam-	Family history, race, stress, obesity, high fat or high sodium diet, tobacco use, oral contraceptive use, sedentary lifestyle, and aging	No symptoms until another serious disease occurs as a result of HBP such as renal failure, an MI, or a stroke	Controlling or eliminating risk factors, yearly blood pressure check are preventive measures	For essential hypertension, regular exercise and a low-fat diet may be all that is needed. In some cases, salt restriction and weight reduction may be necessary also. Treatment

TABLE 12-2	Continued				
Disease	**Special Characteristics**	**Predisposing Factors**	**Some Common Symptoms**	**Prevention/ Control**	**Treatment**
Hypertension (HBP or HT)—Cont'd	age to arteries. BP of 140/90 or below is generally considered "normal"				for secondary hypertension depends on the cause
Coronary Artery Disease (CAD)	Insufficient supply of blood to the heart is usually caused by AS and/or a clot in the coronary arteries	Same as AS	Angina is the classic symptom of CAD; described as a squeezing or tightness in the chest; may also have pain in left arm, neck, jaw, or shoulder blade; nausea, vomiting, fainting, sweating, cold hands or feet; often after physical or emotional stress; may have only one symptom or many of them	Preventive measures are the same as for AS	Treatment is the same as for AS
Myocardial Infarction (MI)	Reduced blood flow to the heart causes ischemia and necrosis. Death occurs in 4–6 minutes if heart stops beating and CPR is not administered	Same as AS	Indigestion may be only sign; more often, pain in center of chest under sternum described as heavy, crushing, or squeezing, which may	Preventive measures are the same as for AS	CPR, drugs, cardioversion, and pacemaker are treatments used, depending on the case

TABLE 12-2	*Continued*				
Disease	**Special Characteristics**	**Predisposing Factors**	**Some Common Symptoms**	**Prevention/ Control**	**Treatment**
Myocardial Infarction (MI)— Cont'd			radiate to left arm, jaw, neck, or shoulder; there may also be vomiting, sweating, and difficulty in breathing; also see symptoms for AS		
Rheumatic Heart Disease	Results from rheumatic fever, which may follow a streptococcal infection in childhood. Months or years after having RF, damage to the heart may be discovered. Exact cause is unknown	Under-nourished children living in crowded conditions are more susceptible; lowered resistance may be involved	Rheumatic fever: joint pain, fever, transient chorea; rheumatic heart disease: inflammation of the heart, congestive heart failure, damage to one or more heart valves	Early antibiotic treatment of any streptococcal infection can prevent rheumatic heart disease	Emphasis is on aggressive treatment of rheumatic fever. Treatment for rheumatic heart disease varies depending on the presenting heart problems.
Congestive Heart Failure	Inability of heart to maintain circulation, usually because of damaged left ventricle. Has many different causes	Myocardial infarct, hypertension, mitral or aortic stenosis, and other conditions that weaken heart	Fatigue, dyspnea, enlarged neck veins, enlarged liver, coldlike symptoms with a dry cough, swelling of ankles	Preventive measures are the same as for AS	Bed rest, diuretics to reduce blood volume, digitalis to strengthen myocardial contractility, and vasodilators to increase cardiac output are used depending on patient's con-

TABLE 12-2	*Continued*				
Disease	**Special Characteristics**	**Predisposing Factors**	**Some Common Symptoms**	**Prevention/ Control**	**Treatment**
Congestive Heart Failure					dition. Once the heart failure is treated, the underlying cause is sought and treated
Thrombo-phlebitis	Inflammation of vein accompanied by formation of a thrombus. Most often occurs in a leg. Involvement of deeper veins more serious as it may lead to embolism, which can travel to lungs and be fatal	Many factors— anything that causes a change in the lining of the vein; may be a result of surgery, childbirth, obesity, heredity, aging, excess of platelets, overproduction of fibrinogen, oral contraceptives, and prolonged bed rest	Heat, pain, swelling, redness, tenderness and hardness along length of vein; possible pain, fever, chills, malaise, and cyanosis for deep vein	Preventive measures are the same as for AS	Bed rest with leg or arm elevated. Anti-coagulants, anti-inflammatory drugs, moist soaks, and anti-embolism stockings may also be prescribed depending on the case
Varicose Veins	Caused by accumulation of blood in veins because of defective valves. Most often in legs but may be in rectal area (hemorrhoids)	Heredity, prolonged standing, varied amounts of pressure (hemorrhoids), pregnancy	May be none or dull aching, fatigability, pain in feet and ankles, cramps at night	Preventive measures are the same as for AS	Antiembolism stockings, prescribed exercise, rest, and elevation of the affected leg; surgery is indicated only in severe cases
Congenital Heart Defects	Any heart abnormality that is present from birth. They include	Cause unknown in over 90% of cases; possible genetic and environ-	Depend on type of defect— cyanosis, tire easily; may be none until	Keeping pregnant women as healthy as possible will help some	Rest, oxygen, and various drugs may offer relief. If not, surgery

TABLE 12-2	*Continued*				
Disease	**Special Characteristics**	**Predisposing Factors**	**Some Common Symptoms**	**Prevention/ Control**	**Treatment**
Congenital Heart Defects— Cont'd	ventricular septal defect, patent ductus arteriosum, artrial septal defect, pulmonary stenosis, coarctation of the aorta, aortic stenosis, and tetralogy of Fallot. Most occur during first trimester	mental; (conditions affecting mother, i.e., rubella, drinking, age)	adult—may be found during surgery for other heart disease	but until a cause is identified, these defects will continue to occur	may be considered and many effective techniques of correcting congenital heart defects have been developed
Cerebro-vascular Accident (Stroke)	Caused by a sudden impairment of circulation in one or more of the blood vessels supplying the brain. Three types include: TIA, progressive, and completed. Third most common cause of death in U.S.	Same as atherosclerosis plus history of TIAs, gout, postural hypotension	May be none; generally sudden unconsciousness, heavy breathing, unequal pupil size, paralysis on one side, sweaty skin, speech disturbances; can be more gradual with headache, vomiting, mental impairment, convulsions, fever, and disorientation	Preventive measures are the same as for AS	Anticonvulsants, stool softeners, corticosteroids, and analgesics are used. Surgery can be done if necessary to improve circulation

QUESTIONS FOR REVIEW

1. What caused the change in emphasis from infectious to noninfectious disease?
2. What route does the blood take in circulating through the heart?
3. What is the pathway for the electrical impulses that cause the heart to beat?
4. What is AS?
5. Which arteries are most frequently affected by AS?
6. What is the reaction to injury theory of atherogenesis?
7. What are the end results of uncontrolled AS?
8. Which risk factors for AS can and cannot be changed?
9. What is the connection between AS and cholesterol?
10. What are the lipoproteins in the blood?
11. How are hypertension, smoking, and diabetes mellitus related to AS?
12. What symptoms may be present in AS?
13. What is the significance of the levels of HDL and LDL in a person's blood?
14. What factors are thought to have a relationship to AS, although more evidence needs to be gathered?
15. What is balloon angioplasty?
16. What is the difference between essential hypertension, secondary hypertension, and malignant hypertension?
17. What damage may occur in the body if a person has untreated hypertension?
18. What are considered safe limits for systolic and diastolic blood pressure readings?
19. What are the risk factors for hypertension?
20. Why do individuals with hypertension often neglect to take their medication?
21. How can blood pressure be lowered without drugs?
22. What is the usual cause of coronary artery disease?
23. What are the symptoms of coronary artery disease?
24. What is the difference between the symptoms of angina and those of an MI?
25. What risk factors are associated with congestive heart failure?
26. Why does rheumatic heart disease occur in some who have had rheumatic fever and not in others?
27. What is the progression from rheumatic fever to rheumatic heart disease?
28. What danger is present when thrombophlebitis occurs in a deep vein?
29. What factors may lead to thrombophlebitis?
30. What factors are associated with varicose veins?
31. What congenital heart defects are covered in this chapter?
32. What might be the cause of each of the heart defects named in response to question 31?
33. What treatments can be used for the heart defects named in response to question 31?
34. What is a CVA?
35. What are the risk factors for CVA?
36. Why is a transient ischemic attack a significant predisposing factor for a stroke?
37. What measures are used in treatment of stroke?

FURTHER READING

Alder, S. J., et al. 1999. Limitations of clinical diagnosis in acute stroke. *The Lancet* 354:1523.

Alderman, Michael H. 1999. Measures and meaning of blood pressure. *The Lancet* 355:159.

Alpert, Joseph S. 1999. Coronary heart disease: Where have we been and where are we going? *The Lancet* 353:1540.

Alpert, Martin A. 1999. Homocyst(e)ine, atherosclerosis, and thrombosis. *Southern Medical Journal* 92:858.

Atherosclerosis risk factor: chlamydia pneumoniae? *American Journal of Nursing* 99:16, 1999.

Benitez, R. Michael. 1999. Atherosclerosis: An infectious disease? *Hospital Practice* 34:79.

Bennett, P. 1999. Intrusive memories, post-traumatic stress disorder and myocardial infarction. *British Journal of Clinical Psychology* 38:411.

Berger, Klaus. 1999. Moderate alcohol consumption may lower risk of ischemic stroke. *American Family Physician* 60:1791.

Berlowitz, D. R., A. S. Ash, E. C. Hickey, et al. 1998. Inadequate management of blood pressure in a hypertensive population. *The New England Journal of Medicine* 339:1957.

Biller, Jose, and William H. Thies. 2000. When to operate in carotid artery disease. *American Family Physician* 61:400.

Bonn, Dorothy. 1999. Plaque detection: the key to tackling atherosclerosis. *The Lancet* 354:656.

Bosch, Xavier. 1999. Mechanism for putative link between atherosclerosis and viruses found. *The Lancet* 354:1976.

Bosetti, C. 1999. Smoking and acute myocardial infarction among women and men. *Prevention Medicine* 29:343.

Bosworth, H. B. 1999. The association between self-rated health and mortality in a well-characterized sample of coronary artery disease patients. *Medical Care* 37:1226.

Brown, Morris. 1999. Do vitamin E and fish oil protect against ischaemic heart disease? *The Lancet* 354:441.

Campbell, Lee Ann, Cho-Chou Kuo, and Thomas J. Grayston. 1998. Chlamydia pneumoniae and cardiovascular disease. *Emerging Infectious Disease* 4.

Campbell, Norman R. C., et al. 1999. Lifestyle changes to prevent and control hypertension: do they work? *Canadian Medical Association Journal* 160:1341.

Cappuccio, Francesco P., et al. 1999. High blood pressure and bone-mineral loss in elderly white women: a prospective study. *The Lancet* 354:971.

"Cardiovascular diseases." American Heart Association. [www.americanheart.org].

Chandra, Nisha C., Roy C. Ziegelstein, William J. Rogers, et al. 1998. Observations of the treatment of women in the United States with myocardial infarction: A report from the National Registry of Myocardial Infarction-I. *Archives of Internal Medicine* 158:981.

Clarke, B., P. Woodhouse, A. Ulvik, et al. 1998. Variability and determinants of total homocysteine concentrations in plasma in an elderly population. *Clinical Chemistry* 44:102.

Danesh, John, and Linda Youngman. 1999. Helicobacter pylori infection and early onset myocardial infarction case control. *British Medical Journal* 7218:1157.

Davidson, Michael. 1998. Confirmed previous infection with chlamydia pneumoniae (TWAR) and its presence in early coronary atherosclerosis. *Journal of the American Medical Association* 280:1972.

de Lorgeril, Michel, Patricia Salen, Francois Paillard, et al. 1998. Lipid-lowering drugs and homocysteine. *The Lancet* 353:209.

Doherty, Terence M., et al. 1999. Coronary heart disease deaths and infarctions in people with little or no coronary calcium. *The Lancet* 353:40.

Dunn, N. R. 1999. Risk of myocardial infarction in young female smokers. *Heart* 82:581.

Edwards, Natalie. 1999. Study shows link between snoring and hypertension in pregnancy. *American Family Physician* 60:1792.

Effect of exercise on coronary endothelial function in patients with coronary artery disease. *New England Journal of Medicine* 342:454, 1999.

Effects of alcohol depend on stroke type in male smokers. *Geriatrics* 55:91, 2000.

Eikelboom, John W., and Eva Lonn. 1999. Homocyst(e)ine and cardiovascular disease: a critical review of the epidemiological evidence. *Annals of Internal Medicine* 131:363.

El-Khairy, L. 1999. Lifestyle and cardiovascular disease risk factors as determinants of total cysteine in plasma: the Hordaland homocysteine study. *American Journal of Clinical Nutrition* 70:1016.

Erbel, Raimund, Michael Haude, Hans W. Hopp, et al. 1998. Coronary artery stenting compared with balloon angioplasty for restenosis after initial balloon angioplasty. *The New England Journal of Medicine* 339:1672.

Feldman, Elaine B. 1998. Nonpharmacologic interventions successfully treat hypertension in older persons. *Nutrition Reviews* 56:341.

Folsom, Aaron R. 1999. Antibiotics for prevention of myocardial infarction. *Journal of the American Medical Association* 281:461.

Fried, Linda P., Richard A. Kronmal, Anne B. Newman, et al. 1998. Risk factors for five year mortality in older adults: The cardiovascular health study. *Journal of the American Medical Association* 279:585.

Gasbarro, Ron. 1998. Hypertension guidelines call for pharmacist monitoring. *American Druggist* 215:42.

Gelenijnse, Johanna M., and Lenore J. Launerr. 1999. Tea flavanoids may protect against atherosclerosis. *Archives of Internal Medicine* 159:2170.

Gershlick, A. H., and R. S. More. 1998. Treatment of myocardial infarction. *British Medical Journal* 316:280.

Giri, S. 1999. Clinical and angiographic characteristics of exertion-related acute myocardial infarction. *Journal of American Medicine* 282:1731.

Goldmuntz, E. 1999. Recent advances in understanding the genetic etiology of congenital heart disease. *Current Opinion Pediatrics* 11:437.

Goldstein, Daniel J., Mehmet C. Oz, and Eric A. Rose. 1998. Implantable left ventricular assist devices. *The New England Journal of Medicine* 339:1522.

Hall, Dallas W. 1999. A rational approach to the treatment of hypertension in special populations. *American Family Physician* 60:156.

Hankey, Graeme J., and Charles P. Warlow. 1999. Treatment and secondary prevention of stroke: evidence, costs, and effects on individuals and populations. *The Lancet* 354:1457.

Horner, T. 1999. Psychosocial profile of adults with complex congenital heart disease. *Mayo Clinic Proc* 75:31.

Husten, Larry. 1999. Women win battle of the sexes in heart failure. *The Lancet* 353:1333.

Hyman, David J., Valory N. Pavlik, Carlos Vallbona, et al. 1998. Blood pressure measurement and antihypertensive treatment in a low-income African-American population. *The American Journal of Public Health* 88:292.

Irvine, J. 1999. Depression and risk of sudden cardiac death after acute myocardial infarction: testing for the confounding effects of fatigue. *Psychosomatic Medicine* 61:729.

Jaagosild, Priit, Neal V. Dawson, Charles Thomas, et al. 1998. Outcomes of acute exacerbation of severe congestive heart failure: Quality of life, resource use, and survival. *Archives of Internal Medicine* 158:1081.

Jiang, P. 1999. Recurrent varicose veins: patterns of reflux and clinical severity. *Cardiovascular Surgery* 17:332.

Jinxiang, Xie. 1998. Hypertension control improved through patient education. *Journal of the American Medical Association* 280:1122.

Kaplan, Robert C., and Bruce M. Psaty. 1999. Blood pressure level and incidence of myocardial infarction among patients treated for hypertension. *American Journal of Public Health* 89:1414.

Khan, J. H. 1999. A 5-year experience with surgical repair of atrial septal defect employing limited exposure. *Cardiology Young* 9:572.

Krieger, James, et al. 1999. Linking community based blood pressure measurement to clinical care: a randomized controlled trial of outreach and tracking by community health workers. *American Journal of Public Health* 89:856.

Larkin, Marilynn. 1999. Benefits of walking should be taken to heart. *The Lancet* 354:134.

Low calcium intake linked to risk of ischemic stroke in women. *Geriatrics* 55:92, 2000.

Lucas, Beverly D. 1999. Antihypertensives not usually the cause of impotence. *Patient Care* 33:15.

MacReady, Norra. 1999. Elderly depression linked to cerebrovascular changes. *The Lancet* 354:1183.

Malinow, Rene M., Paul B. Duell, David L. Hess, et al. 1998. Reduction of plasma homocysteine levels by breakfast cereal fortified with folic acid in patients with coronary heart disease. *The New England Journal of Medicine* 38:1009.

Marciniak, Thomas A., Edward F. Ellerbeck, Martha J. Radford, et al. 1998. Improving the quality of care for Medicare patients with acute myocardial infarction: Results from the cooperative cardiovascular project. *Journal of the American Medical Association* 279:1351.

Markus, Hugh S., and Mike A. Mendall. 1998. *Helicobactor pylori* infection: A risk factor for ischaemic cerebrovascular disease and carotid atheroma. *Journal of the American Medical Association* 279:1238.

Martinelli, I. 1999. Genetic risk factors for superficial vein thrombosis. *Thrombo haemost* 82:1215.

Mead, Gillian E., Helen Shingler, Anne Farrell, et al. 1998. Carotid disease in acute stroke. *Age and Aging* 27:677.

Meleady, Raymond, and Ian Grahm. 1999. Plasma homocysteine as a cardiovascular risk factor: casual, consequential, or of no consequences. *Nutrition Reviews* 57:299.

Mitka, Mike. 1999. AHA addresses atherosclerosis testing. *Journal of the American Medical Association* 282:1991.

Moawad, M. R., and S. D. Blair. 1998. Pulsating varicose veins. *The Lancet* 352:1030.

Morrow, Lee E., and Edwin W. Grimsley. 1999. Long term diuretic therapy in hypertensive patients:

effects on serum homocysteine. *Southern Medical Journal* 92:866.

Ness, J. 1999. Prevalence of coexistence of coronary artery disease, ischemic stroke, and peripheral arterial disease in older persons, mean age 80 years in an academic hospital-based geriatrics practice. *Geriatrics* 47:1255.

Ni, Hanyu, Deirdre J. Nauman, and Ray E. Hershberger. 1998. Managed care and outcomes of hospitalization among elderly patients with congestive heart failure. *Archives of Internal Medicine* 158:1231.

Olson, Robert E. 2000. Is it wise to restrict fat in the diets of children? *Journal of the American Dietetic Association* 100:28.

"On whether to have your homocysteine level measured: Accumulating evidence links homocysteine to heart disease. *Tufts University Health and Nutrition Letter* 16:3, 1998.

Oparil, Suzanne, and David A. Calhoun. 1998. Managing the patient with hard to control hypertension. *American Family Physician* 57:1007.

Ornish, Dean, Larry W. Scherwitz, James H. Billings, et al. 1998. Intensive lifestyle changes for reversal of coronary heart disease. *Journal of the American Medical Association* 280:2001.

Oya, M. 1999. Effects of exercise training on the recovery of the autonomic nervous system and exercise capacity after acute myocardial infarction. *Jpn Circ J* 63:843.

Peteiro, J. 1999. Comparison of treadmill exercise echocardiography before and after exercise in the evaluation of patients with known or suspected coronary artery disease. *Journal of American Society of Echocardiography* 147:237.

Port, Sidney, et al. 1999. Systolic blood pressure and mortality. *The Lancet* 355:175.

Pulse pressure associated with stroke and death in older hypertensives. *Geriatrics* 54:16, 1999.

Rao, V. 1999. Minimally invasive surgery with cardioscopy for congenital heart defects. *Annal Thoracic Surgery* 68:1843.

Ray, Joel G. 1998. Meta-analysis of hyperhomocysteinemia as a risk factor for venous thromboembolic disease. *Archives of Internal Medicine* 158:2101.

Ridker, P. M. 1999. Prospective study of chlamydia pneumoniae IgG seropositivity and risks of future myocardial infarction. *Circulation* 99:1161.

Roivaniene. M. 1999. Enteroviruses and myocardial infarction. *American Heart Journal* 138:S479.

Ross, Russell, and Franklin H. Epstein. 1999. Atherosclerosis—an inflammatory disease. *New England Journal of Medicine* 340:115.

Rothwell, R. M., et al. 2000. Evidence of a chronic systemic cause of instability of atherosclerotic plaques. *The Lancet* 355:19.

Royal College of Physicians of Edinburgh Consensus Conference on medical management of stroke, 26–27 May 1998. *Age and Aging* 27:665, 1998.

Ryan, M. 1999. Preventing stroke in patients with transient ischemic attacks. *American Family Physician* 60:2329.

Saarinen, J. 1999. The incidence and cardiovascular risk indicators of deep venous thrombosis. *Vasa* 28:195.

Sadovsky, Richard. 2000. Walking to work decreases risk of hypertension. *American Family Physician* 61:221.

Sadovsky, Richard. 1999. ACLAs: Risk factors for atherothrombosis. *American Family Physician* 60:2684.

Sadovsky, Richard. 1999. Role of vitamins E and C and carotenoids in stroke risk. *American Family Physician* 60:1843.

Senior, Kathryn. 1999. Worrying trend in hypertension described for USA. *The Lancet* 354:747.

Seppa, N. 1999. High blood pressure is linked to bone loss. *Science News* 156:199.

Seppa, N. 1998. Secondary smoke carries high price. *Science News* 153:36.

Sheifer, S. E. 2000. Prevalence, predisposing factors, and prognosis of clinically unrecognized myocardial infarction in the elderly. *Journal of the American Coll Cariolo* 141:60.

Sherman, S. E. 1999. Comparison of past versus recent physical activity in the prevention of premature death and coronary artery disease. *American Heart Journal* 138:900.

Shor, Allan, and James I. Phillips. 1999. Chlamydia pneumoniae and atherosclerosis. *Journal of the American Medical Association* 282:2071.

Simons, L. A., J. McCallum, Y. Friedlander, et al. 1998. Risk factors for ischemic stroke: Dubbo Study of the elderly. *Stroke* 29:1341.

Stewart, Simon, Sue Pearson, and John D. Horowitz. 1998. Effects of a home-based intervention among patients with congestive heart failure discharged from acute hospital care. *Archives of Internal Medicine* 158:1067.

Stein, J. H. 1999. Purple grape juice improves endothelial function and reduces the susceptibility of DLD cholesterol to oxidation in patients with coronary artery disease. *Circulation* 100:1050.

Sternberg, Daniel, and Antonio M. Gotto. 1999. Preventing coronary artery disease by lowering cholesterol levels. *Journal of the American Medical Association* 282:2043.

Stevens, Roger J.G. 1999. Women's risk of stroke after heart surgery is greater than men's. *Student British Medical Journal* 7:354.

Stiffens, D. C. 1999. Cerebrovascular disease and depression symptoms in the cardiovascular health study. *Stroke* 30:2159.

Stollerman, Gene H., and Alan L. Bisno. 2000. ACE inhibitors for atherosclerotic disease. *Hospital Practice* 35:40.

Stroke prevention. *Geriatrics* 55:24, 2000.

Strong, Jack P., et al. 1999. Prevalence and extent of atherosclerosis in adolescents and young adults. *Journal of the American Medical Association* 281:727.

Tavel, Morton E., Jeffrey A. Breall, and Bernard J. Gersh, 1998. Ischemic heart disease with congestive heart failure: Problems in clinical management. *Chest* 113:1119.

Van Gijn, Jan. 1999. Low doses of aspirin in stroke prevention. *The Lancet* 353:2172.

Vermeulen, E. G. J., et al. 2000. Effect of homosysteine-lowering treatment with folic acid plus vitamin B_6 on progression of subclinical atherosclerosis: A randomized placebo-controlled trial. *The Lancet* 355:517.

Vitamin E supplementation and cardiovascular events in high-risk patients. *New England Journal of Medicine* 342:154, 2000.

Voelker, Rebecca. 1999. Reviving a lifesaver? *Journal of the American Medical Association* 281:123.

Vogel, Robert A. 1999. Cholesterol lowering and endothelial function. *American Journal of Medicine* 107:479.

Wald, Nicholas J., Hilary C. Watt, Malcolm R. Laaw, et al. 1998. Homocysteine and ischemic heart disease: Results of a prospective study with implications regarding prevention. *Archives of Internal Medicine* 158:862.

Wang, Rebecca, Mysore Mouliswar, Susan Denman, et al. 1998. Mortality of the institutionalized old-old hospitalized with congestive heart failure. *Archives of Internal Medicine* 158:2464.

Welch, George N., and Joseph Loscalzo. 1998. Homocysteine and atherothrombosis. *The New England Journal of Medicine* 338:1042.

Whelton, Paul K., Lawrence J. Appel, Mark A. Espeland, et al. 1998. Sodium reduction and weight loss in the treatment of hypertension in older persons: A randomized controlled trial of nonpharmacologic interventions in the elderly (TONE). *Journal of the American Medical Association* 279:839.

Williamson D. R., and C. Pharand. 1998. Statins in the prevention of coronary heart disease. *Pharmacotherapy* 18:242.

Winker, Margaret A. 1999. The emerging epidemic of atherosclerosis. *Journal of the American Medical Association* 281:84.

With lifestyle changes, many patients could halt blood pressure drugs. *Geriatrics* 54:16, 1999.

Workshop on the potential role of infectious agents in cardiovascular disease and atherosclerosis. *Emerging Infectious Diseases* 5:1, 1999.

13

CANCERS WITH THE HIGHEST FATALITY RATES

O B J E C T I V E S

1. *Define the term* cancer.

2. *State the difference between a benign tumor or neoplasm and a malignant tumor or neoplasm.*

3. *Define common terminology used to describe cancer.*

4. *Explain the theory of oncogenesis.*

5. *Identify five ways in which cancer cells differ from normal cells.*

6. *Identify five risk factors for cancer.*

7. *Explain the role of pain in cancer.*

8. *Identify means of primary and secondary prevention for cancer.*

9. *State the traditional methods for treating cancer.*

10. *Describe three newer methods of treating cancer.*

11. *Explain why lung cancer is increasing although smoking rates have dropped.*

12. *State possible reasons for the high rate of colorectal cancer in the United States.*

13. *Distinguish among the four types of mastectomy.*

14. *State the factors that have been found to be linked to breast cancer in women.*

15. *Distinguish between Hodgkin's disease and non-Hodgkin's lymphoma.*

16. *Explain the association between hepatitis B, cirrhosis, and liver cancer.*

17. *Explain the difference in rate of stomach cancer between Americans and some other nations.*

18. *Describe and identify predisposing factors, symptoms, prevention, and treatment for the cancers in this chapter.*

INTRODUCTION

Cancer is the second leading cause of death in the United States. It is estimated that 1 out of 2 men and 1 out of 3 women alive today will develop cancer, and 552,200 Americans are expected to die in 2000 of cancer* (Table 13-1). Our increased longevity has led to an increased incidence of cancer and other disorders that are more common among older adults. But cancer is also a leading cause of death in children, second only to accidental death.

Cancer is not one but many different diseases characterized by an uncontrolled growth and spread

oncogenesis	ONG-ko-JEN-e-sis

TABLE 13-1	**Estimated New Cancer Cases and Deaths by Sex for Selected Sites, United States, 2000***					
	Estimated New Cases			**Estimated Deaths**		
Cancer Sites **All Sites**	**Both Sexes** **1,220,100**	**Male** **619,700**	**Female** **600,400**	**Both Sexes** **552,200**	**Male** **284,100**	**Female** **268,100**
Oral cavity and pharynx	30,200	20,000	10,000	7,800	5,100	2,700
Esophagus	12,300	9,200	3,100	12,100	9,200	2,900
Stomach	21,500	13,400	8,100	13,000	7,600	5,400
Liver and intrahepatic bile duct	15,300	10,000	5,300	13,800	8,500	5,300
Pancreas	28,300	13,700	14,600	28,200	13,700	14,500
Larynx	10,100	8,100	2,000	3,900	3,100	800
Lung and bronchus	164,100	89,500	74,000	156,900	89,300	67,600
Bones and joints	2,500	1,500	1,000	1,400	800	600
Skin (excluding basal and squamous)	56,900	34,100	22,800	9,600	6,000	3,600
Melanoma-skin	47,700	27,300	20,400	7,700	4,800	2,900
Breast	184,200	1,400	182,800	41,200	800	40,800
Uterine cervix	12,800		12,800	4,600		4,600
Uterine corpus	36,100		36,100	6,500		6,500
Ovary	23,100		23,100	14,000		14,000
Prostate	180,400	180,400		31,900	31,900	
Testis	6,900	6,900		300	300	
Urinary bladder	53,200	38,300	14,900	12,200	8,100	4,100
Kidney and renal pelvis	31,200	17,800	12,400	11,900	7,300	4,600
Brain and other nervous system	16,500	9,500	7,000	13,000	7,100	5,900
Hodgkin's disease	7,400	4,200	3,200	1,400	700	700
Non-Hodgkin's lymphoma	54,900	31,700	23,200	26,100	13,700	12,400
Multiple myeloma	13,600	7,300	6,300	11,200	5,800	5,400
Leukemia	30,800	16,900	13,900	21,700	12,100	9,600

*Statistics are from the American Cancer Society's *Cancer Facts and Figures—2000*, unless otherwise indicated.

of cells. Although it may seem at times that no progress has been made against this dreaded disease, there has been a gain in the survival rate when all cancers are considered together. In the early 1900s, a diagnosis of cancer was believed to be a death sentence, and in those days it usually was, because many cancer patients had little hope of survival. During the years since the beginning of the century, advances have been made slowly but surely, and today, the overall survival rate for cancer is 59%. Cancer statistics are generally based on information that is at least five years old and for this reason do not reflect the recent advances in treatment and lifestyle changes. Also, the survival rate for some cancers is less than 59% while others have a survival rate of more than 59%. Although the number of deaths from lung cancer is still increasing, it should start to decrease as more and more people stop smoking and as other carcinogens are identified and removed from the environment.

CANCER TERMINOLOGY

People often believe that the words *neoplasm* and *tumor* are synonymous with cancer, but that is not the case. *Neoplasm* literally means a "new thing formed," and the word *tumor* means "a swelling." Both words are used when referring to cancer, but unless the word *malignant* ("a bad kind") is used with them, it is not cancer. The term *benign* ("a good kind") is used to indicate a noncancerous growth. Figure 13-1 shows *A,* benign, and *B,* malignant growths.

In one sense, benign neoplasms or tumors may not be good at all. They are only good because they are not malignant. However, benign tumors do continue to grow and, depending upon their location, can cause pain and damage. Like malignant tumors, benign tumors can also cause death if they are in an inoperable location. A malignant neoplasm or tumor does mean cancer, but it does not mean certain death.

One main difference between benign tumors and malignant tumors is that malignant tumors **metastasize** (spread) through the circulatory and lymphatic systems and invade surrounding tissue (Figure 13-2). Benign tumors are generally encapsulated and do not spread to other parts of the body, although a benign tumor occasionally may turn into a malignant tumor.

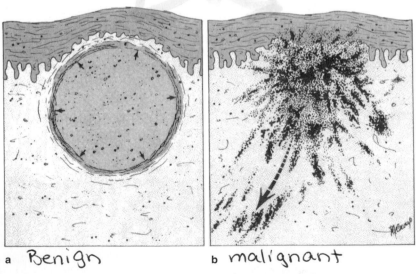

a Benign   b malignant

Figure 13-1

Diagram of benign versus malignant growth. (a) A "typical" benign neoplasm is cohesive, expands from the center, has a smooth border, and is often encapsulated. (b) A malignant neoplasm is less cohesive, has an irregular border, and invades adjacent tissue. Malignant cells are also capable of metastasis (*dotted arrow*).

find out where it will spread - ex Lungs.

oxygenated blood goes to brain.

ex: Breast cancer - goes to bone

if cancer goes to lungs = not called
lung cancer = called a metastasized Breast cancer

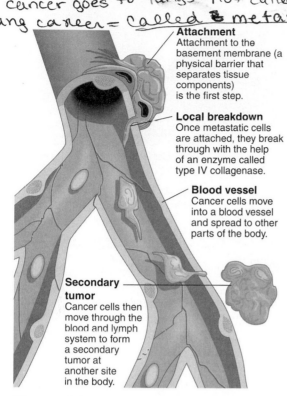

Attachment
Attachment to the basement membrane (a physical barrier that separates tissue components) is the first step.

Local breakdown
Once metastatic cells are attached, they break through with the help of an enzyme called type IV collagenase.

Blood vessel
Cancer cells move into a blood vessel and spread to other parts of the body.

Secondary tumor
Cancer cells then move through the blood and lymph system to form a secondary tumor at another site in the body.

Figure 13-2

How cancer spreads. Movement of cells is integral to the entire process of metastasis. Scientists have identified a protein that causes cancer cells to grow feet, or pseudopodia, enabling them to begin to move to other parts of the body.

Identification of Cancer by Tissue

Malignancies may be classified by the tissue in which they occur or by location and sometimes both, as in osteosarcoma (occurring in the bone). The following terms are used to identify cancers according to the tissue in which they occur.

Carcinoma—Epithelium

Carcinoma arises from the epithelial tissue that forms the outer surface of the body and lines the body cavities and principal tubes and passageways leading to the exterior. About eighty-five percent of all tumors occur in epithelial tissue. A drawing of a cancer is shown in Figure 13-3.

Sarcoma—Connective Tissue

Sarcoma arises from connective tissue cells such as those found in bone, cartilage, and tendons. Only two percent of malignant tumors are of this type.

Melanoma—Skin Cells with Melanin

Melanoma arises from the melanin-containing cells of the skin. This type of cancer has been rare, but it is becoming more common.

Neuroblastoma—CNS

Neuroblastoma originates in immature cells of the central nervous system (CNS). A rare form of cancer, it is found mostly in children.

Adenocarcinoma—Dual Connection

Adenocarcinoma derives from cells from both the epithelium and endocrine glands.

Hepatoma—Liver

Hepatoma originates in cells of the liver; mortality is high.

Leukemia—Blood Cells

Leukemia is a malignant growth of bone marrow cells and blood-forming tissue cells. There are many forms of leukemia, and they are classified by the dominant cell type. Leukemia occurs in both children and adults.

Lymphoma—Lymphatic, Other Immune System Tissues

Lymphoma is a malignant growth of cells in the lymphatic tissues or other immune system tissues.

Grading and Staging

The terms used in classifying tumors are grading and staging. In grading, the tumor cells are classified by grades I to IV, depending on their degree of

metastasize	me-TAS-ta-siz
neuroblastoma	NU-ro-blas-TO-ma
adenocarcinoma	AD-e-no-kar-sin-O-ma

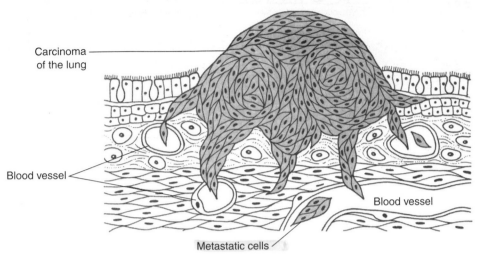

Figure 13-3

Portrait of a cancer. The ball of cells is a carcinoma, developing from epithelial cells lining the interior surface of a human lung. Unless destroyed by the immune system, the mass of cells grows, invading surrounding tissues, eventually penetrating into lymphatic vessels and blood vessels, both of which are plentiful within the lung. These vessels carry metastatic cancer cells.

TABLE 13-2	Cancer Staging—the TNM System*
T = PRIMARY TUMOR	
T0	No evidence of a primary tumor
Tx	Evidence of tumor in some tests but unable to assess because of location, type, etc.
TIS	Tumor in situ (localized)
T1–T4	Increasing degrees of size and involvement
N = NODAL INVOLVEMENT	
N0	No lymph node involvement
N1–N3	Increasing number and range of lymph nodes
Nx	Unable to assess lymph node involvement
M = METASTASES	
M0	No evidence of metastases to distant points
M1–M3	Increasing degrees of metastases, including some to distant nodes

*Staging varies for each specific form of cancer, but these are general principles.

difference from normal cells and growth rate. Staging is often done by the TNM system (Table 13-2) and is used to quantify the extent of the cancer. The staging system allows **oncologists** (physicians who specialize in treating cancer) to discuss patient needs for various types of therapy according to the characteristics of the specific case.

CANCER CELLS

New cells are being produced constantly in each of us. Each cell has a prescribed function, but in the case of cancer, something happens and the cell does not develop in the expected manner. Cancer research today is zeroing in on these "lawless" cells and the genes that may cause their development. A current theory is that within each cell there are a number of proto-oncogenes, which, if altered, could become oncogenes, which in turn activate the development of cancer cells. It is thought that carcinogenic (cancer-causing) substances may convert the proto-oncogenes into oncogenes. There are also tumor suppressor genes in the cells that inhibit cell growth. If they mutate, they may not work correctly. More simply, proto-oncogenes encourage cell growth and tumor suppressor genes inhibit cell growth. Cancer cells differ from normal cells in a number of ways. Some of those ways are:

> They lack cellular cohesiveness. They do adhere to each other to some extent, but it is easier for them to break off and travel.

> They grow and reproduce at an abnormal rate. Normal cells multiply by dividing into two cells, which are each capable of reproducing themselves; cancer cells may divide into three, four, or five different cells in a haphazard way.

> They lack contact inhibition. They do not know when to stop growing as normal cells do.

> They have a higher nutrient demand because they lack the machinery to provide the energy they need.

> They are more likely to survive damage than normal cells in spite of the damage to their genome.

> They have lost specialized function and normal tissue organization but continue to survive in mutated forms.

PREDISPOSING FACTORS

Although the search for the cause and a cure for malignant growths has produced no final answers, we do know many predisposing factors related to cancer, and many carcinogenic substances have been identified in the environment. The best prevention at present lies in avoidance or elimination of these factors and carcinogens in our lives whenever possible. Some genetic factors may increase susceptibility to cancer. Although these cannot be changed, being aware of them can lead to earlier

detection and thus increase the chances of surviving cancer (Box 13-1). Scientists believe that most cancers can be cured if caught in the early stages.

Symptoms
Many associate cancer with pain, but in cancer, pain does not usually occur until the later stages. Approximately twenty percent to forty percent of cancer patients have no pain at all. The amount of pain, the time of onset, and the severity all differ, depending upon the location and size of the cancer and its pattern of growth. For example, a tumor located in the brain has very little space to grow before it compresses nerves and blood vessels. Individuals with cancer become more susceptible to infections, which can also cause pain. Cancer patients also tend to lose interest in eating and may be nauseous because of chemotherapy. For this reason, they become malnourished and lose weight. Most patients also have a mild anemia.

Primary Prevention
The best prevention is a healthy lifestyle and avoidance of environmental carcinogens and the other risk factors associated with cancer. No smoking, a varied diet, moderation in alcohol (if used at all), and staying out of the sun or using a sunscreen are all preventive measures.

Secondary Prevention
For the most part, secondary prevention measures will be dealt with as each type of cancer is discussed. In general, it is important that everyone know cancer's seven warning signals, developed by the American Cancer Society (ACS). They are

1. **C** hange in bowel or bladder habits
2. **A** sore that does not heal
3. **U** nusual bleeding or discharge
4. **T** hickening or lump in breast or elsewhere
5. **I** ndigestion or difficulty in swallowing
6. **O** bvious change in a wart or mole
7. **N** agging cough or hoarseness

If any of these lasts more than five days, a doctor should be consulted immediately.

---

oncologists   ong-KO-logists

BOX 13-1

Factors That May Increase Susceptibility to Cancer

Heredity. If cancer is prevalent in the family history, tests for early detection should be performed at recommended ages and intervals.

Occupation. Certain occupations bring employees into contact with carcinogenic agents and should be avoided.

Tobacco use. Tobacco use can lead to cancer of the mouth, lungs, and bladder. It is believed that the carcinogens in tobacco tar may be responsible for other forms of cancer.

Diet. The American Cancer Society makes the following recommendations on diet:

- Avoid obesity.
- Reduce total fat intake.

- Eat more high fiber foods.
- Include foods rich in vitamins A and C in your daily diet.
- Include cruciferous vegetables (broccoli, cabbage, kale, etc.) in your diet.
- Avoid smoked, salt-cured, and nitrate-cured foods.
- Limit alcohol to moderate consumption.

Sun exposure. Ultraviolet (UV) radiation from the sun or tanning beds can trigger cancer, particularly for people with light complexions. A person who has had a severe burn one or more times has an increased risk of skin cancer. Using sunscreen may help, but it does not always prevent.

Treatment

Traditional treatments for cancer include surgery, chemotherapy, radiation, hormones, immunotherapy, or a combination of these.

Researchers are working all the time to find better methods of treating cancer. One area of study is based on the belief that cancer cells have the ability to inactivate the immune system.

Researchers are also working with monoclonal antibodies to take advantage of their ability to recognize features(antigens) on the surface of cancer cells. Crucial in all antibody-based approaches is selecting an antigen that can selectively target tumor cells while sparing normal cells. The simplest approach for using a tumor-targeting antibody is to activate the body's own immune system. Two such treatments, **Herceptin** for breast cancer and **Mabthera** for lymphoma, have been approved by the FDA. Other approaches involve attaching a radioisotope (radioimmunotherapy) or cytotoxic agent (chemo-immunotherapy) to an antibody in the hope of selectively delivering radiation or a drug, respectively, to the tumor cells. An even more elaborate approach, called *ADEPT* for Antibody-Dependent

Enzyme-Prodrug Therapy, involves attaching an enzyme to an antibody that can activate a prodrug that is administered later. All of these approaches are being explored in clinical trials.

Among the less "scientifically" oriented forms of therapy is the emphasis on the mind-body connection. Most doctors now agree that patients' attitude can make a significant difference in their recovery. One physician who has investigated this area is Dr. Bernie Siegel, a surgeon in the eastern United States who has operated on thousands of cancer patients. He began to wonder not about cancer causation but about why some people considered to be terminally ill somehow survived. Dr. Siegel founded a group called *E-Cap* (an acronym for exceptional cancer patients).

The group soon branched into many groups in many parts of the country. In these groups, newly diagnosed cancer patients are joined by "survivors" who talk about their experiences and encourage the others to express their feelings. Dr. Siegel found that those who survived took their diagnosis as a challenge and had the attitude "I can beat this" rather than accepting it as a death sentence. He believes that patients should use traditional cancer treatments but also attend these groups. Although group leaders think that the groups are beneficial, it would be difficult to prove the benefits of group therapy for cancer because having a control group is not feasible (who could withhold beneficial treatment from a cancer patient?).

SUMMARY OF BASIC INFORMATION ON CANCER

Cancer is the second leading cause of death in the United States. However, cancer is many diseases, not just one. Overall survival rates have improved, and by 1999, sixty percent of those diagnosed with cancer were cured. A number of different words and terms are used to describe cancer, its location, and its severity or spread. These developed so that physicians specializing in cancer (oncologists) could discuss patient needs for treatment.

Cancer cells differ from other cells: they (1) are less likely to survive damage, (2) have a higher nutrient demand, (3) lack cellular cohesiveness, (4) grow and reproduce at a different rate, *quickly* and (5) lack contact inhibition.

Heredity, occupation, tobacco use, diet, and sun exposure are some factors that have been linked to cancer. For many people with cancer, there is no pain, and if pain does occur, the cancer is generally in a late stage.

Primary prevention of cancer is based on reducing or eliminating risk factors. Secondary prevention involves identifying high-risk groups, screening, visiting a doctor if an individual has any of the seven warning signs of cancer, and following guidelines for diagnostic tests for detecting various types of cancer.

The traditional treatments for cancer are surgery, radiation, and chemotherapy, used singly or in combination. New drugs and other methods for treating cancer are being developed. They include boosting the immune system, monoclonal antibodies, emphasis on the mind-body connection, and group therapy. *immunotherapy*

System - everywhere

THE DEADLIEST CANCERS

Of all the diseases labeled with the dreaded name of cancer, the deadliest (Figure 13-4) will be discussed in this chapter and some cancers with lower fatality rates will be covered in Chapter 14. A clinical description and prognosis for each cancer, the predisposing factors, symptoms, prevention measures, and treatment are discussed.

LUNG CANCER

Cancer of the lungs has become the most common killing cancer for both sexes, with 164,100 new cases and 156,900 deaths estimated for 2000. In the past, there were more cases in men than women, but women are catching up quickly; lung cancer now exceeds breast cancer in deaths among women. Figure 13-5 shows an increase in deaths for women and a recent significant decrease in lung cancer deaths for men over an eight-year period. The cancer usually develops in the walls of the bronchial tubes and may appear as an ulcer, nodule, or small flattened lump, or on the surface, blocking air tubes. It may also invade the surface of the tubes and extend to lymphatics and blood vessels (Figure 13-6). The prognosis is poor, with a five-year survival rate of fifty percent when the cancer is still localized but only fourteen percent for all stages combined if the cancer has spread to distant sites. Unfortunately, only fifteen percent of lung cancers are discovered in the early stage.

Predisposing Factors

Of those who develop lung cancer, 87% are smokers, and the chances for persons who smoke to get lung cancer increase with the number of years they have been smoking and the number of cigarettes they smoke per day. There are also carcinogenic agents that many of us are exposed to, such as automobile exhaust gases, residential radon gas and radioactive dust, asbestos, sidestream smoke,

| **herceptin** | her-SEP-tin |

→ Vitamin C — Tumor used vitamin to protect itself from radiation therapy

↑ Systemically

Chemo & Radiation = Kills cells dividing rapidly cells in mouth, throat, stomach (mouth cells) Bone marrow, Hair, Low white BC count / Low RBC count

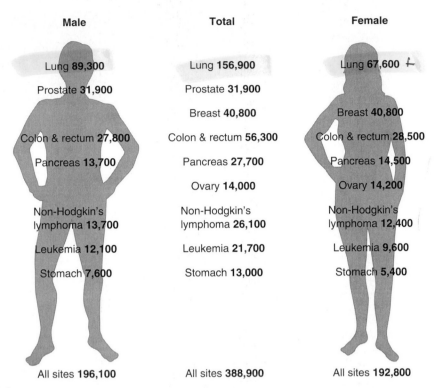

Figure 13-4
Deadliest cancers. Estimated cancer deaths by site and sex for 2000.

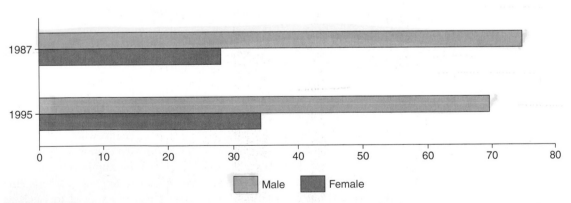

Figure 13-5
Age-adjusted death rates from lung cancer per 100,000 population, 1987 and 1995.

CSF'S Colony stimulating Factors
        drug given to stimulate WBC, RBC, & platelete count
        very expensive - make a big difference
need to take ~~antimedics~~
                antiemetics (p. 342)

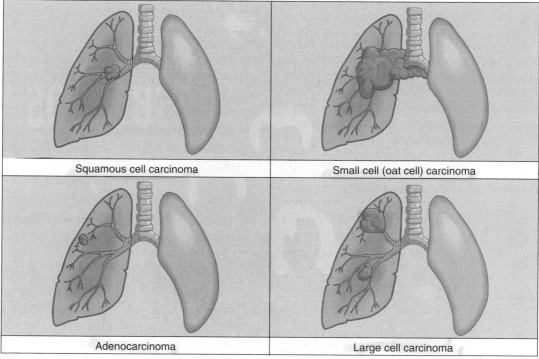

Figure 13-6

Common sites for lung cancer.

and other pollutants in the air (Figure 13-7). Persons who are not or who have never been smokers may develop lung cancer if they have a history of long-time exposure to passive and/or sidestream smoke or environmental/occupational hazards other than tobacco smoke. Moreover, smokers exposed to one or more of these other carcinogens are even more likely to develop lung cancer.

Symptoms

In the early stages there are generally no symptoms. Late-stage symptoms include smoker's cough, wheezing, labored or difficult breathing, coughing up of blood, chest pain, fever, weakness, weight loss, and anorexia. Because lung tumors may alter the production of hormones that regulate body function, many other symptoms can occur including **gynecomastia** and bone and joint pain. Lung cancer metastases may occur in any part of the body but the most frequent sites are the CNS, liver, and bone.

Primary Prevention

Cigarette smokers have up to twenty times or even greater risk than nonsmokers of developing lung cancer. If smoking is discontinued, the chances for exsmokers to develop lung cancer quickly approach those of nonsmokers, providing that the cancer process has not already begun before they stop. Persons working in an industrial situation where they are exposed to particulates in the air should be sure proper measures are taken to prevent inhaling them constantly. A relationship between asbestosis and lung cancer has been proved, and it is suspected that exposure to materials in other industries might also increase the risk of lung cancer.

---

gynecomastia   JI-ne-ko-mas-te-a

83 % of lung cancer patients are smokers

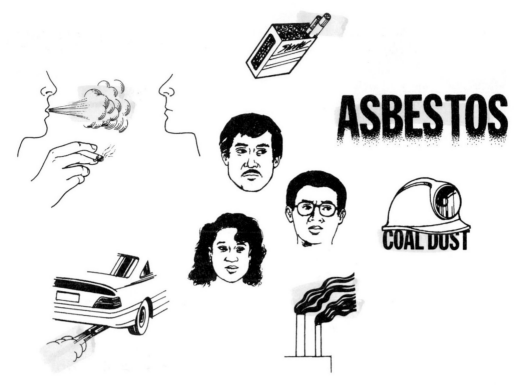

Figure 13-7
Risk factors for lung cancer.

Secondary Prevention

Individuals at high risk for lung cancer should consult their doctor about having a lung X ray exam during routine physicals. Cancer that shows up in an X ray film is usually far advanced, but a lesion can be detected by X ray up to two years before symptoms appear. Analysis of the types of cells in the sputum and fiberoptic examination of the bronchial tubes can also aid in detecting lung cancer.

Treatment

Depending upon the stage of the cancer, treatment could be surgery, radiation, chemotherapy, or a combination of these. Several drugs in combination have been found to induce remission in some kinds of lung cancer. Immunotherapy and laser therapy are both being used experimentally.

COLORECTAL CANCER

For the second most common cancer in the United States, colorectal cancer, 130,200 new cases are predicted for 2000, with an estimated 56,000 deaths for the same year. There has been a decrease in colorectal cancer death rates for both men and women over an eight-year period (Figure 13-8). Colorectal cancer develops slowly and remains localized for a long time. The five-year survival rate is 90% when detected in the localized state. If it has spread regionally, the survival rate is 65% and if there are distant metastases, the rate of survival drops to nine percent. At the present time, only thirty-seven percent are diagnosed in a localized site.

Predisposing Factors

Colorectal cancer is more likely in those with a history of this kind of cancer in the family, polyps

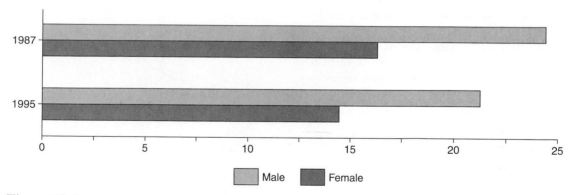

Figure 13-8

Age-adjusted death rates from colon and rectum cancer per 100,000 population, 1987 and 1995.

in the rectum, and/or ulcerative colitis. Until recently it was thought that a high fiber diet would protect us from cancer of the colon and/or rectum, but at least two very large studies* have found no association between dietary fiber intake and the risk of colorectal cancer. It is still wise to include fresh fruits, vegetables, and whole grains in the diet on a regular basis because they are known to be beneficial for other diseases and they contain nutrients necessary for the body's health.

Symptoms

Symptoms of colorectal cancer depend on the location of the tumor, as shown in Figure 13-9.

Primary Prevention

Studies have shown that individuals who are forty percent or more overweight run a substantially higher risk of developing colorectal cancer. Maintaining an ideal weight can reduce the risk of cancer and other chronic diseases.

Secondary Prevention

Digital examination can detect almost fifty percent of the tumors in the anus, rectum, or lower sigmoid, where over fifty percent of the tumors occur. The ACS recommends that everyone over forty years of age should have this exam once a year.

*Charles S. Fuchs, Edward L. Giovannucci, et al., 1999, "Dietary fiber and the risk of colorectal cancer and adenoma in women," *New England Journal of Medicine* 340:169.

Transverse colon
Pain, obstruction, change in bowel habits, anemia

Ascending colon
Pain, mass, change in bowel habits, anemia

Descending colon
Pain, change in bowel habits, bright red blood in stool, obstruction

Rectum
Blood in stool, change in bowel habits, rectal discomfort

Figure 13-9

Sites of colorectal cancers.

A hemoccult or "hidden blood" test can detect blood in the stools. This test can be performed at home and sent to a lab for diagnosis. The ACS recommends this test be performed annually after age fifty.

Proctosigmoidoscopy involves the use of an instrument that can be inserted into the anus,

| proctosigmoidoscopy | PROK-to-SIG-moyd-OS-ko-pe |

allowing the physician to examine the areas of concern. This examination can detect fifty percent of all colorectal cancers. The ACS recommends undergoing this examination every three to five years after the age of fifty. Other procedures may be used to confirm the diagnosis or when there are indications that a problem exists that has not been identified by the above tests. Only a tumor biopsy can verify colorectal cancer.

Treatment

Surgery, sometimes combined with radiation, is the most effective treatment for colorectal cancer, and different procedures are used depending on the location of the tumor. If the surgery requires removal of a part of the colon so that feces cannot travel through the rectum, a **colostomy** may be performed, which involves making an opening in the abdominal wall and attaching a pouch to collect the feces (Figure 13-10).

BREAST CANCER

One in nine women presently living will be diagnosed as having breast cancer. For 1999, 176,300 new cases and 43,700 deaths are estimated. Death rates for women decreased in the eight-year period shown in Figure 13-11. There was also a slight decrease in breast cancer deaths for men during the same period.

Historically, more women have developed breast cancer than any other kind of cancer, and more women have died from breast cancer than any other disease. However, lung cancer has now become the number one killer from cancer for both men and women. Although breast cancer may occur in men, it does so rarely. The distribution of sites for breast cancer is shown in Figure 13-12.

The five-year survival rate for localized breast cancer has improved from seventy-two percent in the 1940s to ninety-seven percent today because of earlier diagnosis and new treatment methods. If the cancer has spread regionally, the survival rate is seventy-seven percent. If metastasis has occurred in distant parts of the body, the survival rate is twenty-two percent. The disease may develop at any time of life, but it is uncommon

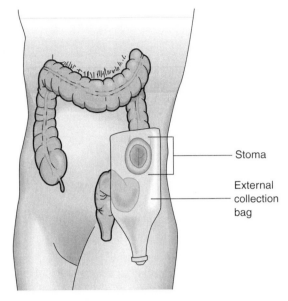

Stoma

External collection bag

Figure 13-10
Colostomy site and pouch.

before thirty-five years of age. Breast cancer occurs more often in the left breast than in the right, and fifty percent occur in the upper outer quadrant. Growth rates can vary. Slow-growing breast cancer can take up to eight years before it can be detected by self-examination.

Predisposing Factors

There are a number of factors that place a woman at *high risk*. These include:

- A family history of breast cancer
- Long menstrual cycles or early menses
- Late menopause (after age fifty)
- First pregnancy (after age thirty)
- History of endometrial, ovarian, or colon cancer
- Higher education and socioeconomic class
- Constant stress or unusual disturbances in home or work life
- Never giving birth, or late age at first live birth
- Obesity (forty percent above normal)

If a woman has been pregnant before the age of twenty, has had multiple pregnancies, is Indian or Asian, and/or is of lower socioeconomic class, she is at a *reduced risk* for developing breast

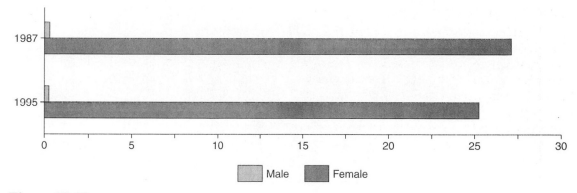

| | Male | Female |

Figure 13-11

Age-adjusted death rates from breast cancer per 100,000 population, 1987 and 1995.

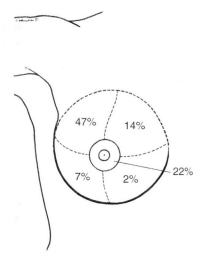

Figure 13-12

Distribution of carcinomas in breast.

cancer. Other factors are being studied including pesticide and chemical exposure, alcohol consumption, weight gain, induced abortion, and physical inactivity. There is also some new genetic research going on that may lead to possible cures or treatment for breast cancer.

Symptoms

A woman is far more likely to discover a sign of breast cancer than is her doctor, because she knows her own body better, and by self-examination at least once a month, she can detect changes.

A lump or mass in the breast that was not there before is one sign. Noncancerous cysts often form in women's breasts, but the only way to be certain is to seek a medical diagnosis. A change in breast symmetry or size is suspect, as is a change in skin temperature or color, such as a small warm, hot, or pink spot. Dimpling or sores on the skin need to be investigated, as does any unusual drainage or bloody discharge from the nipple. Scaliness, pain, or tenderness of the nipple may also indicate cancer. Pain should always be reported to the doctor, but it is generally not a sign of breast cancer unless the tumor is advanced.

Primary Prevention

At present it is thought that a high-fat diet may be a factor in the development of breast cancer. Obesity should be avoided. The planning of pregnancies should take the risk factors into consideration. The rest of the risk factors cannot be controlled now, although any woman who is susceptible because of them needs to take all steps possible to prevent cancer.

Secondary Prevention

The ACS recommends the monthly practice of breast self-examination (BSE) by women twenty years of age and older (Figure 13-13). From ages twenty to forty, a physical examination should be

---

colostomy   ko-LOS-to-me

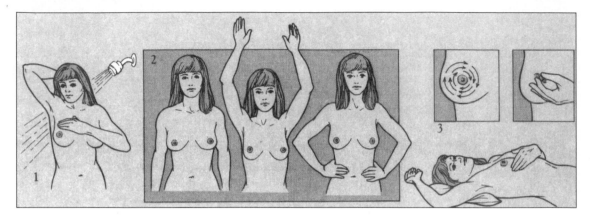

Figure 13-13

Breast self-examination. Breasts can be examined: 1, in a shower, 2, in front of a mirror, or 3, lying down.

done by a doctor at least every three years. A baseline mammogram is recommended for women ages thirty-five to thirty-nine, a mammogram every one to two years between forty and forty-nine years of age, and every year after age fifty. Breast cancer can be detected by a mammogram before self-examination can but both procedures should performed as recommended above.

Treatment

Breast cancer may be treated in a number of ways, depending upon the extent of the cancer. Radiation therapy, chemotherapy, hormone manipulation, or surgery may be used singly or in combination. However, for most breast tumors, surgery would generally be selected, particularly if the tumor has not metastasized to distant locations. Breast reconstruction after surgery for removal of a breast has had good results. There are basically four types of breast surgery or **mastectomy.** They are:

1. *Radical mastectomy,* in which the entire affected breast, the chest muscles underneath, and the lymph nodes in the armpit are removed. If there is any chance that the cancer has spread or metastasized, then this procedure is preferred.
2. *Modified radical mastectomy,* in which the entire affected breast and the lymph nodes in the armpit are removed. However, the chest muscles are left intact.

3. *Total or simple mastectomy,* which involves complete removal of the breast but not the lymph nodes or chest muscles.
4. *Partial or segmental mastectomy* (also called *lumpectomy* or *local excision*), in which only a portion of the breast is removed, including the cancer and a surrounding portion of breast tissue.

Chemotherapy may be used after surgery to eliminate any remaining cancer cells. Treatment by radiation is sometimes used before or after surgery for additional therapy. Other forms of treatment are used, depending upon the individual case and the woman's response to traditional therapies. There is some discussion about using prophylactic bilateral mastectomy for high-risk women because it reduces the incidence of breast cancer. The procedure is still controversial.

PROSTATE CANCER

Cancer of the prostate is among the top three killers of men, with 180,400 new cases and 31,900 deaths estimated for 2000. About one man in ten will develop prostate cancer at some time during his life. Better methods of screening and diagnosis have been a factor in the increased incidence. There has been an increase in the death rates in the eight-year period 1987 to 1995 (Figure 13-14). If

CASE STUDY

Prostate Cancer

A sixty-nine year-old retired professor made an appointment with his doctor because of persistent diarrhea. Upon examination, no cause for the diarrhea was found but a nodule was found in his prostate gland. Ultrasound revealed a lesion in the prostate. Needle biopsy confirmed a malignant growth. Magnetic resonance imaging examinatin (MRI) showed no spread to the lymph nodes. He was entered in a study using new methods of chemotherapy over a four-month period. Twelve months after treatment there was no evidence of recurrence.

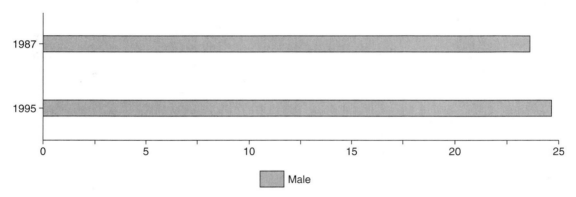

Figure 13-14

Age-adjusted death rates from prostate cancer per 100,000 population, 1987 and 1995.

this cancer is detected while it is localized, the five-year survival rate is 100 percent. The survival rate for all stages combined is 92%. Prostatic cancer does not generally occur until men are over fifty years of age, and over seventy-five percent of all prostate cancers occur in men over sixty-five years of age.

Predisposing Factors

No predisposing factors have been proved to be related to the development of cancer of the prostate. Investigations have centered around possible linkage with androgen, which controls the growth of the prostate. African-American males have the highest rate in the world, but the reason for this is not known. Occurrence is higher in some families, but it is not known whether this is from genetic or environmental influences. The rate is lowest among Asians. An argument for an environmental factor is the fact that men who live in a low-incidence area and move to an area where the rates are high soon have the same risk. One factor could be dietary fat, because international studies have shown that those with prostatic cancer often have high-fat diets. Some recent studies indicate a relationship between vasectomy and cancer of the prostate. Other studies have been unable to find a statistically significant relationship. More research needs to be done in this area.

mastectomy   mas-TEK-to-me

...gns for cancer of the prostate include ... interrupted urine flow; the need to urinate ...uently, especially at night; inability to urinate; blood in the urine; pain or burning on urination; and continuing pain in lower back, pelvis, or upper thighs. These symptoms could also be related to other conditions such as infection or prostate enlargement. Signs that the cancer is spreading include anemia, weight loss, and lumbosacral pain that may radiate to the hips or down the legs.

Primary Prevention

Methods of primary prevention are unknown.

Secondary Prevention

Men fifty years of age or older should have a rectal examination yearly. Ultrasound can also be used and will detect cancers too small to be found with a digital rectal examination. Men at high risk will benefit by the use of ultrasound examinations.

Treatment

Surgery of the testicle to halt the male hormone production helps to control the growth of prostatic cancer. Because of the possibility of impotence, many men refuse this surgery. However, a new procedure for this treatment has led to seventy-two percent of the patients retaining their potency. Administration of the female hormone stilbestrol to counteract the effects of androgen has also led to relief of symptoms and has largely replaced cas-tration. Chemotherapy and radiation may also be used.

PANCREATIC CANCER

The incidence of pancreatic cancer has been increasing steadily over the past twenty years. According to estimates, there will be 28,300 new cases and 28,200 deaths from pancreatic cancer in 2000. Death rates for men have decreased whereas they have stayed about the same for women from 1987 to 1995 (Figure 13-15). Because pancreatic cancer has usually metastasized when found, most patients die within a year of diagnosis, with only three percent surviving more than 5 years.

Predisposing Factors

A number of carcinogens have been suggested as factors in the development of pancreatic cancer. Cigarette smoking, diets high in fat and protein, food additives, exposure to certain industrial chemicals, and chronic alcohol abuse have all been implicated by various studies. A recent study at Harvard suggested that drinking two or more cups of coffee a day may also be a cause. Cancer of the pancreas also appears frequently in diabetics.

Symptoms

Early signs are vague and nonspecific. In the later stages jaundice, weight loss, and abdominal or low back pain are the most common symptoms. Fever,

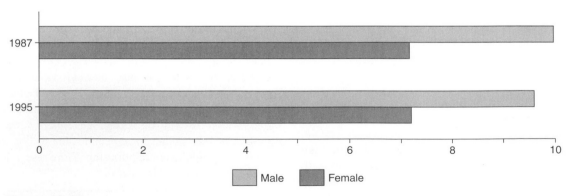

Figure 13-15

Age-adjusted death rates from pancreatic cancer per 100,000 population, 1987 and 1995.

skin lesions (usually on the legs), and emotional disturbances may also be present.

Primary Prevention

Eliminating as many of the risk factors as possible is the best course to follow to minimize the chances of pancreatic cancer. The relationship to smoking has become clear-cut. Smokers who develop the disease do so fifteen years earlier than those who are nonsmokers. Avoiding the carcinogenic substances that have been linked to pancreatic cancer may provide protection against other cancers also.

Secondary Prevention

There is as yet no method to detect pancreatic cancer before symptoms occur.

Treatment

Surgery, radiation, and chemotherapy may be used but are rarely effective. Different surgical techniques have been tried with little success.

LYMPHATIC CANCER

Hodgkin's Disease

This rare form of cancer involves the tissues of the lymphatic system, mainly in the lymph nodes and spleen. There are 7,400 new cases estimated for 2000 and 1,400 deaths. The disease occurs more often in people twenty to forty years of age (average age of thirty-two) and in people between the ages of

fifty-five and seventy. It follows a variable but relentlessly progressive course and is ultimately fatal if untreated, but recent advances in treatment make Hodgkin's disease potentially curable even in advanced cases. The overall five-year survival rate is eighty-two percent when diagnosed in the early stages. Figure 13-16 shows a decrease in death rates for men and women over an eight-year period from 1987 to 1995. The sites that are involved in Hodgkin's disease are shown in Figure 13-17.

Predisposing Factors

The cause of Hodgkin's disease is unknown.

Symptoms

The first sign is usually a painless enlargement of lymph nodes in the neck or armpits. Most of the other symptoms are due to this enlargement and the invasion of other body organs by the proliferating lymphoid tissue or impairment of the effectiveness of the immune system. These symptoms include a feeling of malaise, fever, loss of appetite, weight loss, night sweats, and itching. Other symptoms may occur, depending on which lymph nodes or organs become involved.

Prevention

Preventive measures for Hodgkin's disease are unknown.

Treatment

If the disease is diagnosed in an early stage, radiation may cure it. If it is more advanced and involves many organs, then chemotherapy is usually

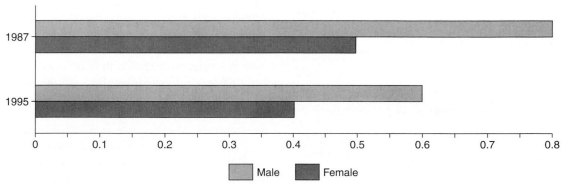

Figure 13-16
Age-adjusted death rates from Hodgkin's disease per 100,000 population, 1987 and 1995.

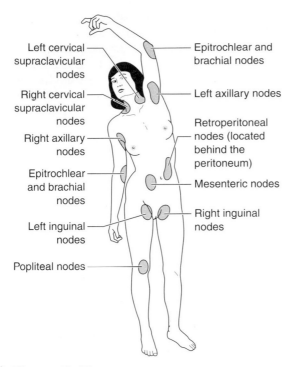

Figure 13-17
Sites for Hodgkin's disease.

recommended. Bone marrow transplants and mono-clonal antibody treatment are being tested.

Non-Hodgkin's Lymphoma

Any cancer of the lymphoid tissue that is not diag-nosed as Hodgkin's disease is referred to as non-Hodgkin's lymphoma. These cancers vary in degree, with some being more dangerous than others, depending on their nature. Figure 13-18 shows a steady increase in death rates from non-Hodgkin's lymphoma from 1987 to 1995. Estimates are 54,900 new cases for 2000, and 26,100 deaths. The peak incidence is higher than that of Hodgkin's disease, with about twenty-five percent occurring between the ages of fifty and fifty-nine and the greatest inci-dence between sixty and sixty-nine years of age.

Predisposing Factors

In most cases, the cause is unknown. Suppression of the immune system, viruses, and chromosomal abnormalities have been suspected. One kind, Burkitt's lymphoma (Figure 13-19), found only in Africa, is thought to be caused by the Epstein-Barr virus, and it is suspected that infection with HIV increases the risk for developing non-Hodgkin's lymphoma. It is also more common in organ trans-plant patients and other patients with autoimmune diseases such as rheumatoid arthritis and systemic lupus **erythematosus.**

Symptoms

There is usually a painless swelling of one or more lymph nodes in the groin or neck areas. There may also be enlargement of the liver and spleen. Other symptoms are abdominal pain, intestinal bleeding, and vomiting of blood. When different organs become involved, the symptoms vary. Spread of the disease impairs the immune system, so the patient may die from infections or an uncontrolled spread of other cancers.

Prevention

Preventive measures are unknown.

Treatment

Radiation, chemotherapy, and bone marrow trans-plants may be used alone or together, depending upon the stage and location of the cancer.

LEUKEMIA

Leukemia is a chronic or acute disease character-ized by unrestrained growth of white blood cells (leukocytes). There are many different types of leukemia, which are classified according to the dominant cell type and severity of the disease. Although leukemia is often thought of as a child-hood disease, it strikes many more adults (28,200 cases per year, compared with 2600 in children). For 2000 it is estimated that there will be 30,800 new cases and 21,700 deaths. Efforts to treat leukemia have been more successful than for most other cancers. The low five-year survival rate of forty-three percent for all types is due to very poor survival for some types whereas the rates have improved significantly for others. For acute lym-phocytic leukemia, the five-year survival rate has improved from thirty-eight percent in the 1970s to

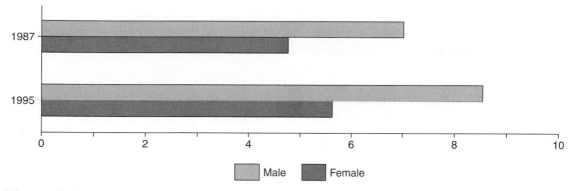

Figure 13-18

Age-adjusted death rates from non-Hodgkin's lymphoma per 100,000 population, 1987 and 1995.

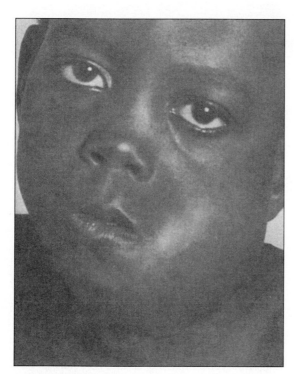

Figure 13-19

Burkitt's lymphoma.

43% in the late 1980s and early 1990s. For children, the five-year survival rate for acute lymphocytic leukemia has improved from fifty-three percent to seventy-eight percent for the same period. Leukemia death rates for males have increased

slightly while they have decreased slightly for females over the eight-year period 1987 to 1995 (Figure 13-20).

Predisposing Factors

The causes of leukemia are unknown. Among the possible factors are viruses, radiation, and certain chemicals.

Symptoms

Cold symptoms that do not clear up within two weeks, fatigue, weight loss, repeated infections, and easy bruising are the warning signs for leukemia.

Prevention

Preventive measures for leukemia are unknown.

Treatment

The traditional treatments for leukemia are chemotherapy and bone marrow transplant.

OVARIAN CANCER

Twenty-three thousand one hundred new cases of ovarian cancer are estimated in the United States for 2000 and 14,000 deaths. Because ovarian cancer is often asymptomatic, it may be far advanced before detection. The five-year survival rate for localized ovarian cancer is ninety-five percent, but

erythematosus   e-ryth-e-ma-TO-sus

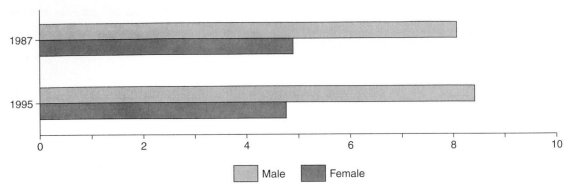

Figure 13-20
Age-adjusted death rates from leukemia per 100,000 population, 1987 and 1995.

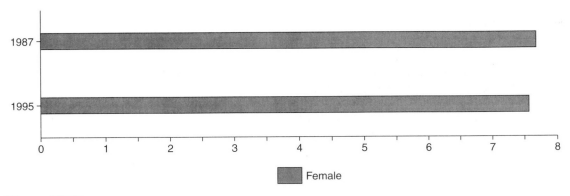

Figure 13-21
Age-adjusted death rates from ovarian cancer per 100,000 population, 1987 and 1995.

that drops to twenty-eight percent when it has spread to distant sites. Over an eight-year period, death rates for ovarian cancer have decreased slightly (Figure 13-21).

Predisposing Factors
Ovarian cancer is rare in women under forty years of age and occurs more in women of higher socioeconomic status and in single women. Women who have never had children are twice as likely to develop ovarian cancer. If a woman has had breast cancer, her chances of developing ovarian cancer double. Risk increases with age, with the highest rates for women over sixty years of age. The highest incidence rates for ovarian cancer come from the industrialized nations, except for Japan where the rates are lower.

Symptoms
As was indicated earlier, ovarian cancer is often symptomless until it is advanced. If symptoms do occur, there may be abdominal swelling and discomfort, vague pain, bloating, nausea, anorexia, or heartburn. These symptoms are related to the location of the cancer in the ovaries. There may also be frequent urination, constipation, pelvic discomfort, distention, and weight loss.

Primary Prevention
Primary preventive measures are unknown.

Secondary Prevention
Yearly pelvic examinations after the age of forty may lead to early detection. With early detection, ninety-five percent live five years or longer.

Treatment

Treatment for ovarian cancer varies a great deal, with different combinations of surgery, chemotherapy, and radiation. If the cancer is only on one side in adolescents or young women, a more conservative approach may be used. In other cases, more aggressive therapy may be used, including hysterectomy and removal of the fallopian tubes and ovaries on both sides, along with multiple biopsies of other organs and lymph nodes. In some cases, remissions have been achieved with drug combinations.

LIVER CANCER

Liver cancer may arise in liver cells or, frequently, be the result of metastasis from other parts of the body. There were 15,300 new cases and 13,800 deaths estimated for cancer of the liver and biliary (bile) system for 2000. For the eight-year period shown in Figure 13-22 there was a steady increase in death rates for both men and women from primary and unspecified cancer of the liver. Cancer of the liver is more prevalent in men, and, as with many cancers, it becomes more common as people get older. The disease is usually fatal within a year.

Predisposing Factors

Exposure to hepatitis B seems to be closely linked to primary liver cancer. This cancer may also be associated with cirrhosis of the liver. Whether cirrhosis leads to cancer or whether alcoholism and the subsequent malnutrition predispose the liver to develop cancer is unclear. Either way, alcoholism is a high- risk factor. There have been some indications that exposure to certain environmental carcinogens may result in liver cancer. These substances include the chemical compound aflatoxin (a mold that grows on rice and peanuts), androgens, and oral estrogens.

Secondary liver cancer
= mestasis

Symptoms

The most common signs of liver cancer are weight loss, loss of appetite, and lethargy. There may also be pain in the upper abdomen. In the later stages of disease there is jaundice and **ascites** (fluid in the abdomen).

Primary Prevention

Avoidance of hepatitis B, not sharing needles used for injections, and use of alcohol in moderation (if at all) reduce the risk of developing cancer of the liver.

Secondary Prevention

A physical exam can detect an enlarged liver, and ultrasound scanning can detect abnormal areas in the liver, but a liver biopsy is the only way to confirm the diagnosis. These tests are not performed routinely.

ascites a-SI-tez

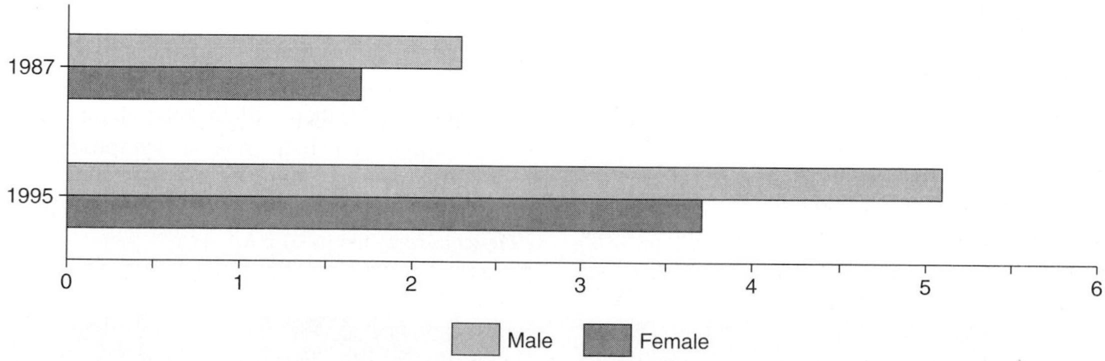

Figure 13-22

Age-adjusted death rates from liver and intrahepatic bile duct cancer per 100,000 population, 1987 and 1995.

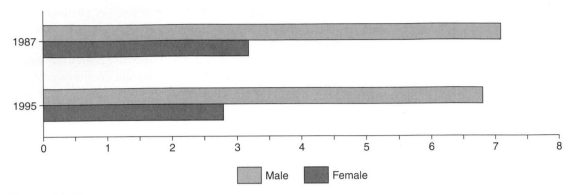

Figure 13-23
Age-adjusted death rates from stomach cancer per 100,000 population, 1987 and 1995.

Treatment

In primary liver cancer, if cirrhosis is not also present and the cancer is in only one lobe of the liver, the tumor can be removed surgically, possibly leading to a cure. A liver transplant may be considered if the disease has not spread, and there is chemotherapy that can help the patient survive longer. There is no cure for secondary liver cancer, but survival can still be prolonged with chemotherapy.

STOMACH CANCER

Stomach cancer develops in the lining of the stomach. It is estimated that there will be 21,500 new cases and 13,000 deaths from stomach cancer in 2000. Stomach cancer usually develops after the age of forty and is twice as common in men as in women. There are geographic variations in incidence, with a very high rate in Japan, Chili, Costa Rica, Hungary, and Poland. In the last fifty years, the incidence of stomach cancer has shown a dramatic decrease worldwide, but the reason for this is unknown. Figure 13-23 shows a slight decrease in death rates from stomach cancer over an eight-year period in the United States.

Predisposing Factors

The cause of stomach cancer is unknown, but it is thought that diet plays a part, and recent research indicates that *Helicobacter* (formerly *Campylobacter*) bacteria may also be involved. Having gastritis, anemia, and belonging to blood group A seem to increase the risk. Eating a great deal of smoked, pickled, or salted food may also be a factor in the development of stomach cancer.

Symptoms

Generally there are no symptoms until the cancer is in an advanced state. When they do appear, they are similar to those for peptic ulcer, and people tend to treat themselves with antacids for the fullness feeling, nausea, and eventual vomiting.

Prevention

Preventive measures are unknown.

Treatment

Gastrectomy, or removing all or part of the stomach, is the only effective treatment. If the condition is inoperable, then radiation therapy and anti-cancer drugs can help relieve symptoms and prolong survival.

Helicobacter	he-le-ko-BAK-tur

SUMMARY

Table 13-3 provides a summary of relevant data concerning the eleven major cancers just discussed.

TABLE 13-3	Cancers with the Highest Fatality Rates*				
Disease	**Special Characteristics**	**Predisposing Factors**	**Common Symptoms**	**Prevention**	**Treatment**
Lung Cancer	Most common cancer in the United States, 171,600 new cases, and most deaths, 158,900 estimated for 1999. Five-year survival 50%. More cases occur in men but women are catching up. In 1987 for the first time, it caused more deaths than breast cancer in women	Cigarette smoking; history of smoking 20 or more years; exposure to certain industrial substances; residential radon exposure; exposure to sidestream smoke	Persistent cough, sputum streaked with blood, chest pain, recurring pneumonia or bronchitis, fever, weakness, weight loss, anorexia, bone and joint pain, gynecomastia (all late stage symptoms)	No smoking; chest X ray; sputum analysis, fiberoptic exam of bronchi	Traditional treatments are used. Immunotherapy and laser therapy are being used experimentally
Colorectal Cancer	Second most common cancer, 124,400 new cases, and second highest number of deaths, 56,000, estimated for 1999. Five-year survival 91%. Develops slowly and remains localized for a long time. Equal number of deaths	Personal or family history of cancer or polyps of colon or rectum; inflammatory bowel disease, high-fat and/or low fiber diet, 40% or more over ideal weight	Pallor, malnutrition, fluid in abdomen, enlarged liver, swollen lymph glands, black tarry stools, cramping, rectal bleeding, and feeling of pressure in abdomen (colon); in the rectum, change in bowel habits with diarrhea or periods of	Maintain ideal weight, low-fat, high-fiber diet, digital exam, hemoccult test, and proctoscopy as recommended by doctor	Surgery is the most effective treatment, colostomy may be necessary

*Five-year survival rates given are for cancer that is localized unless otherwise stated.

TABLE 13-3	*Continued*				
Disease	**Special Characteristics**	**Predisposing Factors**	**Common Symptoms**	**Prevention**	**Treatment**
Colorectal Cancer— Cont'd	among men and women		diarrhea and constipation alternating, blood or mucus in stools, sense of incomplete evacuation; in late stages, pain, feeling of fullness, constant ache in rectal or sacral area		
Breast Cancer	1 in 9 women will develop breast cancer; 176,300 new cases, 43,700 deaths estimated for 1999. Five-year survival 97% Incidence rate has steadily increased but death rate has remained stable with improved treatment methods	Family history of breast cancer; long menstrual cycles; early menses or late menopause; first pregnancy after age 35; Caucasian or middle or upper socioeconomic level; constant stress in home or work life	A lump, thickening, swelling, dimpling, skin irritation, distortion of the breast; retraction, scaliness, pain, or tenderness of the nipple	Stress management, self-examination, mammograms	Radiation therapy, chemotherapy, hormone manipulation, or surgery are standard treatments The four types of mastectomy are: radical, modified radical, total or simple, and partial or segmental (lumpectomy)
Prostate Cancer	Among the top three killers of men; 179,300 new cases and 37,000 deaths for 1999; 93%	Highest in African American males; cause unknown, many possibilities being investigated	Weak or interrupted urine flow, need to urinate frequently, especially at night; blood in urine; pain	Rectal exam yearly for men over 40; ultrasound for men at high risk	Surgery to remove male hormone production site of testicle; 72% retain potency

TABLE 13-3	*Continued*				
Disease	**Special Characteristics**	**Predisposing Factors**	**Common Symptoms**	**Prevention**	**Treatment**
Prostate Cancer— Cont'd	survival if localized		or burning on urination; continuing pain in lower back, pelvis, or upper thighs; symptoms in advanced stages only		Treatments also include administration of female hormone, chemotherapy, and radiation
Pancreatic Cancer	Incidence has been increasing steadily over past 20 years. Over 28,600 new cases and 28,600 deaths estimated for 1999. Five-year survival rate is 3%	Smoking, sex (30% more in men), and race (65% more in blacks); chronic drinking, coffee, diets high in fat and protein, food additives, certain industrial chemicals	No symptoms until advanced stages, then jaundice, weight loss, abdominal or low back pain	No smoking; avoid suspected carcinogens such as coffee, food additives, alcohol, high fat and high protein foods	Traditional treatments are rarely successful
Hodgkin's Disease	Involves lymphatic tissue mainly in lymph nodes and spleen. Fatal if untreated. Recent advances leading to a cure; 7,200 new cases, 1,300 deaths estimated for 1999	Unknown	Enlargement of lymph nodes in the neck or armpits; malaise; fever; loss of appetite; weight loss, night sweats	Unknown	Treatment includes radiation or chemotherapy (bone marrow transplant and monoclonal antibodies are being tested)
Non-Hodgkin's Lymphoma	Any cancer of lymphoid tissue other	Unknown	Swelling of lymph nodes in groin or	Unknown	Traditional treatment is used

Table 13-3	*Continued*				
Disease	**Special Characteristics**	**Predisposing Factors**	**Common Symptoms**	**Prevention**	**Treatment**
Non-Hodgkin's Lymphoma —Cont'd	than Hodgkin's disease; 56,800 new cases, 25,700 deaths estimated for 1999		neck; enlarged liver and spleen; abdominal pain, intestinal bleeding, vomiting of blood		
Leukemia	Unrestrained growth of white blood cells. Many different types exist. Survival has improved dramatically for some types. Estimate for 1999 new cases— 30,200; deaths— 22,100	Unknown, possibly a virus, radiation, or heredity	Cold symptoms that last beyond 2 weeks, fatigue, weight loss, repeated infections, easy bruising	Unknown	Chemotherapy and bone marrow transplant are the treatments used
Ovarian Cancer	Estimate of 25,200 new cases and 14,500 deaths for 1999. Usually in advanced stages at detection	Rare in women under 40; more in higher socioeconomic status and in single women; twice as likely in women who have never had children and in those who have had endometrial cancer; risk increases	Often none until advanced—if symptoms, abdominal swelling and discomfort, vague pain, bloating, nausea, anorexia, heartburn	Yearly pelvic exams after age of 40	Different combinations of surgery, chemotherapy, and radiation are used. May include hysterectomy and removal of the fallopian tubes and ovaries on both sides. Remissions have occurred with combi-

TABLE 13-3	*Continued*				
Disease	**Special Characteristics**	**Predisposing Factors**	**Common Symptoms**	**Prevention**	**Treatment**
Ovarian Cancer— Cont'd		with age, highest in women 65–84			nations of drugs.
Liver	Estimate of 14,500 new cases and 13,600 deaths for 1999. More prevalent in men and incidence increases with age. Usually fatal within a year	Exposure to hepatitis B, alcoholism, exposure to certain environmental carcinogens	Weight loss, loss of appetite, lethargy, pain in upper abdomen, jaundice, ascites	Avoidance of hepatitis B, moderation in use of alcohol	Treatment includes surgical removal of involved tissue, chemotherapy, and possibly a liver transplant
Stomach Cancer	Develops in lining of stomach; 21,900 new cases and 13,500 deaths estimated for 1999. Incidence has increased dramatically in last 50 years	Cause unknown, diet, and bacteria may be factors; gastritis, anemia, and belonging to blood group A may also be factors	A feeling of fullness, nausea, and vomiting in last stages	Unknown	Gastrectomy is the only effective treatment. If inoperable, chemotherapy and radiation therapy are used to relieve symptoms and prolong survival

QUESTIONS FOR REVIEW

1. How does cancer compare with heart disease in number of deaths?

2. What is the survival rate for cancer today?

3. Why is the number of deaths from lung cancer increasing when there are fewer people smoking today?

4. Define the following: neoplasm, tumor, benign neoplasm, malignant tumor.

5. Identify each step in the theory of cancer development stated in the text.

6. Define the following: carcinoma, sarcoma, melanoma, neuroblastoma, adenocarcinoma, hepatoma, leukemia, lymphoma.

7. What is meant by staging a cancer, and why is it done?

8. In what five ways do cancer cells differ from regular cells?

9. What factors can increase the susceptibility to cancer, and how can they be changed?

10. What is the significance of pain as a symptom of cancer?

11. What are the best means of primary prevention for cancer?

12. What are the seven warning signals for cancer developed by the ACS?

13. What traditional methods are used to treat cancer?

14. What other methods of treating cancer are being studied scientifically?

15. What is meant by the mind-body connection in reference to curing cancer (or any other disease)?

16. What does *E-Cap* stand for, and how did the group get started?

17. Why is it difficult to research some alternative cancer treatments scientifically?

18. Why is the prognosis for lung cancer so poor?

19. What two factors have helped to improve the five-year survival rate for colorectal cancer?

20. What surgery may be performed for advanced stages of colorectal cancer?

21. What percentage of women who are alive today will develop breast cancer if the present rates continue?

22. Why is a woman more likely to discover a sign of breast cancer than a doctor or nurse?

23. Describe the four types of breast surgery used for cancer.

24. What races have the highest and lowest incidence of prostatic cancer? What theories can be given for the cause of this?

25. Which men should have a digital rectal exam and which should have ultrasound screening for prostatic cancer?

26. What kind of treatment may be used for prostatic cancer?

27. Why is the five-year survival rate for pancreatic cancer so low?

28. What is Hodgkin's disease?

29. What is non-Hodgkin's lymphoma?

30. What are some of the unique characteristics of stomach cancer?

31. Why is stomach cancer generally not diagnosed until an advanced stage?

32. What is leukemia?

33. When efforts to treat leukemia are considered so successful, why is the five-year survival rate still so low?

34. What is the treatment for leukemia?

35. Why is the death rate high for ovarian cancer?

36. For the cancers in this chapter, identify predisposing factors and symptoms.

37. What primary prevention procedures are there for lung, colorectal, breast, and pancreatic cancers?

38. What secondary prevention procedures are available for lung, colorectal, breast, prostate, and ovarian cancers?

FURTHER READING

Alavanja, M. C. R., et al., 1999. Residential radon exposure and risk of lung cancer in Missouri. *American Journal of Public Health* 89:1042.

Barber, M. D. 1999. The effect of an oral nutritional supplement enriched with fish oil on weight-loss in patients with pancreatic cancer. *British Journal of Cancer* 81:80.

Barkin, J. S., and J. A. Goldstein. 1999. Diagnostic approach to pancreatic cancer. *Gastroenterol Clinic of North America* 28:709.

Bennett, William P., and C. R. Michael. 1999. Environmental tobacco smoke, genetic susceptibility, and risk of lung cancer in never-smoking women. *Journal of the National Cancer Institute* 91:2009.

Bhatia, S., et al. 1999. Family history of cancer in children and young adults with colorectal cancer. *Medical Pediatric Onco* 33:470.

Bociek, R. G., and J. O. Armitage. 1999. Hodgkin's disease and non-Hodgkin's lymphoma. *Current Opinion Hematology* 6:205.

Bostwick, D. G., and C. S. Foster. 1999. Predictive factors in prostate cancer; current concepts from the 1999 College of American Pathologists conferences on solid tumor prognostic factors and the 1999 WHO second international consultation on prostate cancer. *Seminar Urol Oncol* 17:222.

Braithwaite, K. L., and P. H. Rabbits. 1999. Multi-step evolution of lung cancer. *Seminars in Cancer Biology* 9:255.

Brenner, H. 1999. Helicobacter pyloric infection among offspring of patients with stomach cancer. *Gastroenterology* 118:31.

Brown, Kenneth G. 1999. Lung cancer and environmental tobacco smoke: Occupational risk to nonsmokers. *Environmental Health Perspectives Supplements* 107:885.

Brown, N. L. et al. 1999. Obtaining long-term disease specific costs of care: application to Medicare enrollees diagnosed with colorectal cancer. *Medical Care* 37:1249.

Buchholz, T. A., et al. 1999. Tumor suppressor genes and breast cancer. *Radiation Oncology Investigations* 7:55.

Burach, R. C., and D. P. Wood, Jr. 1999. Screening for prostate cancer. The challenge of promoting informed decision making in the absence of definitive evidence of effectiveness. *Med Clin North America* 83:1423.

Camilleri-Brennan, J., and R. J. Steele. 1999. A comparative study of knowledge and awareness of colorectal and breast cancer. *Eur J Surg. Oncol* 25:580.

"Cancer facts and figures 2000." American Cancer Society, www.cancer.org.

Carpenter, C. L., et al. 1999. Mentholated cigarette smoking and lung-cancer risk. *Annals of Epidemiology* 9:114.

Cohen, Jennifer H., and Alan R. Kristal. 1999. Fruit and vegetable intakes and prostate cancer risk. *Journal of the National Cancer Institute* 92:61.

Cohen, M. M., and E. Strass. 1999. Statement of the American society of human genetics on genetic testing for breast and ovarian cancer predisposition. *American Journal of Human Genetics* 55:1.

Colditz, G. A. 1999. Hormones and breast cancer: Evidence and implications for consideration of risks and benefits of hormone replacement therapy. *Journal of Women's Health* 8:347.

Colorectal cancer screening. *CA:A Cancer Journal for Clinicians* 49:2, 1999.

Cooper, G. S., et al. 1999. Colorectal carcinoma screening attitudes and practices among primary care physicians in counties at extremes of either high or low cancer case-fatality. *Cancer* 86:1669.

Cooperman, A. M., et al. 1999. Nutritional and metabolic aspects of pancreatic cancer. *American Academy of DE* 3:17.

Daniell, H. W., et al. 1999. Progressive osteoporosis during androgendeprivation therapy for prostate cancer. *Journal of Urology* 163:181.

Determinants of long term survival after surgery for cancer of the lung: a population based study. *Cancer* 86:2229, 1999.

Dillman, R. O. 1999. Perceptions of herceptin registered: a monoclonal antibody for the treatment of breast cancer. *Cancer Biotherapy and Radiopharmaceuticals* 14:5.

Donaldson, L., et al. 1999. Association between outcome and telomere DNA content in prostate cancer. *Urology* 162:1788.

Donnell, R. F. 1999. Prostate cancer: A challenge for screening. *Surgical Oncology Clinic in North America* 8:693.

Earnest, F., et al. 1999. Suspected non-small cell lung cancer: incidence of occult brain and skeletal metastases and effectiveness of imaging for detection—pilot study. *Radiology* 211:137.

Environmental Health Perspective Supplements 107:885.

Epstein, J. I., et al. 1999 The significant of prior benign needle biopsies in men subsequently diagnosed with prostate cancer. *Urology* 162:1649.

Fendrick, Mark A., Michael E. Chernew, Richard A. Hirth, et al. 1999. Clinical and economic effects of population based *Helicobacter pylori* screening to prevent gastric cancer. *Archives of Internal Medicine* 159:142.

Ferrell, R. E., et al. 1999. A genetic linkage study of familial breast ovarian cancer. *Cancer Causes Control* 38:241.

Friedenberg, W. R., et al. 1999. Multi-drug resistance in chronic lymphocytic leukemia. *Leukemia & Lymphoma* 34:171.

Fuchs, Charles S., Edward L. Giovanucci, et al. 1999. Dietary fibre and the risk of colorectal cancer and adenoma in women. *New England Journal of Medicine* 340:169.

Gauderman, W. J., and J. L. Morrison. 1999. Evidence for age-specific genetic relative risks in lung cancer. *American Journal of Epidemiology* 151:41.

Green, L. M., et al. Childhood leukemia and personal monitoring of residential exposures to electric and magnetic fields in Ontario, Canada. *Cancer Causes & Control* 10:233.

Guzman, R. C., et al. 1999. Hormonal prevention of breast cancer: Mimicking the protective effect of pregnancy. *Proceedings of the National Academy of Sciences* 96:2520.

Habermann, T. M. 1999. Non-Hodgkin's lymphoma: Present status and future prospects. *Hospital Practice* 34:81.

Hadden, J. W. 1999. The immunology and immunotherapy of breast cancer: An update. *International Journal of Immunopharmacology* 21:79.

Hansson, L. E. 1999. Survival in stomach cancer is improving: Results of a nationwide population based Swedish study. 230:162.

Harlow, B. L., and D. W. Cramer. 1999. Self reported use of antidepressants or benzoidiazepine tranquilizers and risk of epithelial ovarian cancer: Evidence from two combined case-control studies. *Cancer Causes Control* 6:130.

Hart, A. R. 1999. Pancreatic cancer: Any prospects for prevention? *Postgraduate Medical Journal* 75:521.

Hart, K. B., et al. 1999. The impact of race on biochemical disease-free survival in early-stage prostate cancer patients treated with surgery or radiation therapy. *International Journal of Radiat Oncol Biology Phys* 45:1235.

Helm, J. F., and R. S. Sandler. 1999. Colorectal cancer screening. *Medical Clinic of North America* 83:1403.

Hoffman, Philip C., and Ann M. Mauer. 1999. Lungs, cancer, treatment: Small cell lung cancer. *The Lancet* 355:479.

Howard, J. M. 1999. Development and progress is resective surgery for pancreatic cancer. *World Journal of Surgery* 23:901.

Hsing, A. W., et al. 1999. International trends and patterns of prostate cancer incidence and mortality. *International Journal of Cancer* 85:60.

Humphreys, M. J., et al. 1999. The potential of gene therapy in pancreatic cancer. *International Journal of Pancreatology* 26:5.

Interferon-alfa and survival in metastatic renal carcinoma: Early results of a randomized controlled trial. *The Lancet* 353:14, 1999.

Jacobs, Timothy W., Celia Byrne, et al. 1999. Radial scars in benign breast biopsy specimens and the risk of breast cancer. *New England Journal of Medicine* 340:430.

Jaklitsch, M. T., et al. 1999. New surgical options for elderly lung cancer patients. *Chest* 116:480S.

Jarrett, R. F., and J. MacKensie, 1999. Epstein-Barr virus and other candidate viruses in the pathogenesis of Hodgkin's disease. *Semin Hematol* 36:260.

Johnson, Brett A. 1999. Flexible sigmoidoscopy: Screening for colorectal cancer. *American Family Physician* 59:313.

Kamel, O. W., et al. 1999. A population based, case control study of non-Hodgkin's lymphoma in patients with rheumatoid arthritis. *Journal of Rheumatology* 26:1676.

Kernan, G. J., et al. 1999. Occupational risk factors for pancreatic cancer: A case control study based on death certificates from 24 U.S. states. *American Journal of Industrial Medicine* 36:260.

Kneket, Paul, Ritva Jarvinen, Lyly Teppo, et al. 1999. Role of various carotenoids in lung cancer prevention. *Journal of the National Cancer Institute* 91:182.

Kobayashi, K., et al. 1999. Surgical treatment for both pulmonary and hepatic metastases from colorectal cancer. *Journal of Thoracic Cardiovascular Surgery* 118:1090.

Kristal, A. R., et al. 1999. Vitamin and mineral supplement use is associated with reduced risk of prostate cancer. *Cancer Epidemiol Biomarkers Prev* 8:887.

Kumar, S., et al. 2000. Epstein-Barr virus-positive primary gastrointestinal Hodgkin's disease: Association with inflammatory bowel disease and immunosuppression. *American Journal Surg Pathol* 24:66.

Kushi, Lawrence H., Pamela J. Mink, Aaron R. Folsom, et al. 1999. Prospective study of diet and ovarian cancer. *American Journal of Epidemiology* 149:21.

Langman, M. J. 1999. Prospective, double-blind, placebo-controlled randomized trial of cimetidine in gastric cancer. *British Journal of Cancer* 81:1356.

Larkin, Marilyn. 1999. Breast cancer risk much reduced by prophylactic bilateral mastectomy. *The Lancet* 353:301.

Larkin, Marilyn. 1999. Sex differences in lung—cancer susceptibility explained. *The Lancet* 355:121.

Lash, T. L., and A. Aschengrau. 1999. Active and passive cigarette smoking and the occurrence of breast cancer. *American Journal of Epidemiology* 149:5.

Lenner, P., et al. 1999. Serum antibodies against p53 in relation to cancer risk and prognosis in breast cancer: A population-based epidemiological study. *British Journal of Cancer* 79:927.

Lipsett, M., and S. Campleman. 1999. Occupational exposure to diesel exhaust and lung cancer: A meta-analysis. *American Journal of Public Health* 89:1009.

Litwin, M. S., et al. 1999. Defining an international research agenda for quality of life in men with prostate cancer. *Prostate* 41:58.

Loge, J. H., et al. 1999. Hodgkin's disease survivors more fatigued than the general population. *Journal of Clinical Oncology* 17:253.

Lowenfels, A. B., et al. 1999. Chronic pancreatitis and other risk factors for pancreatic cancer. *Gastroenterol Clinic of North America* 28:673.

Lowry, W. S., and R. J. Atkinson. 1999. Tumor suppressor genes and risk of metastasis on ovarian cancer. *British Medical Journal* 307:542.

Lubin, Jay H. 1999. Estimating lung cancer risk with exposure to environmental tobacco smoke. *Environmental Health Perspectives Supplements* 107:879.

McConkey, D. J., and J. Chandra. 1999. Protease activation and glucocorticoid-induced apoptosis in chronic lymphocytic leukemia. *Leukemia & Lymphoma* 33:421.

McCunney, R. J. 1999. Hodgkin's disease, work, and the environment. A review. *Journal of Occupational Environment Medicine* 41:36.

Midgeley, R., and D. Kerr. 1999. Colorectal cancer. *The Lancet* 353:391.

Miller, Karl E. 1999. Pesticide exposure and non-Hodgkin's lymphoma. *American Family Physician* 60:622.

Murray, P. G., et al. 1999. Effect of Epstein-Barr virus infection on response to chemotherapy and survival in Hodgkin's disease. *Blood* 94:442.

Nasu, Y., et al., 1999. Prostate cancer gene therapy: Outcome of basic research and clinical trials. *Tech Uro* 5:185.

Nelson, J. E., and R. E. Harris. 1999. Inverse association of prostate cancer and non-steroidal anti-inflammatory drugs (NSAIDs): Results of a case-control study. *Oncol Rep* 7:169.

Ohsawa, Masahiko, et al. 1999. Risk of non-Hodgkin's lymphoma in patients with hepatitis C virus infection. *International Journal of Cancer* 80:237.

Ohtsubo, H., et al. 1999. Epstein-Barr virus involvement in T-cell malignancy: significance in adult T-cell leukemia. *Leukemia & Lymphoma* 33:451.

Okabe, S. 1999. Mechanistic aspects of green tea as a cancer preventive: effect of components on human stomach cancer cell lines. *Japan Journal of Cancer* 90:733.

Pandian, S. S., et al. 1999. Fatty acids and prostate cancer: Current status and future challenges. *Journal R. Coll. Surg. Edinb* 44:352.

Persson, B., and M. Fredrikson. 1999. Some risk factors for non-Hodgkin's lymphoma. *International Journal of Occupational Medicine and Environmental Health* 12:135.

Petersen, G. M., et al. 1999. Genetic testing and counseling for hereditary forms of colorectal cancer. *Cancer* 86:2540.

Portlock, Carol S. 1999. Greater curability in advanced Hodgkin's disease. *Cancer Journal* 5:264.

Prescott, E., et al. 1999. Alcohol intake and risk of lung cancer: Influence of type of alcoholic beverage. *American Journal of Epidemiology* 149:463.

Provencio, M., et al. 1999. Comparison of the long term mortality in Hodgkin's disease patients with that of the general population. *Annals of Oncology* 10:1199.

Recent findings underscore new trends in colorectal cancer research. *CA:A Cancer Journal for Clinicians* 49:3, 1999.

Reynolds, Peggy. 1999. Epidemiologic evidence for workplace ETS as a risk factor for lung cancer. *Environmental Health Perspectives Supplements* 107:865.

Risch, H. A., et al. 1999. Dietary lactose intake, lactose intolerance, and the risk of epithelial ovarian cancer in southern Ontario (Canada). *Cancer Causes Control* 5:540.

Ritchie, J. P. 1999. Anti-androgens and other hormonal therapies for prostate cancer. *Urology* 54:15.

Rustum, Y. M., and S. Cao. 1999. New drugs in therapy of colorectal cancer: Preclinical studies. *Seminar Oncology* 26:612.

Scheitel, S. M., et al. 1999. Colorectal cancer screening: A community case-control study of proctosigmoidoscopy, barium enema radiography, and fecal occult blood test efficacy. *Mayo Clinical Procedure* 74:1207.

Smalley, Walter, and Wayne A. Ray. 1999. Use of non-steroidal anti-inflammatory drugs and incidence of colorectal cancer. *Archives of Internal Medicine* 159:161.

Smith, J. A. Jr., et al. 1999. Complications of advanced prostate cancer. *Urology* 54:8.

Sohayda, C. J., et al. 1999. Race as an independent predictor of outcome after treatment for localized prostate cancer. *Urology* 162:1331.

Stanford, J. L., et al. 1999. Vasectomy and risk of prostate cancer. *Cancer Epidemiol Biomarkers Prev* 8:881.

Travis, Lois B., Eric J. Holowaty, Kjell Bergfeldt, et al. 1999. Risk of leukemia after platinum based chemotherapy for ovarian cancer. *The New England Journal of Medicine* 340:351.

Vallisa, D., et al. 1999. Association between hepatitis C virus and non-Hodgkin's lymphoma and effects of viral infection on histologic subtype and clinical course. *American Journal of Medicine* 106:556.

Van Veldhuizen, P. J., et al. 1999. Treatment of vitamin D deficiency in patients with metastatic prostate cancer may improve bone pain and muscle strength. *Journal of Urology* 163:187.

Vellenga, E., et al. 1999. Peripheral blood cell transplantation as an alternative to autologous marrow transplantation in the treatment of acute myeloid leukemia? *Bone Marrow Transplantation* 23:1279.

Verfaillie, C. M., et al. 1999. Gene therapy for chronic myelogenous leukemia. *Molecular Medicine Today* 5:359.

Villeneuve, P. J., et al. 1999. Risk factors for prostate cancer: Results from the Canadian National Enhanced Cancer Surveillance System. The Canadian Cancer registries epidemiology research group. *Cancer Causes Control* 10:355.

Woodson, K., et al. 1999. Association between alcohol and lung cancer in the alpha-tocopherol, beta-carotene cancer prevention study in Finland. *Cancer Causes & Control* 10:219.

Wu, Anna H. 1999. Exposure misclassification bias in studies of environmental tobacco smoke and lung cancer. *Environmental Health Perspectives Supplements* 107:873.

Wunsch, Hannah. 1999. Link between fibre and colorectal cancer debunked in largest-ever study. *The Lancet* 353:385.

Yu, H., et al. 1999. Enhanced prediction of breast cancer prognosis by evaluating expression of p53 and prostate specific antigen in combination. *British Journal of Cancer* 81:490.

Zahm, S. H., et al. 1999. Occupational physical activity and non-Hodgkin's lymphoma. *Medical Science Sports Exercise* 31:566.

Zhang, Shumin, and David J. Hunter. 1999. Dietary fat and protein in relation to risk of non-Hodgkin's lymphoma among women. *Journal of the National Cancer Institute* 91:1751.

OTHER CANCERS

OBJECTIVES

1. *State the connection between multiple myeloma and the immune system.*
2. *Identify measures that can be used in secondary prevention of uterine and cervical cancer.*
3. *Compare squamous cell and basal cell cancer with malignant melanoma.*
4. *Explain the "ABCD method" for identifying malignant melanoma.*
5. *State the way in which tobacco may lead to oral cancer.*
6. *Describe and give symptoms, predisposing factors, prevention, and treatment for the types of cancer in this chapter.*

CANCER OF THE CENTRAL NERVOUS SYSTEM

About 16,500 new cases and 13,000 deaths for cancers of the central nervous system (brain and spinal cord) were estimated for 2000. Because tumors of the spinal cord are rare, they will not be discussed, and the following material deals with brain cancer, unless stated otherwise. Cancer in the brain may be a primary growth arising from tissues within the brain or a secondary growth (metastasis) spread by the bloodstream or lymph from cancer elsewhere in the body, most often the lungs or breasts. People around the age of fifty and children are the most common victims. Figure 14-1 shows a slight decrease in death rates from brain cancer over an eight-year period.

Predisposing Factors
Predisposing factors for these cancers are unknown.

Symptoms
Depending upon the location of the tumor, there may be muscle weakness, loss of vision, speech difficulties, epileptic seizures, headache, vomiting, visual disturbances, impaired mental functioning, personality changes, loss

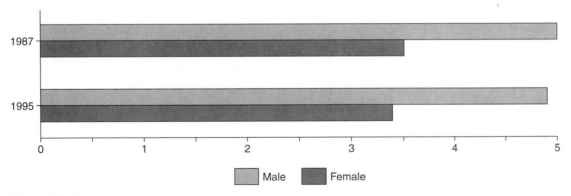

Male	Total	Female
Esophageal **9,400**	Esophageal **12,200**	Esophageal **2,800**
Bladder **8,100**	Bladder **12,100**	Bladder **4,000**
CNS **7,200**	CNS **13,100**	CNS **5,900**
Kidney **7,200**	Kidney **11,900**	Kidney **4,700**
Multiple myeloma **5,800**	Multiple myeloma **11,400**	Multiple myeloma **5,600**
Testicular **300**	Uterus **11,200**	Uterus **11,200**
Oral **5,400**	Oral **8,100**	Oral **2,700**
Melanoma **4,600**	Melanoma **7,300**	Melanoma **2,700**
Laryngeal **3,300**	Laryngeal **4,200**	Laryngeal **900**
Bone **800**	Bone **1,400**	Bone **600**
Thyroid **500**	Thyroid **1,200**	Thyroid **700**
All sites **52,600**	All sites **94,400**	All sites **41,800**

Death rates of other cancers.

Figure 14-1

Age-adjusted death rates from brain and other central nervous system cancers per 100,000 population, 1987 and 1995.

of coordination, and **hydrocephalus.** These symptoms are insidious and vary depending on site, size, and method of expansion.

Prevention

Preventive measures are unknown.

Treatment

When possible, removal of the tumor through surgery is the best treatment, but many malignant tumors in the brain are inaccessible, or surgery may be too invasive to allow removal. Chemotherapy and radiation may be used, and corticosteroids may be prescribed to reduce swelling and relieve symptoms. Treatment is mostly symptomatic, and if the growth cannot be removed completely, one-year survival is less than twenty percent.

ESOPHAGEAL CANCER

About 12,300 new cases and 12,100 deaths for **esophageal** cancer are estimated for 2000. There was a large increase in death rates for males and a small decrease for females (Figure 14-2) for the period 1987 through 1995. The disease occurs mostly in people over fifty years of age and is more common in men than in women, and in blacks than in whites.

Predisposing Factors
The cause of cancer of the esophagus is unknown, but high alcohol consumption and smoking are thought to be factors.

Symptoms
Initially the symptoms are nonspecific—a vague sense of pressure and fullness, and indigestion. Difficulty in swallowing, first with solids and later with fluids, occurs and becomes progressively worse until it is even difficult to swallow saliva. When food cannot pass, vomiting and weight loss occur (forty to fifty pounds in two to three months), but, as with most cancers, there is no pain until the disease is far advanced. The spilling over of vomited food into the trachea leads to frequent respiratory infections and some hoarseness.

Primary Prevention
Moderation in alcohol consumption and no smoking may reduce the risk of esophageal cancer.

Secondary Prevention
Tests to determine cancer of the esophagus would be performed only if a problem is suspected. They include a barium swallow and X-ray examinations, **endoscopy,** and biopsy.

Treatment
Removal of the esophagus provides the best hope of cure, but it involves radical surgery. Most of the esophagus is removed, and the stomach, or sometimes part of the colon, is pulled up into the chest to connect to the remaining upper portion of the esophagus. When the patient is too old or debilitated to survive this surgery, or the disease has spread, radiation and chemotherapy can cause regression of the cancer, relief of some of the symptoms, and occasionally a cure. Sometimes a tube is inserted into the stomach through the abdomen to allow the person to take in liquid or semisolid food.

BLADDER CANCER

The ACS estimated 53,200 new cases of bladder cancer and 12,200 deaths for 2000. Over an eight-year period (Figure 14-3) death rates remained fairly constant for both men and women. Bladder

| esophageal | e-SOF-a-JE-al |
| endoscopy | en-DOS-co-pe |

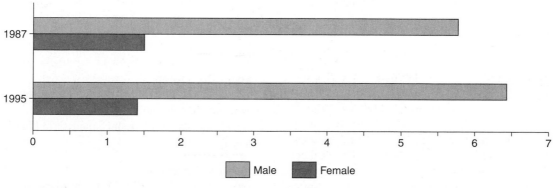

Figure 14-2
Age-adjusted death rates from esophageal cancer per 100,000 population, 1987 and 1995.

CASE STUDY

Esophageal Cancer

A thirty-nine year-old man went to his doctor for a physical exam and was referred to an oncologist. His symptoms were three to four years of heartburn that he treated with over-the-counter drugs, and difficulty swallowing for the past three months. Food seemed to get "hung up" in his throat. He also complained of pain below the sternum that was "gnawing or burning." In the past six or seven months he had lost weight and been bothered by a cough at night. Results of an endoscopy, biopsy, and barium swallow led to a diagnosis of gastroesophageal cancer. Because of the delay in getting to a doctor, the cancer was in an advanced stage. Radiation therapy, chemotherapy and surgery were used but the disease recurred and the patient died shortly after treatment.

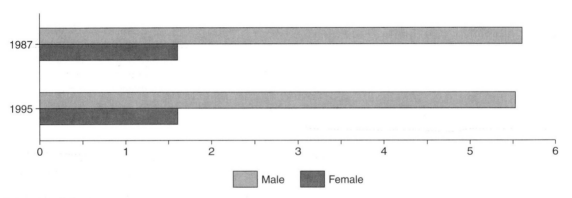

Figure 14-3
Age-adjusted death rates from urinary bladder cancer per 100,000 population, 1987 and 1995.

cancer occurs more often in people over fifty years of age and at an increasing rate as people get older. It has been more common in men than in women but this is changing.

Predisposing Factors

Smoking is considered to be the greatest risk factor, with smokers experiencing twice the risk of nonsmokers. Other environmental carcinogens may be risk factors for bladder cancer. Among these are 2-naphthylamine, benzidine, tobacco, nitrates, saccharin, alcohol, and coffee. Rubber workers, cable workers, weavers, aniline dye workers, hairdressers, petroleum workers, spray painters, and leather finishers are all at risk.

Symptoms

Generally the first symptom is blood in the urine, usually unaccompanied by pain. There may also be bladder irritability, urinary frequency, nocturia (increased urination at night), and dribbling.

Primary Prevention

Selecting a job that does not entail exposure to known carcinogens and avoidance of other carcinogenic agents greatly reduce the risk of bladder cancer.

Secondary Prevention

Bladder cancer can be diagnosed by the use of a cystoscope. This is a slender tube that has a lens and light, and it can be inserted through the urethra and into the bladder to enable the physician to examine the bladder wall.

Treatment

Traditional cancer treatments are used. For a more advanced case, a **cystectomy** (bladder removal) may be performed, and urine collected through a stoma (mouthlike opening) in the abdomen.

KIDNEY CANCER

Tumors of the kidney usually occur in older adults and may affect either one or both kidneys. With early detection, five-year survival rates are 88%. However, about thirty percent are not diagnosed until the cancer has metastasized. Kidney cancer death rates have been increasing in males faster than in females (Figure 14-4). For 2000, 31,200 new cases and 11,900 deaths are estimated.

Predisposing Factors

The cause of kidney cancer is unknown, but exposure to environmental pollutants may be a factor. It is twice as common in men as in women and usually strikes after age forty, with most of the cases being detected between the ages of fifty and sixty.

Symptoms

Hematuria (blood in the urine) is the most common early sign of kidney cancer. In some individuals, pain or a palpable mass may be the first symptom. Most patients do not have all three. Other symptoms include fever, hypertension, **hypercalcemia,** and urinary retention. When the disease is more advanced, weight loss, edema in the legs caused by the enlargement of lymph nodes, nausea, and vomiting occur.

Primary Prevention

Methods of primary prevention are unknown.

Secondary Prevention

The best prevention is a yearly cancer check after age forty. A doctor should be consulted at the first sign of hematuria, unusual pain, or a lump.

Treatment

Surgery to remove the affected parts is the only chance of relieving symptoms or being cured. Anticancer drugs and radiation have had little effect on this cancer. The individual can survive with one kidney, providing the noncancerous one is healthy, and there is the possibility of a transplant if both kidneys are diseased.

MULTIPLE MYELOMA

Multiple myeloma is a malignancy of plasma cells in the bone marrow. These cells are a type of B lymphocyte that function in making antibodies. When

cystectomy	sis-TEK-to-me
hematuria	hem-a-TU-re-a
hypercalcemia	hi-per-kal-SE-me-a

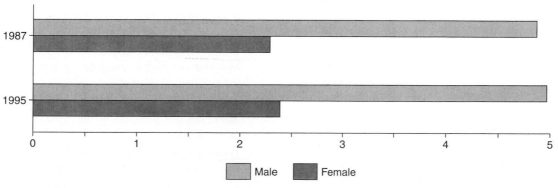

Figure 14-4

Age-adjusted death rates from kidney and renal pelvis cancer per 100,000 population, 1987 and 1995.

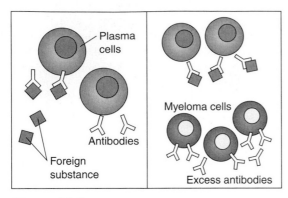

Figure 14-5
Multiple myeloma.

the cancerous cells begin to proliferate, they produce excessive amounts of one kind of antibody whereas production of the other antibodies is impaired (Figure 14-5). Thus the individual becomes particularly susceptible to infection. There has been a steady increase in multiple myeloma death rates as shown in Figure 14-6. For 2000 the estimates were 13,600 new cases and 11,200 deaths. Only about twenty percent of patients survive for four years or longer from the time of diagnosis.

Predisposing Factors
Predisposing factors for multiple myeloma are unknown.

Symptoms
Severe, constant back pain is the earliest symptom of multiple myeloma. Exercise causes an increase in the pain. There may also be arthritic symptoms, fever, malaise, anemia, and pathologic fractures. As the disease worsens, the patient is particularly susceptible to infection; there may also be a decrease in renal function or renal failure along with other symptoms of vertebral compression.

Prevention
No preventive measures are known.

Treatment
Chemotherapy and radiation are the treatments used for this cancer. Bone marrow transplant has been effective in some cases.

SKIN CANCER

Most skin cancers are either basal cell carcinoma or squamous cell carcinoma, which are highly curable. Skin cancer is the most common of all cancers. Approximately 1.3 million new cases of basal cell and squamous cell carcinoma are reported each year. One in every seven Americans is affected. Malignant melanoma is a more dangerous form of skin cancer and can spread swiftly throughout the body if untreated, resulting in death. About 43,700 Americans develop malignant melanoma each year with about 7,700 deaths annually. The five-year survival rate is 95% for melanoma that is discovered early. If it has metastasized regionally, five-year survival drops to 58%, and distant metastasis results in only a 13% survival rate. There has been a steady increase in melanoma death rates each year going back to the 1950s and continuing during the eight-year period shown in Figure 14-7. There has been a steady decrease in death rates from skin cancers other than melanoma during the same period.

Predisposing Factors
Risk factors for skin cancer include excessive exposure to ultraviolet radiation, fair skin, and occupational exposure to coal, tar, pitch, and creosote. Most of the 1,000,000-plus new cases diagnosed each year are due to sun exposure.

Symptoms
The ACS has developed an "ABCD method" for identifying malignant melanoma:

A symmetry, or one-half does not match the size or color of the other half.

B order irregularity (edges of the mole are irregular, notched, blurred, or ragged).

C olor changes or variation (melanomas are often mottled with various shades of brown, black, tan, red, blue, and white occurring on a single mole).

D iameter greater than six mm (larger than the size of a common pencil eraser).

These various characteristics of melanoma are illustrated in Figure 14-8.

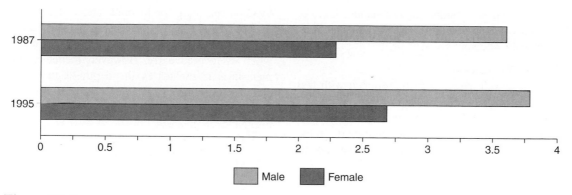

Figure 14-6

Age-adjusted death rates from multiple myeloma per 100,000 population, 1987 and 1995.

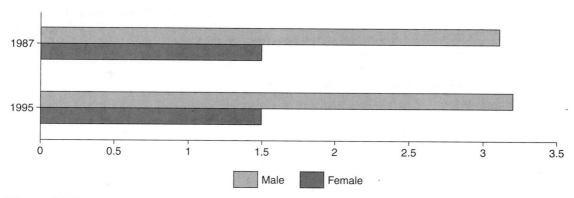

Figure 14-7

Age-adjusted death rates from melanoma of the skin, per 100,000 population, 1987 and 1995.

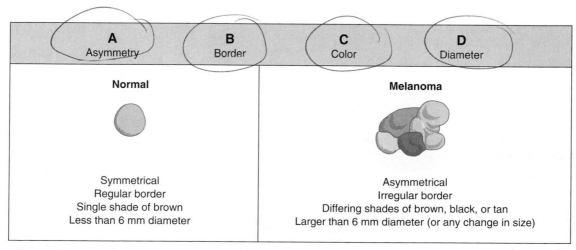

Figure 14-8

Melanoma characteristics.

Any unusual lesions on the hands, face, or other parts of the body that do not heal should be checked by a doctor.

Primary Prevention

The risk of skin cancer can be reduced with less exposure to the sun and by using sunscreens, umbrellas, and hats with wide brims or visors. Exposure to the sun between 10 a.m. and 3 p.m., when the sun's rays are strongest, should be avoided. Tanning beds should not be used because they deliver the same kind of ultraviolet rays. The damage is not immediately apparent, so overexposure occurs more easily. Check for moles regularly and note original size and color of any moles.

Secondary Prevention

Skin cancer is completely curable when treated in its earliest stages. A doctor should examine any mole that changes in size, shape, or color, or becomes ulcerated and does not heal. A dry scaly patch or pimple that persists, an inflamed area with a crusting center, or a waxy, pearly nodule are all considered to be warning signs.

Treatment

There are four methods of treatment for skin cancer: surgery, radiation therapy, **electrodesiccation** (tissue destruction by heat), or cryosurgery (tissue destruction by freezing). Melanoma generally occurs in places where it is visible and easily removed. In some cases, it may occur between the toes, on the scalp, or in other areas of the body where it is not easily seen. Surgery is the basic treatment because the lesions are easy to excise when discovered early. However, the chance of metastasis is greater as the depth of the lesion increases. Removal of nearby lymph nodes is sometimes necessary. Plastic surgery may be needed for large areas.

ORAL CANCER

Cancerous growths may appear on the lips, tongue, or anywhere else in the mouth. They may appear benign in early stages as just a small lump, but they develop into sores that do not heal and if not removed will metastasize. For 2000 it is estimated that there will be 30,200 new cases of oral cancer (including of the pharynx) and 7,800 deaths. The eight-year trend shown in Figure 14-9 shows a decrease in death rates of oral cancer.

Predisposing Factors

Smoking is considered a major factor, especially in combination with alcohol. Loose dentures are also associated with oral cancer, but a great threat today is the increased use of smokeless tobacco, particularly by those under twenty-one years of age. There are three forms of smokeless tobacco, plug, leaf, and snuff. It is the "dipping snuff" that is now causing the greatest concern. This product is made by processing tobacco into a coarse, moist

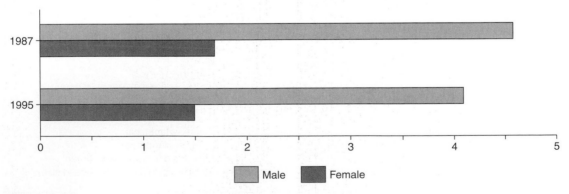

Figure 14-9

Age-adjusted death rates from oral cancer per 100,000 population, 1987 and 1995.

powder that is placed between the cheek and gum. The nicotine and other carcinogenic substances are absorbed through the oral tissue. According to the ACS, oral cancer occurs several times more frequently among those using smokeless tobacco, and the risk may increase fifty times for those who are long-time users.

Symptoms

A sore on the lip, tongue, or any other part of the mouth that does not heal within two weeks, painful whitish plaques, or velvety red lumps all could indicate a potential cancerous growth.

Primary Prevention

No one should use tobacco, and there should be only moderate use of alcohol, if any. Loose-fitting dentures need to be corrected immediately.

Secondary Prevention

Dentists should check for any warning signs during annual checkups. Physicians should check the oral cavity during visits.

Treatment

Cancerous lesions in the oral cavity take a long time to develop and should be recognized before metastasizing. If diagnosed early, most can be removed by surgery, never to occur again. Unfortunately, because the public does not receive adequate health education or because doctors fail to examine patients thoroughly, the cancer has sometimes infiltrated nearby tissue or spread to other parts of the body before it is diagnosed.

UTERINE CANCER (CORPUS OR BODY OF UTERUS)

Uterine cancer is primarily a postmenopausal disease with a median age at diagnosis of sixty-one years. It is the most common invasive cancer of the female genital tract. The cancer begins in the lining of the uterus (endometrium) and generally spreads to the cervix and vagina as well as other parts of the body through the lymphatic system. Thirty-six thousand one hundred new cases and 6,500 deaths were estimated for 2000. The death rates for uterine cancer decreased steadily during the eight years shown in Figure 14-10. The five-year survival rate is ninety-six percent if discovered in an early stage.

Predisposing Factors

Uterine cancer seems linked to a number of predisposing factors. These include:

Multiple sex partners
Never had children
History of infertility
Early menarche
Late menopause
Obesity
Family history of endometrial cancer
Failure to ovulate

electrodesiccation	e-LEK-tro-des-i-ka-shun

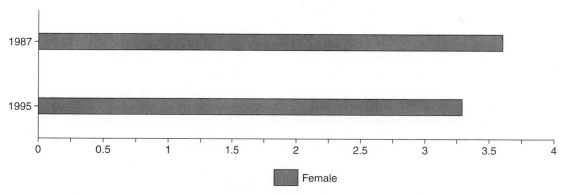

Figure 14-10
Age-adjusted death rates from uterine cancer (cervix not included) per 100,000 population, 1987 and 1995.

History of uterine polyps

Tamoxifen or unopposed estrogen therapy

Women with one or more of these factors have an increased chance of developing uterine cancer, but none has been identified as the underlying cause of the disease.

Symptoms
A bloody discharge at any time other than the menstrual period may be a sign of uterine cancer. The discharge could be watery and blood-streaked at first but gradually becomes more bloody. Other symptoms such as weight loss and pain do not occur until the cancer is in an advanced stage.

Primary Prevention
There is a greater risk of developing cancer of the endometrium if unopposed estrogen therapy is used to allay the symptoms of menopause. Women should maintain their ideal weight, which reduces the risk not only for cancer of the uterus but also for diabetes and many other disorders.

Secondary Prevention
The Pap smear is highly effective for diagnosing cancer of the uterine cervix but only partially effective in detecting cancer of the body of the uterus. The ACS advises an annual test for women who have reached the age of eighteen years and over. Women forty years of age and over should have an annual pelvic exam, and if they are at high risk for endometrial cancer, an endometrial tissue sample should be evaluated.

Treatment
Depending on the extent of the disease when diagnosed, treatment generally involves surgery or radiation or both. Hormonal therapy may be used if there are precancerous endometrial changes.

CERVICAL CANCER (NECK OF UTERUS)

Cervical cancer usually occurs between thirty and fifty years of age. Until the advent of the Pap test, it was the most common cancer of the female genitalia. For 2000, 12,800 new cases and 4,600 deaths are expected. Deaths from cervical cancer decreased steadily from 1987 to 1995 (Figure 14-11). The five-year survival rate is 91% for localized cancer.

Predisposing Factors
Multiple sex partners, multiple pregnancies, intercourse at a young age, smoking, herpes simplex virus Type II, human **papillomavirus,** and other bacterial or viral infections have been related to the development of cervical cancer.

Symptoms
Depending on the type of cancer, there may be no symptoms, or there may be vaginal bleeding, vaginal discharge, and pain and bleeding after intercourse. Symptoms for advanced stages include pelvic pain, anorexia, weight loss, painful urination, lower extremity edema, and anemia.

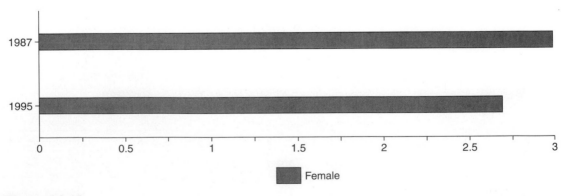

Figure 14-11
Age-adjusted death rates from cervical cancer per 100,000 population, 1987 and 1995.

Primary Prevention

Long-lasting monogamous sexual relationships, planned family size, deferral of intercourse until young adulthood, and avoidance of genital herpes and other viral or bacterial infections that affect the reproductive system are the best measures for prevention.

Secondary Prevention

The ACS recommends a Pap test every year for females who have been or are sexually active or over the age of eighteen years. If the test is negative for three consecutive years, the frequency of the exam should be left to the discretion of the physician.

Treatment

The treatment for cervical cancer depends upon the stage of the cancer. If there is no indication of spread, the treatment may include removing the cancerous part by surgery, using a laser to destroy it, or performing cryosurgery (subjecting tissues to extreme cold). Hysterectomy is performed only if the cancer has metastasized. If the cancer has metastasized, chemotherapy may be added to the treatment regimen.

LARYNGEAL CANCER

Cancer of the larynx is approximately five times more common in males than in females. Malignant tumors of the larynx are classified as intrinsic (within the larynx) and extrinsic (outside the larynx). Ninety-five percent of the latter are squamous cell carcinomas, although any kind of carcinoma or sarcoma may occur in or on the larynx. For 1999, 10,600 new cases and 4,200 deaths were expected. The eight-year trend shows no change in death rates for women, but a steady decrease for men (Figure 14-12). In the United States laryngeal cancer does not generally occur until the fourth decade and occurs most often in individuals over the age of sixty years.

Predisposing Factors

The exact cause of laryngeal cancer is unknown but more occurs in those who smoke and are heavy drinkers. An increased incidence of exposure to asbestos has also been discovered in those with cancer of the larynx. Other environmental factors may also play a part in its development.

Symptoms

Persistent hoarseness is often the first symptom and may be followed by pain, difficulty in swallowing, and coughing up blood. The symptoms are dependent upon the location of the cancer on or in the larynx. If it is on the vocal cords, there may be symptoms before it has had a chance to spread. However, if the cancer occurs in another location, symptoms may not appear until it has grown large enough to cause symptoms.

Primary Prevention

To prevent this disease, people should not use tobacco in any form and drink moderately, if at all.

tamoxifen	TA-mok-si-fun
papillomavirus	PAP-i-lo-ma-vi-rus

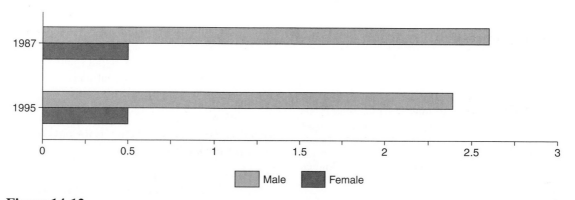

Figure 14-12

Age-adjusted death rates from laryngeal cancer per 100,000 population, 1987 and 1995.

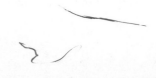

Older buildings need to be checked for asbestos and, if found, this should be removed immediately (this is occurring in most states). Any environmental substances known to be carcinogenic should be avoided.

Secondary Prevention

If hoarseness continues for more than a week with no known cause, a doctor should be consulted. A **laryngoscopy** can be performed to check the vocal cords.

Treatment

If the lesion is identified early, there is an eighty-five percent to ninety percent chance of cure by radiation alone. If it is found during the later stages, partial or total removal of the larynx may be necessary. Radiation and surgery together have increased the five-year survival rate by fifty percent. Chemotherapy may also be used in combination with the other two therapies. Treatment is aimed at eliminating the cancer and preserving speech. If speech is lost, the patient is taught how to speak by use of a stoma, or hole, in the neck. Figure 14-13 shows the relationship of such a stoma to the normal structures.

BONE CANCER

Bone cancer is rare. Less than one percent of all cancers are found in the bone, and most of these are metastases from other sites. The most common form, osteosarcoma, is found most often in the leg bones of children and young adults. Two thousand five hundred new cases and 1,400 deaths from bone cancer were estimated for 2000.

Predisposing Factors

The cause of primary bone cancer is unknown.

Symptoms

Symptoms are dependent on the location of the affected bones. One of the most common signs is pain that may not be disabling but becomes worse at night.

Prevention

Preventive measures for bone cancer are unknown.

Treatment

Treatment includes radiation, chemotherapy, and surgery (amputation may be necessary).

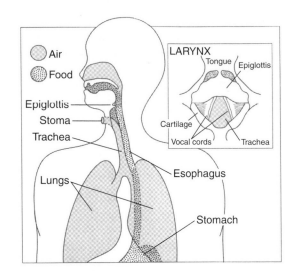

Figure 14-13
Location of stoma in larynx.

THYROID CANCER

This cancer is also rare, accounting for just over one percent of all cancers. The cause is generally unknown, although this kind of cancer has been associated with high doses of radiation. The estimate for 2000 is 18,400 new cases and 1,200 deaths. Cancer of the thyroid gland occurs more than twice as often in women.

Predisposing Factors

Predisposing factors are unknown except for radiation exposure.

Symptoms

A nodule on the neck is generally the first sign. Routine examination cannot distinguish a benign from a malignant growth, and other techniques such as imaging, biopsy, or actual removal of the nodule for microscopic examination are necessary for diagnosis.

Prevention

Avoiding exposure to radiation is the only preventive measure known.

Treatment

Cancer of the thyroid has one of the highest cure rates of all cancers. Physicians differ on the best treatment to use, but traditional forms of therapy (radiation, chemotherapy, and surgery) are used alone or in combination.

TESTICULAR CANCER

About 7,400 males, generally between ages 15 and 40, are afflicted with testicular cancer annually, and there are approximately 300 deaths. The 5-year survival rate is 96% if the cancer is localized. If it has metastasized, the 5-year survival rate is only 54%. Although the number of new cases per year and the death rate are among the lowest now, the incidence of this kind of cancer has been increasing in recent years. It is the leading cancer killer for boys and men in the 15- to 40-year age group.

Predisposing Factors

The cause of testicular cancer is unknown except that the incidence is higher in men with undescended testicles and in male children of women exposed to exogenous estrogen (diethylstilbestrol) during pregnancy. The relationship remains even if there has been surgery to correct the condition.

Symptoms

Self-examination or examination by a physician can lead to the detection of a lump that may range in size from a pea to a grapefruit. As with many cancers, there is no pain, although there may be a feeling of heaviness. If the tumor produces hormones, there may be gynecomastia and nipple tenderness. In the later stages, there may be urethral obstruction, shortness of breath, weight loss, and fatigue.

Primary Prevention

Unknown.

Secondary Prevention

The most common and effective means of early detection is self-examination. Young men should be educated on how to detect a tumorous growth in the testicles.

Treatment

Traditional cancer treatment is used. The intensity of the treatment depends upon the stage and type of the tumor. Most surgeons remove just the testis(es) involved and leave the scrotum to be used for a prosthetic testicular implant at a later date, if desired.

laryngoscopy	lar-in-GOS-ko-pe

SUMMARY

Table 14-1 summarizes relevant data concerning the forms of cancer discussed in this chapter.

TABLE 14-1	**Other Cancers**				
Site	**Special Characteristics**	**Predisposing Factors**	**Common Symptoms**	**Prevention**	**Treatment**
Brain	16,800 new cases, 13,100 deaths estimated for 1999; often a metastasis; people	Unknown for primary brain cancer	Depend upon location; may be muscle weakness, loss of vision,	Unknown for primary brain cancer	Treatment is surgical removal of the tumor if possible, chemotherapy,

TABLE 14-1	Continued				
Site	**Special Characteristics**	**Predisposing Factors**	**Common Symptoms**	**Prevention**	**Treatment**
Brain—Cont'd	around age of 50 and children most common victims		speech problems, epilepsy, headache, vomiting, visual disturbances, impaired mental function, hydrocephalus		radiation, and possibly corticosteroids to reduce swelling and relieve symptoms. Many brain tumors are inaccessible or too far advanced when diagnosed to be curable
Esophagus	12,500 new cases and 12,200 deaths estimated for 1999; more in men than in women, in blacks than in whites	Cause unknown, high alcohol consumption and smoking may be factors	Difficulty in swallowing, vomiting, weight loss, and pain when in the later stages	No smoking, moderation in drinking	Treatment includes surgery, radiation, and chemotherapy depending upon the stage of the cancer and the condition of the patient
Bladder	Occurs more often in people over 50; 54,200 new cases and 12,100 deaths estimated for 1999	Tobacco, coffee, nitrates, and other environmental chemicals; many occupations cause exposure to risk factors	Blood in urine, pain, urinary frequency, nocturia, dribbling	Job selection, no tobacco, moderation in coffee drinking	Treatment is surgery that may involve removal of the bladder and replacing it by an opening in the abdomen for urine to be collected externally. Radiation and chemotherapy may also be used

TABLE 14-1	*Continued*				
Site	**Special Characteristics**	**Predisposing Factors**	**Common Symptoms**	**Prevention**	**Treatment**
Kidney	Usually occurs in older adults; 30,000 new cases and 11,900 deaths estimated for 1999; 5-year survival rate is 89%; twice as common in men; usually strikes between ages 50 and 60	Cause unknown; exposure to environmental pollutants may be a factor	Blood in urine, pain or a palpable mass, fever, hypertension, hypercalcemia, urinary retention; more advanced symptoms: weight loss, edema in the legs, nausea, vomiting	Avoidance of environmental pollution	Treatment is surgery to remove tissue involved or whole kidney. Chemotherapy is not effective in kidney cancer. Patient can survive on one kidney; possibility of kidney transplant if both are affected.
Bone Marrow (Multiple Myeloma)	Cancer of plasma cells in bone marrow; 13,700 new cases, 11,400 deaths for 1999	Unknown	Severe, constant back pain; arthritic symptoms; fever, malaise; pathologic fractures	Unknown	Treatment is chemotherapy and radiation
Skin	Basal cell and squamous cell most common, malignant melanoma most deadly; most new cases due to sun exposure; 54,000 new cases estimated for 1999 and 9,200 deaths;	Excessive sun exposure, fair skin, exposure to coal, tar, pitch, and creosote	Asymmetry; border irregularity; color changes or variation; diameter greater than 6 mm; any lesion that does not heal	Less sun exposure, sunscreens, hats with wide brims, umbrellas; no tanning beds, check moles; check with doctor if A, B, C, or D occur	Surgery is generally successful. Radiation and/or chemotherapy may be used if metastasis has occurred

TABLE 14-1 *Continued*

Site	Special Characteristics	Predisposing Factors	Common Symptoms	Prevention	Treatment
Skin—Cont'd	44,200 of the new cases and 7,300 of the deaths from melanoma; 5-year survival rate for melanoma 54%				
Oral Cavity	Cancers on lips, tongue, mouth, or pharynx; 29,800 new cases and 8,100 deaths estimated for 1999	Smoking; use of smokeless tobacco; excess use of alcohol; dentures	A sore that bleeds easily and does not heal; a red or white patch; a lump or thickening; difficulty in chewing, swallowing, moving tongue or jaw (late changes)	No tobacco use. Moderation in use of alcohol; regular dental checkups for early detection; good oral hygiene	Surgery is successful if cancer identified early; radiation and/or chemotherapy if metastasized
Uterus	Usually affects post-menopausal women between ages of 50 and 60; 37,400 new cases, 6,400 deaths for 1999; 5-year survival 96%	Early age at first intercourse; never had children; abnormal uterine bleeding; obesity; family history of endometrial cancer; history of uterine polyps; unopposed estrogen therapy	Bloody discharge between periods	No estrogen therapy if possible, maintain ideal weight, avoid diabetes; endometrial biopsy; regular pelvic exams	Treatment is removal of uterus (hysterectomy) and other involved structures. Radiation and hormonal therapy are used to inhibit recurrence and lengthen survival time
Cervix	Steady decrease; 12,800 new	Multiple sex partners; multiple	May be none or may be vaginal bleeding,	Long-lasting monogamous sexual	Treatment is removal of involved

TABLE 14-1	*Continued*				
Site	**Special Characteristics**	**Predisposing Factors**	**Common Symptoms**	**Prevention**	**Treatment**
Cervix— Cont'd	cases and 4,800 deaths estimated for 1999; 5-year survival 91%	pregnancies; intercourse at a young age; herpes virus II and other genital infections	vaginal discharge, and pain and bleeding after intercourse	relations, planned family size, deferral of intercourse until young adulthood, avoidance of genital herpes and other genital infections, use of condoms	tissue or hysterectomy if metastasized. Cryosurgery or destruction of tissue by laser may be tried
Larynx	Nine times more common in males; may be intrinsic or extrinsic; most are squamous cell; 10,600 new cases and 4,200 deaths espected for 1999; most often in individuals over 60	Unknown; More in smokers and heavy drinkers	Persistent hoarseness, followed by pain, difficulty swallowing, and coughing up blood	No tobacco use, moderation in drinking if at all; carcinogens in environment removed or avoided	Treatment is radiation if discovered early, surgery and chemotherapy for lesions that have metastasized
Bone	Rare—most are metastases from other sites; 2,600 new cases and 1,400 deaths estimated for 1999	Unknown	Dependent on location; may have pain that gets worse at night	Unknown	Treatment is radiation, chemotherapy, and/or surgery
Thyroid	Rare— associated with high doses of	Unknown except for radiation connection	Nodule on neck	Avoid exposure to radiation	Radiation, chemotherapy, and surgery are

TABLE 14-1	*Continued*				
Site	**Special Characteristics**	**Predisposing Factors**	**Common Symptoms**	**Prevention**	**Treatment**
Thyroid— Cont'd	radiation; 18,100 new cases and 1,200 deaths estimated for 1999				standard treatments
Testis	About 7,400 men between 20–34 diagnosed annually, 300 deaths; incidence is increasing; 96% survival when found early	Unknown	Heaviness or a lump	Self-examination	Surgery, radiation, and chemo-therapy are usual treatments

QUESTIONS FOR REVIEW

1. Why was the development of the Pap test so important?
2. What recommendation does the ACS make for taking the Pap test?
3. What group of women are most likely to have cancer of the uterus?
4. Describe the treatment for esophageal cancer.
5. At what age is bladder cancer more likely to occur?
6. What surgical technique may be performed for advanced cases of bladder cancer?
7. What is multiple myeloma?
8. What are the two most common types of skin cancer?
9. Why is malignant melanoma the most dangerous type of skin cancer?
10. Why does oral cancer have a high number of new cases each year but a comparatively low death rate?
11. For what kind of lesions on the lips, tongue, or in the mouth should a doctor or dentist be consulted?
12. Why is laryngeal cancer more common in males?
13. What is meant by intrinsic or extrinsic in reference to cancer of the larynx?
14. What surgery may be performed if laryngeal cancer is not diagnosed in an early stage?
15. What treatment may be used for bone cancer?
16. What is often the first sign of cancer of the thyroid?
17. For the cancers in this chapter, identify predisposing factors and symptoms.
18. What primary prevention procedures are there for esophageal, urinary bladder, kidney, skin, oral, uterine, laryngeal, and thyroid cancer?
19. What secondary prevention procedures are there for esophageal, urinary bladder, skin, oral, uterine, and laryngeal cancer?

FURTHER READING

Askling, Johan, and Per Sorensen. 1999. Is history of squamous cell skin cancer a marker of poor prognosis in patients with cancer? *Annals of Internal Medicine* 131:655.

Aslan, T., et al. 1999. Patients with multiple myeloma may safely undergo autologous transplantation despite ongoing RSV infection and no ribavirin therapy. *Bone Marrow Transplantation* 24:505.

Barbalias, G.A., et al. 1999. Adenocarcinoma of the kidney: nephron-sparing surgical approach vs radical nephrectomy. *Journal of Surgical Oncology* 72:156.

Battista, G., et al. 1999. Mortality due to asbestos-related causes among railway carriage construction and repair workers. *Occupational Medicine* 49:536.

Belldegrun, A., et al. 1999. Efficacy of nephron-sparing surgery for renal cell carcinoma: analysis based on the new 1997 tumor-node-metastatsis staging system. *Journal of Clinical Oncology* 17:2868.

Bhatia, S., et al. 1999. Second primary tumors in patients with cutaneous malignant melanoma. *Cancer* 86:2014.

Blade, Joan, Patricia Fernandez-Llama, Frances Bosch, et al. 1998. Renal failure in multiple myeloma: Presenting features and predictors of outcome in 94 patients from a single institution. *Archives of Internal Medicine* 158:1889.

Blecker, D., et al. 1999. Melanoma in the gastrointestinal tract. *American Journal of Gastroenerology* 94:3427.

Bomb tests and thyroid cancer—screening program not recommended. *Journal of Environmental Health* 61:42, 1998.

Bonn, Dorothy. 1998. Study finds low cancer risk from 131I. *The Lancet* 352:294.

Branicki, Frank J. 1998. Quality of life in patients with cancer of the esophagus and gastric cardia: A case for palliative resection. *Journal of the American Medical Association* 279:1930.

Buller, David B., and Ron Borland. 1999. Skin cancer prevention for children: a critical review. *Health Education and Behavior* 26:317.

Burton, R. C., C. Howe, L. Adamson, et al. 1998. General practitioner screening for melanoma: Sensitivity, specificity, and effect of training. *Journal of Medical Screening* 5:156.

Can sunscreens reduce skin cancer? *American Journal of Nursing* 99:14, 1999.

Cantor, K. P., et al. Drinking water source and chlorination by products in Iowa, Illinois. Risk of brain cancer. *American Journal of Epidemiology* 150:552.

Cantuaria, G., et al. 1999. Primary malignant melanoma of the uterine cervix: a case report and review of the literature. *Gynocology Oncology* 75:170.

Carew, John F., and Jatin P. Shah. 1998. Advances in multi-modality therapy for laryngeal cancer. *CA—A Cancer Journal for Clinicians* 48:211.

Carson, John J., Louis H. Gold, et al. 1998. Fatality and interferon alpha for malignant melanoma. *The Lancet* 352:1443.

Chomchai, J.S., et al. 1999. Prognostic significance of p53 gene mutations in laryngeal cancer. *Laryngoscope* 109:455.

Cirasino, Lorenso, et al. 1999. Images in clinical medicine. *New England Journal of Medicine* 341:1582.

Clarke, R. 1999. A population based survey of the management of women with cancer of the cervix. *British Journal of Cancer* 80:1958.

Cocco, P., et al. 1999. Occupational risk factors for cancer of the central nervous system among U.S. women. *American Journal of Industrial Medicine* 36:70.

Cocco, Pierluigi, and Mustafa Dosmeci. 1998. Brain cancer and occupational exposure to lead. *Journal of Occupational and Environmental Medicine* 40:937.

Costa, C. M., B. de Camargo, R. Bagietto, et al. 1998. Abdominal recurrence of osteogenic sarcoma: A case report. *Journal of Pediatric Hematology Oncology* 20:271.

Danpanich, E., and B. L. Kasiske. 1999. Risk factors for cancer in renal transplant recipients. *Transplantation* 68:1859.

Davidowitz, S., et al. 1999. The epidemiology of malignant melanoma in Louisiana and beyond. *Journal of Louisiana Medical Society* 151:493.

Dosemeci, M., et al. 1999. Gender differences in risk of renal cell carcinoma and occupational exposures to chlorinated aliphatic hydrocarbons. *American Journal of Industrial Medicine* 36:54.

Do you routinely screen your patients for oral cancer? *Journal of the American Dental Association* 130:1699, 1999.

Faure, I., et al. 1999. Multiple myeloma in two HIV-infected patients. *AIDS* 13:1797.

Fillmore, C.M., et al. 1999. Cancer mortality in women with probable exposure to silica: a death certificate study in 24 states of the U.S. *American Journal of Industrial Medicine* 36:122.

Floderus, B., et al. 1999. Occupational magnetic field exposure and site-specific cancer incidence: a Swedish cohort study. *Cancer Causes Control* 10:323.

Forbes, R. B., and M. S. Eljamel. 1998. Meningeal chondrosarcomas, a review of 31 patients. *British Journal of Neurosurgery* 12:461.

Freedberg, K.A., et al. 1999. Screening for malignant melanoma: a cost effectiveness analysis. *Journal of the American Academy of Dermatology* 41:738.

Gago-Dominguez, M., et al. 1999. Increased risk of renal cell carcinoma subsequent to hysterectomy. *Cancer Epidemiology Biomakers Prevention* 8:999.

Gago-Dominguez, M., et al. 1999. Regular use of analgesics is a risk factor for renal cell carcinoma. *British Journal of Cancer* 81:542.

Gahrton, Gosta. 1999. Treatment of multiple myeloma. *The Lancet* 353:85.

Gilbert, Ethel S., Robert Tarone, Andre Bouville, et al. 1998. Thyroid cancer rates and [SUP 131]I doses from Nevada atmospheric nuclear bomb tests. *Journal of the National Cancer Institute* 90:1654.

Gollub, M.J., and J.C. Prowda. 1999. Primary melanoma of the esophagus: radiologic and clinical findings in six patients. *Radiology* 213:97.

Goodman, M., et al. 1999. Cancer in asbestos-exposed occupational cohorts: a meta-analysis. *Cancer Causes Control* 10:453.

Griggs, Heidi, and Sue K. Cammarata. 1998. Acute mental changes in a 64 year old man with bladder cancer. *Chest* 114:621.

Grofeld, J. L. 1999. Risk-based management: current concepts of treating malignant solid tumors of childhood. *Journal of American Coll Surgery* 189:407.

Gross, Edward, A. 1999. Nonmelanoma skin cancer: clues to early detection, keys to effective treatment. *Consultant* 39:829.

Harada, K., et al. 1999. Telemerase activity in central nervous system malignant lymphoma. *Cancer* 86:1050.

Harrigan, Peter. 1998. Melanoma vaccine promise increases. *The Lancet* 352:40.

Hart, D. N. J., and G.R. Hill. 1999. Dendritic cell immunotherapy for cancer: application to low-grade lymphoma and multiple myeloma. *Immunology and Cell Biology* 77:451.

Hernberg, M., et al. 1999. Regimens with or without interferon-alpha as treatment for metastatic melanoma and renal cell carcinoma: an overview of randomized trials. *Journal of Immunotherapy with Emphasis on Tumor Biology* 22:145.

Hill, David. 1999. Efficacy of sunscreens in protection against skin cancer. *The Lancet* 354:699.

Holowaty, Philippa, Anthony B. Miller, Tom Rohan, et al. 1999. Natural history of dysplasia of the uterine cervix. *Journal of the National Cancer Institute* 91:252.

Hurst, R., et al. 1999. Brain metastasis after immunotherapy in patients with metastatic melanoma or renal cell cancer: is craniotomy indicated? *Journal of Immunotherapy with Emphasis on Tumor Biology* 22:356.

Hwang, Mi, et al. 1999. The importance of a pap test. *Journal of the American Medical Association* 281:1666.

Hwang, Mi Young, Richard M. Glass, et al. 1999. Detecting skin cancer. *Journal of the American Medical Association* 281:676.

Incidence of uterine cancer in U.S. women age 50 and older. *Journal of the National Cancer Institute* 91:1713, 1999.

Jiang, W., et al. 1999. P53 protects against skin cancer induction by UV-B radiation. *Oncogene* 18:4247.

Joanna, M. 1999. Oral cancer. *British Medical Journal* 318:1051.

Karagas, Margaret R., Tor D. Tosteson, et al. 1998. Design of an epidemiological study of drinking water arsenic exposure and skin and bladder cancer risk in a US population. *Environmental Health Perspectives Supplement* 106:1047.

Kawai, A., G. F. Muschler, J. M. Lane, et al. 1998. Prosthetic knee replacement after resection of a malignant tumor of the distal part of the femur. Medium to long term results. *Journal of Bone and Joint Surgery, American Volume* 80:636.

Kelsen, David P., Robert Ginsberg, Thomas F. Pajak, et al. 1998. Chemotherapy followed by surgery compared with surgery alone for localized esophageal cancer. *The New England Journal of Medicine* 339:1979.

Kerawala, C.J. 1999. Oral cancer, smoking and alcohol: the patients' perspective. *British Journal of Oral Maxillofactory Surgery* 37:374.

Key, Sandra W., and Michelle Marble. 1998. Scientists spot cancer killing cells in patients. *Cancer Weekly Plus*:18.

Kidney and renal pelvis cancer rates. *Journal of the National Cancer Institute* 90:964, 1998.

King, R., et al. 1999. Metastatic malignant melanoma resembling malignant peripheral nerve sheath tumor: report of 16 cases. *American Journal of Surgical Pathology* 23:1499.

Kinouchi, T., et al. 1999. Incidence rate of satellite tumors in renal cell carcinoma. *Cancer* 86:2331.

Kirsner, R.S., et al. 1999. Skin cancer screening in primary care: prevalence and barriers. *Journal of American Academy of Dermatology* 41:564.

Kmietowicz, Zosia. 1998. Neutron beam therapy targets brain cancer. *British Medical Journal* 317:1176.

Krieg, R., and R. Hoffman. 1999. Current management of unusual genitourinary cancers. Part 2: urethral cancer. *Oncology* 13:1511.

Laryngeal cancer. *CA—A Cancer Journal for Clinicians* 48:141, 1998.

Larkin, Marilynn. 1999. Low-dose thalidomide seems to be effective in multiple myeloma. *The Lancet* 354:925.

Larkin, Marilynn. 1999. Thalidomide continues to look promising as an anticancer agent. *The Lancet* 354:1705.

Le, K., and R.M. Tyszko. 1999. A presentation of a conjunctival malignant melanoma. *Journal of American Ophthalmology Association* 70: 653.

Lecouvet, F. E., B. C. Vande Berg, L. Michaux, et al. 1998. Development of vertebral fractures in patients with multiple myeloma: Does MRI enable recognition of vertebrae that will collapse? *Journal of Computer Assisted Tomography* 22:430.

Lerut, T., et al. 1999. Treatment of esophageal carcinoma. *Chest* 116:463S.

Levi, Fabio, and Lalao Randimbison. 1998. Non-melanomatous skin cancer following cervical, vaginal, and vulvar neoplasms: Etiologic association. *Journal of the National Cancer Institute* 90:1570.

Lohmann, C.P., et al. 1999. Severe loss of vision during adjuvant interferon alfa-2b treatment for malignant melanoma. *The Lancet* 353:1326.

Majeski, J. 1999. Bilateral breast masses as initial presentation of widely metastatic melanoma. *Journal of Surgical Oncology* 72:175.

Mannetje, A., 1999. Smoking as a confounder in case control studies of occupational bladder cancer in women. *American Journal of Industrial Medicine* 36:75.

Mejean, A., et al. 1999. Mortality and morbidity after nephrectomy for renal cell carcinoma using a transperitoneal anterior subcostal incision. *European Urology* 36:298.

Menck, Herman R., Kirby I. Bland, et al. 1998. Clinical highlights from the National Cancer Data Base, 1998. *CA—A Cancer Journal for Clinicians* 48:134.

Mihara, S., et al. 1999. Early detection of renal cell carcinoma by ultrasonographic screening—based on the results of 13 years screening in Japan. *Ultrasound Medical Biology* 25:1033.

Mintz, Arlan Pinzer, and J. Gregory Cairncross. 1998. Treatment of a single brain metastasis. *The Journal of the American Medical Association* 280:1527.

Miyoshi, Y., et al. 1999. Telmerase activity in oral cancer. *Oral Oncology* 35:283.

Muglia, J.J., et al. 1999. Skin cancer screening: a growing need. *Surgical Oncology Clinic of North America* 8:735.

Patchell, Roy A., Phillip A. Tibbs, et al. 1998. Postoperative radiotherapy in the treatment of single metastases to the brain. *Journal of the American Medical Association* 280:1485.

Patel, B. C., C. A. Egan, R. W. Lucius, et al. 1998. Cutaneous malignant melanoma and oculodermal melanocystosis (nevus of Ota): Report of a case and review of the literature. *Journal of the American Academy of Dermatology* 38:862.

Petralia, S.A., et al. 1999. Cancer mortality among women employed in health care occupatons in 24 U.S. states. *American Journal of Industrial Medicine* 36:159.

Pommer, W., et al. 1999. Urothelial cancer at different turmor sites: role of smoking and habitual intake of analgesics and laxatives. Results of the Berlin urothelial cancer study. *Nephrology Dialysis Transplant* 14:2892.

Robins, Perry. 1998. How to examine your skin for suspicious moles. *Consultant* 38:1959.

Robinson, C.F., and J.T. Walker. 1999. Cancer mortality among women employed in fast-growing U.S. occupations. *American Journal of Industrial Medicine 36:186.*

Rossing, M.A., et al. 2000. Risk of papillary thyroid cancer in women in relation to smoking and alcohol consumption. *Epidemiology* 11:49.

Sansom, Clare. 1999. New drug lines up in fight against brain cancer. *The Lancet* 353:472.

Scanlan, M.J., et al 1999. Antigens recognized by autologous antibody in patients with renal-cell carcinoma. *International Journal of Cancer* 83:456.

Schwatz, Stephen M., Janet R. Daling, David R. Doody, et al. 1998. Oral cancer risk in relation to sexual history and evidence of human papillomavirus infection. *Journal of the National Cancer Institute* 90:1626.

Settimi, L., et al. 1999. Cancer risk among female agricultural workers: a multi-center case-control study. *American Journal of Industrial Medicine* 36:135.

Shah, Keerti V. 1998. Do human papillomavirus infections cause oral cancer? *Journal of the National Cancer Institute* 90:1585.

Shillitoe, E. J., et al. 1999. Effects of herpes simplex virus on human oral cancer cells, and potential use of mutant viruses in therapy of oral cancer. *Oral Oncology* 35:326.

Simple new therapy for skin cancer. *Modern Medicine* 66:9, 1998.

Singhal, Seema, et al. 1999. Antitumor activity of thalidomide in refractory multiple myeloma. *New England Journal of Medicine* 341:1565.

Skin cancer screenings infrequent in primary care. *Geriatrics* 55:90, 2000.

Spencer, K.R., et al. 1999. The use of titanium mandibular reconstruction plates in patients with oral cancer. *International Journal of Maxillofactory Surgery* 28:288.

Suganuma, M., et al. 1999. Green tea and cancer chemoprevention. *Mutation Research* 428:339.

Sunscreens do protect against melanoma, says skin cancer specialist. *Oncology* 12:1328, 1998.

Syrigos, K.N., et al. 1999. Use of monoclonal antibodies for the diagnosis and treatment of bladder cancer. *Hybridoma* 18:219.

Talamini, Renato, Carlo La Vecchia, Fabio Levi, et al. 1998. Cancer of the oral cavity and pharynx in non-smokers who drink alcohol and in non-drinkers who smoke tobacco. *Journal of the National Cancer Institute* 90:1901.

U.S. urinary bladder cancer death rates. *Journal of the National Cancer Institute* 91:1362, 1999.

Vaiana, R., et al. 1999. Hyperthyroidism and concurrent thyroid cancer. *Tumori* 85:247.

van der Meijden, Adrian P. M. 1998. Bladder cancer. *British Medical Journal* 317:1366.

Voelker, Rebecca. 1999. Copper and cancer. *Journal of the American Medical Association* 283:994.

Vogelzang, Nicholas J., and Walter M. Stadler. 1998. Kidney cancer. *The Lancet* 352:1691.

Walling, Anne, D. 1999. Sunscreen and beta-carotene for preventing skin cancer. *American Family Physician* 61:841.

Wasef, W.R., and J.K. Roberts. 1999. Primary malignant melanoma of the cervix uteri. *Journal of Obstetrics & Gynecology* 19:673.

Wassberg, C., et al. 1999. Cancer risk in patients with earlier diagnosis of cutaneous melanoma in situ. *International Journal of Cancer* 83:314.

Wehrwein, Peter. 1998. Genetics of brain cancer yields to study. *The Lancet* 352:40.

Winn, Deborah M., Scott R. Diehl, et al. 1998. Scientific progress in understanding oral and pharyngeal cancers. *Journal of the American Dental Association* 129:713.

Wright, C.D. 1999. Multimodality therapy of esophageal cancer. *Chest* 116:461S.

Yellowitz, Janet, Alice M. Horowitz, et al. 1998. Knowledge, opinions and practices of general dentists regarding oral cancer: A pilot survey. *Journal of the American Dental Association* 129:579.

Yilmaz, T., S. Hoysal, G. Gedikoglu, et al. 1998. Prognostic significance of depth of invasion in cancer of the larynx. *Laryngoscope* 108:764.

CHRONIC RESPIRATORY, DIGESTIVE, AND EXCRETORY DISEASES

OBJECTIVES

1. *Describe the diseases that are included in chronic obstructive pulmonary disorder (COPD).*

2. *State predisposing factors for peptic ulcer.*

3. *Identify preventive measures for gastric ulcer.*

4. *State the basic preventive measures for hiatal hernia.*

5. *Explain the dangers that result from cirrhosis of the liver.*

6. *State the degree to which the predisposing factors for cirrhosis of the liver play a part.*

7. *State predisposing factors for gallbladder disease.*

8. *Compare the symptoms of peptic ulcer, hiatal hernia, cirrhosis of the liver, and gallbladder disease.*

9. *Describe the treatment for the respiratory and digestive diseases discussed in this chapter.*

10. *Identify predisposing factors for chronic renal failure.*

11. *Explain the symptoms of chronic renal failure.*

12. *State means of reducing the risk of chronic renal failure.*

13. *Identify predisposing factors, symptoms, and prevention for kidney stones.*

14. *State predisposing factors for irritable bowel syndrome.*

15. *Compare the symptoms for irritable bowel syndrome and diverticular disease.*

16. *Explain the theory of the cause of diverticular disease.*

17. *Distinguish between diverticulosis and diverticulitis.*

18. *Describe the treatment for diseases of the excretory system discussed in this chapter.*

RESPIRATORY DISEASES

There is nothing so terrifying as the inability to fill the lungs with air. The lodged object in the wind-pipe, the smothering effect of thick smoke, and the inability of the drowning victim to gain air are all experiences that cause terror because of insufficient oxygen. Thousands of people are stricken every year with chronic lung diseases that can produce the terror of suffocation. As with many chronic diseases, most common disorders of the respiratory system could be prevented with changes in lifestyle and the environment. Figure 4-1 shows the structures of the respiratory system.

Chronic bronchitis and emphysema cause years of suffering for their victims that may lead to constant discomfort, overwhelming disability, and, eventually, death. Asthma, which was discussed in Chapter 3, results in much of the same kind of suffering because of the inability of the victim to get enough air. However, asthma differs from chronic bronchitis and emphysema because there is no strong relationship between asthma and smoking as there is for chronic bronchitis and emphysema. These three disorders are often grouped under the acronym COPD, for chronic obstructive pulmonary disease, or COLD, for chronic obstructive lung disease, and two or more may be present in the same person at the same time. Each disorder interferes with the functioning of the respiratory system, making it increasingly difficult for the individual to breathe.

Normal respiration requires efficient action of the diaphragm, a clear route to the lungs, healthy bronchial tubes, and effective diffusion of gases. Oxygen that is inhaled must be diffused across the alveolar-capillary membrane into the blood, and at the same time, carbon dioxide must be diffused from the blood across the same membranes, into the lungs for exhalation.

Air usually enters the body through the nose. During periods of exertion, it may enter through the mouth, but the nose is a preferable point of entry for several reasons. First, the cilia (fine hairs in the nasal passages) protect against dust and other particles from the air. Next, particles that may slip through the cilia are caught in the thick, sticky, mucous lining of the nasal passages, allowing only clean air to pass to the lungs. Third, air is warmed in the nasal cavity, and, finally, moisture is added.

Air passes from the nose backward and downward through the pharynx to the larynx. The larynx contains the vocal cords, which the air passes through on its way to the trachea. The trachea branches into the right and left bronchial tubes, which in turn branch into bronchioles, which ultimately end in alveolar sacs.

The two chronic diseases discussed in this section of the chapter involve processes that cannot function or fail to function efficiently because of a respiratory disorder.

Chronic Bronchitis

When a productive cough is present for at least three months of two successive years with no other cause, the diagnosis is chronic bronchitis. The cough is the result of irritation and inflammation of the bronchial tubes, leading to excess production of mucous and the inability of the cilia, paralyzed by pollutants, to remove the irritants. Figure 15-1 shows the damage that can occur in chronic bronchitis.

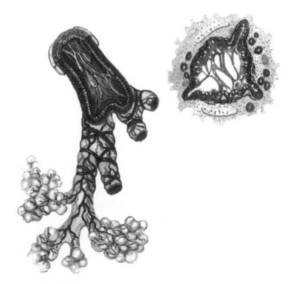

Figure 15-1
Airway obstruction caused by chronic bronchitis.

CASE STUDY

Emphysema

Fred was a sixty-two year-old retired postman. He had been a pack-a-day smoker since his twenties. He had been retired only two years when he started having trouble with shortness of breath—periodically at first, until it became constant. Soon he started coughing up mucus and finally went to see his doctor. After taking his history, the doctor examined his heart and lungs and gave him a spirometry (breathing test).

Fred had emphysema. He was told to stop smoking, begin a prescribed exercise program, have pneumonia and flu shots each year, and get immediate treatment for any lung infection. If he followed the treatment schedule, he could still have many good years although, with no care, the condition would gradually get worse until he had to be on oxygen all the time as long as he lived.

Predisposing Factors

Chronic bronchitis is caused by, and progresses because of, environmental pollutants (waste of factories, carbon and tar of smoke—household or tobacco), infections, and allergies. Smoking is by far the most important factor. In a smoker, the cilia become paralyzed and are unable to sweep the impurities and foreign particles from the bronchi. Smoking also causes increased mucus production, destruction of alveolar walls, and an abnormal formation of fibrous tissue around the bronchioles.

Symptoms

A productive cough and shortness of breath on exertion are the first signs of chronic bronchitis. Most individuals have no symptoms until middle age. The coughing gradually gets worse and the amount of mucous secretion increases. Environmental pollutants lead to **hyperplasia** of the mucous glands, **hypertrophy** of smooth muscle, and increased thickening of the bronchial wall. The excess secretion of mucous leads to plugging of the small airways. Residual lung volume increases, vital capacity decreases, and there is wheezing and shortness of breath. As the symptoms worsen, the increased demands on the heart from lack of sufficient oxygen lead to death from *cor pulmonale* (failure of right ventricle caused by disorders of the lungs, pulmonary vessels, or chest wall).

Prevention

The best means of prevention are nonuse of tobacco products, living and working where there is low exposure to environmental pollutants, and treatment of allergies.

Treatment

A person with chronic bronchitis should not smoke, and if living or working in an area of high environmental pollution, relocation is advisable. Bronchodilators and/or expectorants may be used to relieve bronchospasm and help to remove excess mucus. Ultrasonic and mechanical **nebulizers** may be used to loosen secretions, diuretics can be given for edema, and oxygen for difficulty in breathing.

Emphysema

Emphysema is sometimes divided into four different types according to its anatomic location in one or both lungs. The term will be used loosely in this discussion to apply to all types. In emphysema, the walls of the alveoli are destroyed, causing an

hyperplasia	hi-per-PLA-ze-a
hypertrophy	hi-PER-tro-fe
nebulizer	NEB-u-li-zer
cor pulmonale	cor pul-mon-A-le

enlargement of total air space as alveoli coalesce to form one saccule. The alveoli also lose their elasticity, and the process of breathing becomes exceedingly difficult as air exchange becomes more and more difficult. The destruction of alveoli that occurs in emphysema is pictured in Figure 15-2. Because of the struggle to breathe, the chest becomes barrel shaped, respiratory movements are diminished, and expiration is difficult and prolonged. It is a dreaded disease because those with emphysema do not die quickly but live for years, fighting for every breath.

Predisposing Factors
Smoking and a deficiency of **alpha-antitrypsin** (hereditary) are the major predisposing factors for emphysema. The hereditary factor is rare, but if present, the trypsin may digest lung tissue, or so it is believed.

Symptoms
The disease has an insidious onset. Labored breathing and gasping for breath are the most common symptoms. Long-term signs include a chronic cough, anorexia, weight loss, "barrel chest," **hypoxemia** (too little oxygen in the blood), and heart failure (*cor pulmonale*).

Prevention
No smoking and avoidance of other environmental pollutants as much as possible reduce the risk of getting emphysema. Once a person is diagnosed with emphysema, recommended changes are (1) eliminating as many respiratory irritants in the environment as possible by changing occupation (if there is exposure to these substances), and (2) moving to a part of the country that has less air pollution.

Treatment
Bronchodilators, **mucolytic** agents, weight reduction if obesity is present, oxygen for easier breathing, *no smoking,* and avoidance of air pollutants are included in the treatment. In some cases a process of massaging and pressure applied to the chest (chest physiotherapy) is used to help mobilize the mucus. Vaccination for influenza and pneumonia is advisable.

DIGESTIVE DISORDERS

From one meal to the next, our digestive systems function without ceasing and without our awareness until something goes wrong. As long as we ingest a well-balanced, nutritious diet, the process of digestion, which begins in the mouth, generally takes place efficiently and quietly. (For a theory about indigestion, see Did You Know? in this chapter.) But when a disease or disorder occurs in some part of the digestive tract (the mouth, esophagus, stomach, and intestines) or the organs that secrete digestive juices, the pleasure that most find in eating can change to discomfort, pain, and suffering. Figure 15-3 shows the structure of the gastrointestinal tract.

The teeth and tongue start the process of digestion by cutting, tearing, and kneading the food, while saliva adds lubrication and enzymes begin to break down starches. By the time the food is swallowed, it is a soft ball called a bolus. The bolus passes down the pharynx to the esophagus,

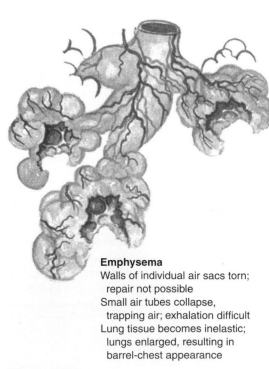

Emphysema
Walls of individual air sacs torn; repair not possible
Small air tubes collapse, trapping air; exhalation difficult
Lung tissue becomes inelastic; lungs enlarged, resulting in barrel-chest appearance

Figure 15-2
Airway obstruction caused by emphysema.

Nonimaginary Digestive Discomfort

Many individuals with ulcer symptoms may be victims of nonulcer **dyspepsia,** or in simpler terms, indigestion. This does not explain why, for some people, the symptoms occur after every meal. One theory has been that some people may be more sensitive to internal events, picking up messages that most people don't get.

The first evidence of this theory was published in 1991 by researchers at the Autonomous University of Barcelona. A device was used that has an inflatable bag that can be passed into the stomach; also present were electronic sensors that can detect how much pressure a given volume of inflation creates and how tense the stomach wall becomes. The researchers discovered that patients with nonulcer dyspepsia were far more sensitive than others to what was taking place in their stomachs. Those with nonulcer dyspepsia reported feeling pain when at a level of inflation that produced no symptoms at all in the control group.

This discovery did not produce a cure for nonulcer dyspepsia, but at least those suffering with it now know that there is a reason for their discomfort, and they are not imagining it.

---

where peristalsis moves it downward to the stomach.

The upper part of the stomach, or fundus, holds the food as it is delivered gradually to the lower part, or antrum. There the food is churned and mixed with enzymes and acids that continue the digestive process until the contents are reduced to a sticky liquid called **chyme.**

The chyme is released gradually into the first section of the small intestine, the duodenum, through the pyloric sphincter. The entry of the acid chyme into the duodenum brings about the discharge of bile from the gallbladder and the secretion of pancreatic juice by the pancreas.

The nutrients are absorbed into the blood from the small intestine, and the indigestible part of the chyme passes through the large intestine. Liquid is extracted along the way, and the remaining feces pass on out of the body. The disorders of the digestive system that will be discussed in this chapter occur in the stomach, intestines, liver, gallbladder, and pancreas.

Peptic Ulcer

A peptic ulcer is a break or ulceration (sore) in the mucosal membrane (lining) of the lower esophagus, stomach, or upper part of the small intestine. About eighty percent of peptic ulcers are in the duodenum (duodenal ulcers), and most of the rest

are in the stomach (gastric ulcers). It is now known that infection with a bacterium, *Helicobacter pylori,* is a major cause of duodenal ulcers. In addition, the use of NSAIDs (Nonsteroidal antiinflammatory drugs) and **hypersecretory** disorders may also be factors. Figure 15-4 shows a deep ulcer in the wall of the duodenum.

Predisposing Factors

Duodenal Ulcers In addition to infection with *H. pylori,* people with duodenal ulcers tend to secrete excess acid and pepsin, respond more to stimuli of acid secretion, and have more rapid gastric emptying. The rapid emptying of the stomach's contents into the duodenum (through the pyloric valve) may result in exposing the duodenal mucosa to greater acidity.

Other factors include smoking and a decrease in the secretion of bicarbonate from the mucosa. There is no evidence that stress causes ulcers as once thought, however, stress, anxiety, and fatigue

alpha-antitrypsin   al-fa an-ti-TRIP-sin
hypoxemia   hi-poks-E-me-a
mucolytic   mu-ko-LI-tik
dyspepsia   dis-PEP-se-a
chyme   kime
Helicobacter pylori   hel-i-ko-BAK-tur pi-LOR-e
hypersecretory   hi-per-SEK-re-tory

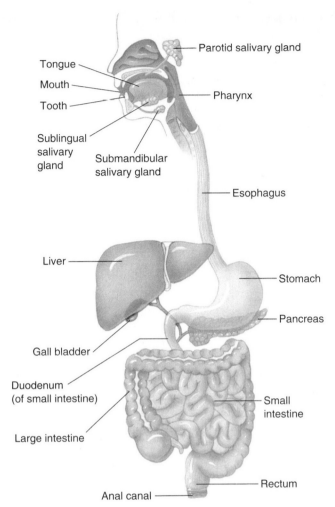

Figure 15-3

Location of the organs of the digestive system.

have been known to reactivate or aggravate an ulcer. Smoking, aspirin, and other NSAIDs have been implicated in ulcer formation, but there is not enough evidence to confirm this, although they are known irritants and, as with stress, may aggravate or reactivate an ulcer that is or has been present.

Gastric Ulcers

People with gastric ulcers tend to have lower levels of gastric acid than normal. It is thought that these individuals may have a primary defect in their gastric mucosa, making it more susceptible to lesions. In sixty percent to eighty percent of the

cases, gastritis is present along with an ulcer. Interestingly enough, when the ulcer heals, the gastritis persists, suggesting that the gastritis is primary and the ulcer secondary. Another theory is that the pyloric sphincter (lower valve of the stomach) may be weakened, allowing bile to reflux into the stomach. Cigarette smoking also decreases the effectiveness of the resting sphincter, increasing bile reflux. It is possible that bile acids seeping back into the stomach could damage the mucosal barrier, lead to chronic gastritis, cause increased acid penetration, and eventually ulcers. Exogenous agents, in addition to smoking, that have

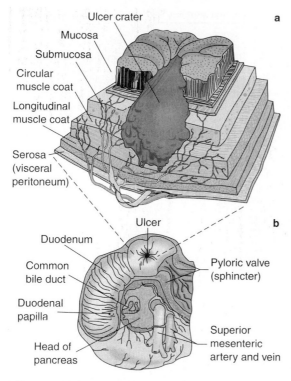

Ulcer crater
Mucosa
Submucosa
Circular muscle coat
Longitudinal muscle coat
Serosa (visceral peritoneum)
a

Ulcer **b**
Duodenum
Common bile duct
Duodenal papilla
Head of pancreas
Pyloric valve (sphincter)
Superior mesenteric artery and vein

Figure 15-4

Duodenal ulcer. The illustration shows a deep ulceration in the duodenal wall, extending as a crater through the entire mucosa and into the muscle layers. **a,** A cut-away segment of the duodenal wall showing an ulcer crater. **b,** The position of the ulcer in the duodenum.

been implicated in the formation of gastric ulcers are aspirin and other NSAIDs, chronic alcohol consumption, caffeine, corticosteroids, and other drugs.

Symptoms

Heartburn, indigestion, and pain are the typical symptoms of peptic ulcers. For a gastric ulcer, the pain is in the left epigastrium and accompanied by a feeling of fullness immediately after eating. A duodenal ulcer causes discomfort in the mide-pigastrium two to four hours after eating; this is relieved by eating. Individuals with gastric ulcers tend to lose weight, because eating a large meal stretches the gastric wall, causing discomfort and pain. On the other hand, eating relieves the discomfort and pain from duodenal ulcers, and suf-

ferers eat more in an effort to feel better. In both kinds of peptic ulcer, the symptoms range from none to severe back pain. An untreated ulcer may suddenly rupture and hemorrhage.

Prevention *Tylenol*

Avoiding the use of nicotine, caffeine, alcohol, and aspirin-containing compounds and learning to manage stress are the best means of prevention. Medical advice should be sought for any persistent pain, heartburn, or indigestion.

Treatment

The treatment for peptic ulcer depends upon the severity of the symptoms. Antacids are sometimes sufficient to clear up the condition. Newer drugs are now available to help reduce the secretion of acid. If complications occur, surgery may be performed. Even after the ulcer is healed, renewed stress or alcohol use may lead to recurrence.

Hiatal Hernia *Not on Final*

When an organ protrudes or projects through the tissues that usually contain it, this protrusion is called a hernia. A **hiatal hernia** occurs when a defect in the diaphragmatic hiatus allows part of the stomach to protrude into the chest cavity at the **gastroesophageal** junction. The hernia may be direct or "sliding," **paraesophageal,** or "rolling," or mixed. Figure 15-5 shows a type of hiatal hernia.

Predisposing Factors

Hiatal hernias increase in incidence with age and are more prevalent in women than in men. They usually result from muscle weakness that is common with aging or other factors, including esophageal cancer, trauma, surgical procedures, or congenital weakness of the diaphragmatic hiatus. Intraabdominal pressure, which may be from pregnancy, obesity, coughing, bending, straining, or extreme physical exertion, creates the conditions that allow the stomach to rise into the chest. This

hiatal hernia	hi-A-tal HER-ne-a
gastroesophageal	gas-tro-e-SOF-a-JE-al
paraesophageal	par-a-e-sof-a-JE-al

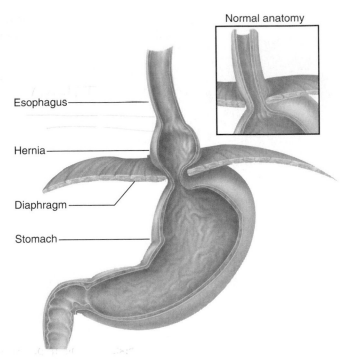

Normal anatomy

Esophagus

Hernia

Diaphragm

Stomach

Figure 15-5
A hiatal hernia with a portion of the stomach protruding through the diaphragm into the thoracic cavity.

may be accompanied by reflux of stomach acids, which leads to the familiar condition of heartburn.

Symptoms

Many individuals with hiatal hernia never have symptoms. If there are symptoms they could include heartburn from one to four hours after eating and chest pain (retro- or substernal). Complications such as difficulty in swallowing, bleeding, severe pain, and shock may also occur.

Prevention

Because a number of different factors may lead to hiatal hernia, there is no single means of prevention. Avoidance of excessive weight gain during pregnancy and maintaining an ideal weight throughout life may reduce the risk, as would avoidance of other factors that cause intraabdominal pressure.

Treatment

Treatment is aimed at minimizing symptoms and avoiding complications. Surgery is not recommended initially because the hernia often recurs

after surgery. The individual is given **antiemetics** and cough suppressants and told to avoid constrictive clothing, adjust the diet to ensure easy bowel movements, stop smoking if a smoker, use antacids, lose weight if overweight, and elevate the head of the bed. Drug therapy is also used to strengthen the cardiac sphincter tone. If these measures do not control the symptoms or if complications occur, surgical repair may be necessary.

Cirrhosis of the Liver

The liver has an amazing capacity to repair itself after all kinds of damage. A healthy liver is shown in Figure 15-6 and cirrhosis of the liver in a sixty-five-year-old man in Figure 15-7. The widespread destruction of cells and fibrotic regeneration that occur in cirrhosis lead to permanent loss of function. There are also many complications that can occur. Resistance to blood flow in the portal vein leads to portal hypertension. To allow blood to reach the heart without going through the liver, the

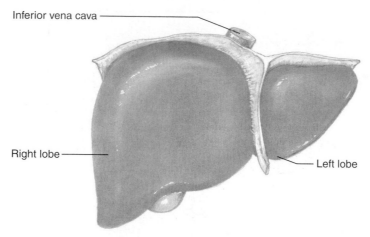

Inferior vena cava

Right lobe

Left lobe

Figure 15-6
Anterior view of the liver structure.

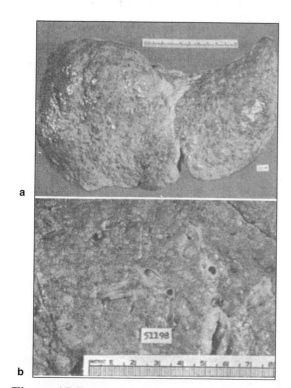

a

b

Figure 15-7
Cirrhosis of the liver. **a,** Liver showing alcoholic cirrhosis in a 65-year-old man. **b,** Cut surface of liver showing damage caused by cirrhosis.

body opens up other pathways called collateral circulation. These new veins are often in the lower part of the esophagus, and as the pressure builds up, tend to hemorrhage, resulting in a life-threatening situation.

Predisposing Factors
The causes of cirrhosis of the liver can be identified as follows:

> Alcoholism—thirty percent to fifty percent
>
> Bile duct disease—fifteen percent to twenty percent
>
> Various types of hepatitis—ten percent to thirty percent
>
> Miscellaneous disorders—five percent to ten percent
>
> Unknown cause—ten percent

Symptoms
The early symptoms include anorexia, indigestion, nausea, vomiting, and **hepatomegaly.** There may be no symptoms, but a doctor can detect an

antiemetics	an-ti-e-MET-iks
hepatomegaly	hep-a-to-MEG-a-le

CONTEMPORARY CONCERNS

When Too Much of a Good Thing Is Bad

Excess amounts of vitamin A can be deadly, and individuals taking it to improve their health wind up damaging their health instead. In one study, forty-one patients who had no other evident reason for liver disease were found to have abnormalities known to result from too much vitamin A. Seventeen had cirrhosis, eighteen showed milder damage, and six died of liver failure.

Too much vitamin A can also cause itching, hair loss, dry skin and mouth, irritability, nausea or vomiting, bone and joint pains, fatigue, and chronic headache. Children are more sensitive to excess amounts than adults, and no one should take more than the recommended daily amount unless prescribed by a doctor.

enlarged liver. There may also be vascular hemangiomas, gynecomastia, and testicular atrophy. Later symptoms include edema, splenomegaly, hemorrhoids, esophageal **varices,** collateral veins about the umbilicus, and jaundice. As the disease continues, widespread damage to the body occurs, and death most frequently comes as a result of hepatic coma.

Prevention

Eating regular nutritious meals and using alcohol in moderation, if at all, greatly reduce the risk for developing cirrhosis of the liver. In addition, if there are any symptoms of disease such as nausea, indigestion, anorexia, and/or vomiting that are persistent, the individual should see a physician. (Contemporary Concerns in this chapter discusses liver damage from excess ingestion of vitamin A.)

Treatment

Therapy depends upon the cause and severity of the disease. The goal is to remove or alleviate the underlying cause and prevent further liver damage or treat complications.

Gallbladder Disease

Gallbladder disease is one of the most common causes of hospitalization among adults. It is usually caused by calculi or gallstones, which may irritate the gallbladder and/or clog the bile duct, causing pain and discomfort on the right side.

Figure 15-8 shows the location of the gallbladder, liver, and pancreas.

Predisposing Factors

Gallstones are formed from cholesterol, bilirubin, and calcium. They appear to arise because of a sluggish gallbladder, which may be caused by pregnancy, oral contraceptives, diabetes mellitus, celiac disease, cirrhosis of the liver, and pancreatitis. Or they may be the result of too much cholesterol in the bile (synthesized by the liver). Fasting for long periods may lead to the development of gallstones by causing bile to stagnate in the liver. Gallstones generally occur during middle age and are more common in women. Recent evidence indicates that heredity affects the formation of gallstones, and there is a strong correlation between gallstones and obesity. High levels of estrogens, use of oral contraceptives, and having many children also increase the risk.

Symptoms

Gallbladder disease may be asymptomatic. However, symptoms may occur, particularly after eating a fatty meal. These may range from acute, sharp pain on the right side radiating to the back with nausea and vomiting, to mild discomfort in the abdominal area. The pain may be so severe that emergency room treatment is sought.

Prevention

No preventive measures are known.

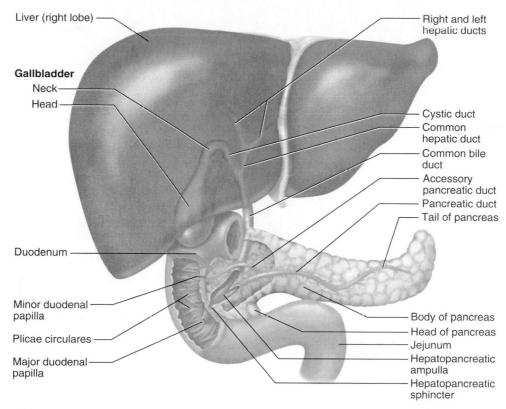

Figure 15-8
Location of the liver, gallbladder, and pancreas, which are necessary organs of digestion.

Treatment

Because it is believed that the gallbladder is not necessary to health, elective surgery is generally the treatment. Most doctors have felt that when there are gallstones present, the gallbladder should be removed. In a few short years, removal of the gallbladder by laparoscopy has largely taken the place of major surgery. Although some physicians were afraid that complications might occur in a procedure that was so new, a study of 1518 **laparoscopic cholecystectomies** found that fewer complications were present using the new method than had been reported in previous studies of conventional gallbladder removal. Laparoscopic gallbladder surgery is referred to as "bandaid" surgery, because only a few "keyhole" incisions are necessary for the procedure.

EXCRETORY DISORDERS

Kidney Disease

The kidneys are part of the urinary tract, which contains the two kidneys, a ureter connected to each one, the bladder, and the urethra, which leads to the outside of the body (Figure 15-9). An individual can survive with only one kidney, but if both kidneys fail, the waste products of metabolism will build up in the blood, leading to discomfort, suffering, and, ultimately, death. The kidneys

varices   VAR-i-sez
laparoscopic cholecystectomies
lap-ar-OS-ko-pik ko-le-sis-TEK-to-me

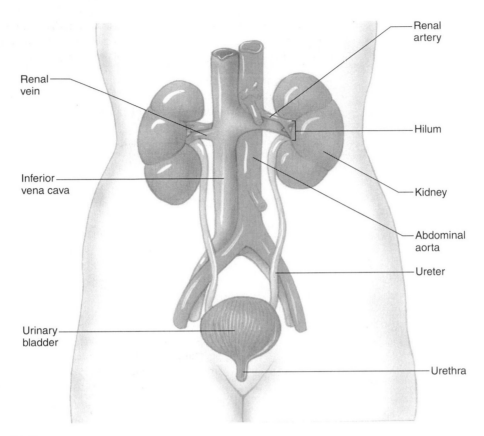

Renal artery

Renal vein

Hilum

Inferior vena cava

Kidney

Abdominal aorta

Ureter

Urinary bladder

Urethra

Figure 15-9

Organs of the urinary system.

perform the life-sustaining functions of removing fluid and waste products from the blood and regulating internal body chemistry by selectively excreting or retaining various compounds.

Within each kidney is an intricate mechanism to provide the filtering, reabsorption, and excretion functions. Over a million nephrons perform the operation; the actual filtering of the blood takes place in a glomerulus within each nephron. Blood flows from the aorta into the nephrons through the renal arteries and, after passing through the maze of tubules and other structures, returns to the lower vena cava through the renal veins. The liquid wastes extracted from the blood are carried by the ureter to the bladder for excretion through the urethra. When the glomeruli or other parts of the kidney do not function as they should, then kidney disease is the result.

Chronic Renal Failure

Chronic renal failure is usually the end result of a gradually progressive loss of renal function that can be due to one or more different diseases. Occasionally, it is the result of a rapidly progressive disease of sudden onset. Few symptoms develop until after more than seventy-five percent of glomerular filtration is lost. Then the remaining normal tissue deteriorates progressively, and symptoms worsen as renal function decreases. If the condition continues unchecked, uremic toxins accumulate and produce potentially fatal physiologic changes in all major organ systems.

Predisposing Factors

Chronic glomerular disease (**glomerulonephritis**), chronic infections, congenital defects, vascular diseases, kidney stones, systemic diseases such as lupus erythematosus, drug overdose, and endocrine diseases can be factors leading to kidney failure.

Symptoms

Symptoms arise from the major changes that occur in all body systems. These include:

Cardiovascular—hypertension, dysrhythmias, and congestive heart failure

Respiratory—increased susceptibility to infection, pulmonary edema, and pleurisy

Gastrointestinal—ulcers, colitis, and pancreatitis

Skin—yellow-bronze color, dry, scaly, itchy; thin, brittle fingernails

Neurologic—restless legs syndrome, pain, burning, and itching in legs and feet, muscle cramping, shortened memory span, and drowsiness

Blood—anemia and easy bruising

Skeletal—calcium-phosphorus imbalance, demineralization, and fractures

Prevention

Although some of the predisposing factors cannot be changed, attending to any infectious conditions when they occur and controlling hypertension could help avoid kidney problems in later years. Proper nutrition, avoiding the use of drugs, and a healthy lifestyle in general could also reduce the chances of chronic renal failure.

Treatment

Dialysis can eliminate or markedly decrease most symptoms. However, some may remain. A low-protein diet may be prescribed, fluid balance must be maintained, and a regular stool analysis may be required. Drug therapy often relieves some of the symptoms, and careful monitoring of serum potassium levels is necessary. Kidney transplant is also an option.

Kidney Stones

A stone or calculus that forms in the kidney usually consists of two or more of the following: uric acid, oxalates, and calcium phosphate. In the United States, kidney stones are more common in men and are rare in blacks and children.

Predisposing Factors

Infections, as well as irritation and disease of the parathyroid glands, may cause the formation of stones. Other risk factors are a family history of kidney stones, dehydration, certain medications, and metabolic factors such as too much uric acid in the blood and diet.

Symptoms

The usual symptom is pain, which can be excruciating. Depending on the location of the stone, the pain may be in the back, legs, or abdomen, and it may be dull or severe. Nausea and vomiting often accompany severe pain. There may also be chills and fever.

Prevention

Particular attention to diet and medications is important if there is a family history of kidney stones. A physician should be consulted if a stone occurs to determine any underlying cause that can be eliminated to prevent recurrence.

Treatment

If the stone is not too large to pass through the urinary tract, then measures are taken to promote natural passage. If the stone is not in the lower pelvic area, it can be crushed with a laser. If it is in the urethra, a **cystoscope** (tube with a light and crushing device attached) can be inserted to destroy the stone. Ultrasonic **lithotripsy** has been used in recent years. In this process, an ultrasonic probe is used through a telescopic tube to help break up the stones. And a shockwave can be focused on the stones from outside the body, causing their disintegration. If these methods cannot be used because of placement or size of the stone, analgesics are administered to relieve pain, and surgery may be necessary.

glomerulonephritis	glo-mer-u-lo-ne-FRI-tis
cystoscope	SIST-o-skop
lithotripsy	lith-o-TRIP-se

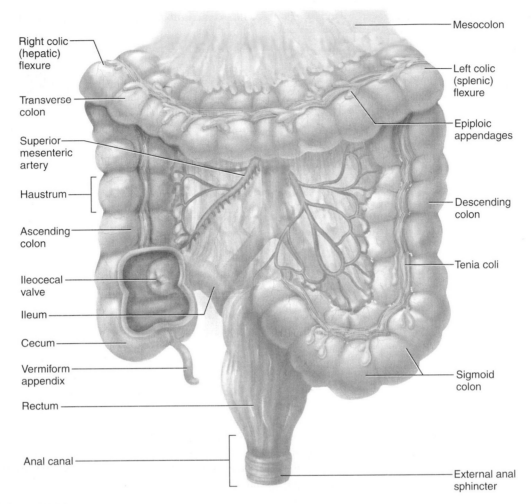

Figure 15-10
Divisions of the large intestine.

Irritable Bowel Syndrome

Irritable bowel syndrome is the most common disorder of the intestines, accounting for more than half of the patients seen by **gastroenterologists.** The condition is associated with psychological stress, but it may also result from physical factors. It is twice as common in women as in men.

Predisposing Factors
Although irritable bowel syndrome is associated with psychological stress, it may also be due to physical factors such as **diverticular** disease (to be discussed next), lactose intolerance, abuse of laxatives, food poisoning, or colon cancer.

Symptoms
In addition to the abdominal pain, diarrhea, and constipation, there may be mucus in the feces, a sense of incomplete evacuation of the bowels, excessive gas, and symptoms aggravated by certain foods.

Prevention
No preventive measures are known.

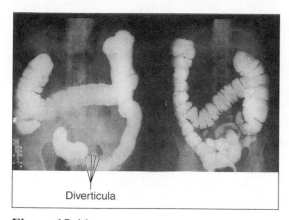

Diverticula

Figure 15-11

Multiple diverticula in a section of the colon.

Treatment

High-fiber foods may be prescribed for the constipation, and an antispasmodic drug to relieve muscular spasm. Antidiarrheal drugs may be given briefly if the diarrhea is prolonged. This treatment can ease the symptoms, but there is no known cure.

Diverticular Disease

There are two kinds of diverticular disease, diverticulosis (an increased number of diverticula) and diverticulitis (inflammation of the diverticula). In each case, small sacs form in the intestines, most commonly in the sigmoid colon (Figure 15-10).

Figure 15-11 shows multiple diverticula in a section of the colon. In the United States, over half the population have diverticular disease by the time they are eighty years of age.

Predisposing Factors

The sacs may be formed when there is excess pressure on weak areas in the walls of the intestine; lack of fiber in the diet is thought to be a factor.

Symptoms

If symptoms are present in diverticulosis, they tend to be the same as for irritable bowel syndrome. In diverticulitis, there may be fever, pain, tenderness, and rigidity of the abdomen over the intestine area that is involved.

Prevention

Eating a diet high in fiber is thought to lower the risk of diverticular disease.

Treatment

For cramps, a high-fiber diet, fiber supplements, and antispasmodic drugs may relieve the symptoms. Bed rest and antibiotics will usually take care of diverticulitis. If the symptoms are severe, treatment may include a liquid diet, intravenous feeding, or surgery to remove the diseased section of the intestine.

gastroenterologists	gas-tro-en-ter-OL-o-jists
diverticular	di-ver-TIK-u-lar

SUMMARY

Table 15-1 summarizes relevant data on the chronic respiratory, digestive, and excretory diseases discussed in this chapter.

TABLE 15-1	Diseases of the Systems Involved with Respiration, Digestion, and Excretion				
Disease	**Special Characteristics**	**Predisposing Factors**	**Common Symptoms**	**Prevention**	**Treatment**
RESPIR-ATORY DISORDERS					
Chronic Bronchitis	Presence of a productive cough for at least 3 months of 2 successive years; middle age, older people, smokers, and those exposed to excess industrial and environ-mental pollu-tants; part of COPD with emphysema and asthma	Smoking, industrial and enviorn-mental pollutants, respiratory infections, allergies	Productive cough, shortness of breath, which gradually gets worse, heart failure, (cor pulmonale)	No smoking, living and working environment as free from pollution as possible, treatment for allergy	No smoking, avoidance of air pollution, broncho-dilators, nebulizers, diuretics, and oxygen as needed
Emphysema	Walls of alveoli destroyed; alveoli lose elasticity; chest becomes bar-rel shaped with struggle for breath; do not die quickly	Smoking, air pollution, and deficiency of alpha-antitrypsin (hereditary)	Labored breath-ing, gasping for breath; chronic cough, anorexia, weight loss, "barrel chest," hypoxemia, and heart failure (cor pumonale)	No smoking, avoidance of environmen-tal pollutants	Broncho-dilators, mucolytic agents, normal weight, oxy-gen, no smoking, avoidance of air pollutants, chest physio-therapy
DIGESTIVE DISORDERS					
Peptic Ulcer	May be in the stomach (gastric) or in the duodenum; a lesion in the mucous	Cause of origi-nal lesion is unknown, may be an inherited fac-tor; theories include	Indigestion, heartburn, and pain in left epigas-trium for gastric ulcer and	Avoiding use of nicotine, caf-feine, alcohol or aspirin and stress management	Antacids, drugs, surgery

TABLE 15-1	*Continued*				
Disease	**Special Characteristics**	**Predisposing Factors**	**Common Symptoms**	**Prevention**	**Treatment**
Peptic Ulcer— Cont'd	membrane; 80% are duo denal; more likely in males; acid may be dumped into duodenum through pyloric valve	infection with bacteria, overactive vagus nerve, hyperacidity of gastric juice, inade- quate mucosal blood flow, hormonal stimulation; duodenal ulcers more frequent with blood type O, gastric more frequent with blood type A	midepigastri- um for duodenal ulcer; feeling of fullness immediately after eating for gastric ulcer (lose weight); nausea and pain 2-4 hours after eating for duodenal ulcer (gain weight); if untreated, may rupture and hemor- rhage or penetrate pancreas; can cause severe back pain		
Hiatal Hernia	Defect in the diaphrag- matic hiatus allows part of stomach to protrude into chest cavity; may be a sliding or rolling hernia or a combi- nation of the two	More in women than in men; result from muscle weakness that may be congenital or brought on by trauma; any condition producing intraabdomi- nal pressure may cause the hernia; may be accompanied by reflux that	May be none, or may be heartburn and chest pain 1-4 hours after eating	Because excess weight can cause intra- abdominal pressure, maintaining ideal weight may reduce risk	Antiemetics, cough suppressants, avoid move- ments that strain the intra- abdominal area, no smoking, antacids, weight con- trol, abdomi- nal, elevation of head of bed, drugs to strengthen cardiac sphincter,

TABLE 15-1	*Continued*				
Disease	**Special Characteristics**	**Predisposing Factors**	**Common Symptoms**	**Prevention**	**Treatment**
Hiatal Hernia—Cont'd		leads to heartburn			surgery (hernia often returns)
Cirrhosis of the liver	Destruction of cells and fibrotic regeneration leads to permanent loss of liver function; many complications can occur	Alcoholism (30%-50%), bile duct disease, hepatitis are the main factors	Anorexia, indigestion, nausea, vomiting, and hepatomegaly; sometimes asymptomatic; liver enlarged; later symptoms, edema, splenomegaly, hemorrhoids, esophageal varices, jaundice	Good nutrition, little alcohol if at all	Removal or alleviation of underlying cause
Gall Bladder Disease	Caused by calculi or gallstones that may irritate the gallbladder or clog the bile duct; one of most common conditions requiring surgery	Appears to be due to a sluggish gall bladder, which can be caused by pregnancy, oral contraceptives, diabetes mellitus and other conditions; may be hereditary factor, linked to obesity and high levels of estrogen	May be asymptomatic; symptoms range from mild discomfort in abdominal area, acute sharp pain on right side radiating to the back with nausea and vomiting	Unknown	Laparoscopic surgery now used most of the time rather than the conventional gallbladder surgery

TABLE 15-1	*Continued*				
Disease	**Special Characteristics**	**Predisposing Factors**	**Common Symptoms**	**Prevention**	**Treatment**
DISORDERS OF THE EXCRETORY ORGANS					
Chronic Renal Failure	Due to gradually progressive loss of renal function caused by one or more disorders of the kidneys; 75% of glomerular function lost before most symptoms develop; if untreated, progresses until fatal	Glomerulo-nephritis, chronic infections, congenital defects, vascular diseases, kidney stones, some systemic and endocrine diseases; arterio-sclerosis	Symptoms in all body systems when disease is in late stages; early symptoms include nausea, drowsiness, vomiting, breathlessness, and decrease in amount of urine output; 75% loss of function	Treatment for kidney infections, control of HBP, proper nutrition, avoiding use of drugs, and a healthy lifestyle in general	Dialysis, low-protein diet, maintenance of fluid balance and potassium levels, regular stool analysis, drugs, kidney transplant
Kidney Stones	Usually consist of uric acid, oxalates, or calcium phosphate (2 or more)	Infections, irritation and disease of parathyroid glands, family history, dehydration, certain medications and diet	Pain in back, legs, or abdomen, which may be dull or severe; nausea, vomiting, chills, fever, may accompany severe pain	Attention to diet and medication if there is a family history	Promotion of natural passage of stone if possible, laser, cystoscope, ultrasonic lithotripsy, analgesics, surgery
Irritable Bowel Syndrome	Most common disorder of the intestines; twice as common in women as in men	Psychological stress and certain physical factors	Abdominal pain, diarrhea, constipation, and sometimes mucus in the feces; sense of	None known	High-fiber diet, antispasmodic drugs, antidiarrheal drugs if necessary

Disease	Special Characteristics	Predisposing Factors	Common Symptoms	Prevention	Treatment
Irritable Bowel Syndrome— Cont'd Diverticular Disease	2 kinds— diverticulosis and diverticulitis; in U.S., over half have it by the time they are 80	Pressure on weak areas in walls of intestines and lack of roughage in diet	incomplete evacuation, gas Diverticulosis symptoms same as irritable bowel syndrome if present; in diverticulitis, fever, pain, tenderness, and rigidity of abdomen over area of intestine involved	Diet high in fiber may lower risk	High-fiber diet, fiber supplements, antispasmodic drugs, bed rest, antibiotics; may need a liquid diet, intravenous feeding, or surgery if severe

TABLE 15-1 *Continued*

QUESTIONS FOR REVIEW

1. What are the differences between chronic bronchitis, asthma, and emphysema?

2. What are the possible causes for peptic ulcers?

3. What measures can be taken to prevent a gastric ulcer?

4. What conditions may predispose a person to hiatal hernia?

5. What happens to the liver in cirrhosis, and what are the consequences?

6. To what extent are alcoholism, hepatitis, and bile duct disease factors in cirrhosis of the liver?

7. What factors may determine whether a person gets gallbladder disease?

8. How do the symptoms of peptic ulcer, hiatal hernia, cirrhosis of the liver, and gallbladder disease differ?

9. What is the treatment for chronic bronchitis, asthma, and emphysema?

10. What is the treatment for peptic ulcer, hiatal hernia, cirrhosis of the liver, and gallbladder disease?

11. What conditions may lead to chronic renal failure?

12. What are the symptoms for chronic renal failure?

13. How can the risk of chronic renal failure be reduced?

14. What are the predisposing factors, symptoms, and prevention for kidney stones?

15. What factors are linked to irritable bowel syndrome?

16. How do the symptoms for irritable bowel syndrome and diverticular disease differ?

17. What is the difference between diverticulosis and diverticulitis?

18. What is the treatment for chronic renal failure, kidney stones, irritable bowel syndrome, and diverticular disease?

FURTHER READING

Bateson, Malcolm. 1999. Gallbladder disease. *British Medical Journal* 318:1745.

Bensoussan, Alan, and Nick J. Talley. 1998. Treatment of irritable bowel syndrome with Chinese herbal medicine. *Journal of the American Medical Association* 280:1585.

Brunetto, M. R., F. Oliveri, et al. 1998. Effect of interferon-alpha on progression of cirrhosis to hepatocellular carcinoma: A retrospective cohort study. *The Lancet* 351:1535.

Cameron, A.J. 1999. Barrett's esophagus: prevalence and size of hiatal hernia. *American Journal of Gastroenterology* 94:2054.

Caselli, M., et al. 1999. *Helicobacter pylori* and chronic bronchitis. *Scandinavian Journal of Gastroenterology* 34:828.

Cazzola, M., et al. 1999. Comparative study of dirithromycin and azithromycin in the treatment of acute bacterial exacerbations of chronic bronchitis. *Journal of Chemotherapy* 11:119.

Delaney, Brendan C., and F. D. R. Hobbs. 1998. Commentary: *Helicobacter pylori* eradication in primary care. *British Medical Journal* 316:1654.

Drossman, Douglas A. 1999. Do psychosocial factors define symptom severity and patient status in irritable bowel syndrome? *American Journal of Medicine* 107:51S.

Duggan, A. E., and K. Tolley, et al. 1998. Varying efficacy of *Helicobacter pylori* eradication regimes: Cost effectiveness study using a derision analysis model. *British Medical Journal* 316:1648.

Elsenbruch, S. 1999. Subjective and objective sleep quality in irritable bowel syndrome. *American Journal of Gastroenterology* 94:2447.

Erkinjuntti-Pekkanen, R., et al. 1999. IgG antibodies, chronic bronchitis, and pulmonary function values in farmer's lung patients and matched controls. *Allergy* 54:1181.

Everhart, J.E. 1999. Prevalence and ethnic differences in gallbladder disease in the United States. *Gastroenterology* 117:632.

Farmer, C. K. T. 1998. Individual kidney function before and after renal angioplasty. *The Lancet* 352:288.

Fass, R., S. Fullerton, B. Naliboff, et al. 1998. Sexual dysfunction in patients with irritable bowel syndrome and non-ulcer dyspepsia. *Digestion* 59:79.

Francis, P., A. Prior, P. J. Whorwell, et al. 1998. *Chlamydia trachomatis* infection: Is it relevant in irritable bowel syndrome? *Digestion* 59:157.

Furr, Allen L. 1998. Psycho-social aspects of serious renal disease and dialysis: A review of the literature. *Social Work in Health Care* 27:97.

Gelb, A.F., et al. 1999. Lung function 4 years after lung volume reduction surgery for emphysema. *Chest* 116:1608.

Goh, S.K., et al. 1999. A prospective study of infections with atypical pneumonia organisms in acute exacerbations of chronic bronchitis. *Annal Academy of Medicine Singapore* 28:476.

Gold, B.D. 1999. Current therapy for *helicobacter pylori* infection in children and adolescents. *Canadian Journal of Gastroenterology* 13:571.

Hawkey, C. J., Z. Tulassay, et al. 1998. Randomized controlled trial of *Helicobacter pylori* eradication in patients on non-steroidal anti-inflammatory drugs: HELP NSAIDS study. *The Lancet* 352:1016.

Health, John M. 1998. Chronic bronchitis: Primary care management. *American Family Physician* 57:2365.

Huffman, Grace B. 1998. Pulmonary function in cases of stable chronic bronchitis. *American Family Physician* 57:2253.

Jarrett, M., M. Heitkemper, K. C. Cain, et al. 1998. The relationship between psychological distress and gastrointestinal symptoms in women with irritable bowel syndrome. *Nursing Research* 47:154.

Jones, K.L., and R.A. Robbins. 1999. Alternative therapies for chronic bronchitis. *American Journal of Medicine Science* 318:96.

King, T. S., M. Elia, et al. 1998. Abnormal colonic fermentation in irritable bowel syndrome. *The Lancet* 352:1187.

Koenig, Clint J. 1999. Accuracy of hematuria in diagnosing kidney stones. *Journal of Family Practice* 48:912.

Kyohler, L., D. Rixen, and H. Troidl. 1998. Laparoscopic colorectal resection for diverticulitis. *International Journal of Colorectal Disease* 13:43.

Laitinen, L.A., and K. Koskela. 2000. Chronic bronchitis and chronic obstructive pulmonary disease: Finnish national guidelines for prevention and treatment 1998-2007. *Respiratory Medicine* 93:297.

Lansoprazole prevents gastric ulcer recurrence safely. *Modern Medicine* 66:16, 1998.

Lewis, C. 1999. Every breath you take. Preventing and treating emphysema. *FDA Consumer* 33:9.

Lucas, Beverly, and Lawrence Agodoa. 1999. Chronic renal failure: slowing the onset, changing the course. *Patient Care* 33:76.

Masand, Prakash S., Sanjay Gupta, et al. 1998. Irritable bowel syndrome (IBS) and alcohol abuse or dependence. *American Journal of Drug and Alcohol Abuse* 24:513.

Mason, Andrew L., Lizhe Xu, et al. 1998. Detection of retroviral antibodies in primary biliary cirrhosis and other idiopathic biliary disorders. *The Lancet* 351:1620.

Mentor, S.J., and S.J. Swanson. 1999. Treatment of patients with lung cancer and severe emphysema. *Chest* 116:477S.

Miller, John D. 1999. Emphysema sufferers breathe easier. *Canadian Medical Association Journal* 161:1140.

Mooney, M. J., P. L. Elliott, D. B. Galapon, et al. 1998. Hand assisted laparoscopic sigmoidectomy for diverticulitis. *Diseases of the Colon and Rectum* 41:630.

Naoumov, Nikolai V., Elena P. Petrova, et al. 1998. Presence of a newly described human DNA virus (TTV) in patients with liver disease. *The Lancet* 352:195.

New treatment for acute exacerbations of chronic bronchitis. *Modern Medicine* 66:43, 1998.

Niederman, M.S., et al. 1999. Treatment cost of acute exacerbations of chronic bronchitis. *Clinical Therapy* 21:576.

Ohguro, N. 1999. Corneal endothelial changes in patients with chronic renal failure. *American Journal of Ophthalmology* 128:234.

Pak, Charles Y. C. 1998. Kidney stones. *The Lancet* 351:1797.

Paterson, William G., et al. 1999. Recommendations for the management of irritable bowel syndrome in family practice. *Canadian Medical Association Journal* 161:154.

Peura, David. 1998. *Helicobacter pylori*: Rational management option. *American Journal of Medicine* 105:424.

Ransom, Kenneth J. 1998. Laparoscopic management of acute cholecystitis with subtotal cholecystectomy. *American Surgeon* 64:955.

Rose, Verna L. 1998. Combined triple therapy for *H. pylori* infection. *American Family Physician* 58:1691.

Schmulson, Max W., and Lin Chang. 1999. Diagnostic approach to the patient with irritable bowel syndrome. *American Journal of Medicine* 107:20S.

Serna, D.L., et al. 1999. Survival after unilateral versus bilateral lung volume reduction surgery for emphysema. *Journal of Thoracic Cardiovascular Surgery* 118:1101.

Serum ascorbic acid levels related to reduced gallbladder disease in women. *Modern Medicine* 66:13, 1998.

Simon, Joel A., and Esther S. Hudes. 1998. Serum ascorbic acid and other correlates of gallbladder disease among US adults. *American Journal of Public Health* 88:1208.

Smart, Reginald G., Robert E. Mann, et al. 1998. Changes in liver cirrhosis death rates in different countries in relation to per capita alcohol consumption. *Journal of Studies on Alcohol* 59:245.

Smith, A.B. 1999. Pressure overload induced sliding hiatal hernia in power athletes. *Journal of Clinical Gastroenterology* 28:352.

Sperber, A.D. 1999. Fibromyalgia in the irritable bowel syndrome: studies of prevalence and clinical implications. *American Journal of Gastroenterology* 94:3541.

Strasser, S.I. 1999. Cirrhosis of the liver in long-term marrow transplant survivors. *Blood* 93:3259.

Thamer, M., N. F. Ray, S. C. Henderson, et al. 1998. Influence of the NIH Consensus Conference on *Helicobacter pylori* on physician prescribing among a medical population. *Medical Care* 36:646.

Triple ulcer therapy. *Geriatrics* 53:19, 1998.

Utz, J. P., R. D. Hubmayr, and C. Deschamps. 1998. Lung volume reduction surgery for emphysema: Out on a limb without a NETT. *Mayo Clinic Proceedings* 73:552.

Van Dulmen, A. M., J. F. M. Fennis, et al. 1998. Towards effective reassurance in irritable bowel syndrome: The importance of attending to patients' complaint related cognitions. *Psychology, Health and Medicine* 3:405.

Wang, Xiaorong, and Eiji Yano. 1999. Pulmonary dysfunction in silica-exposed workers: a relationship to radiographic signs of silicosis and emphysema. *American Journal of Industrial Medicine* 36:299.

Wilson, R., et al. 1999. Five-day moxifloxacin therapy compared with 7-day clarithromycin therapy for the treatment of acute exacerbations of chronic bronchitis. *Journal of Antimicrobiology Chemotherapy* 44:501.

Wood, Hugh M., and Cynthia Wark. 1999. Screening for *Helicobacter pylori* and nonsteroidal anti-inflammatory drug use in Medicare. *Archives of Internal Medicine* 159:149.

16

CHRONIC SKIN AND MUSCULOSKELETAL DISORDERS

OBJECTIVES

1. *Identify basic skin lesions.*
2. *Describe common disorders of the skin.*
3. *Evaluate treatments for acne.*
4. *Explain the reason for the symptoms of psoriasis.*
5. *Distinguish between osteoarthritis and rheumatoid arthritis (Chapter 2).*
6. *State the suspected cause of gout.*
7. *Explain what causes the symptoms of gout.*
8. *Identify the predisposing factors for fibromyalgia.*
9. *Explain how carpal tunnel syndrome occurs.*
10. *Distinguish between tendinitis and bursitis.*
11. *Discuss the symptoms of osteoporosis.*
12. *State the best treatment for osteoporosis.*
13. *Identify the best means of prevention for back problems.*
14. *Distinguish among lordosis, kyphosis, and scoliosis.*

SKIN DISORDERS

The skin is the largest organ of the body. This tough, resilient, protective barrier against environmental threats contains body fluids, regulates body temperatures, and plays a part in the production of vitamin D. The skin also contains touch and pressure receptors that provide sensations. The functions of the skin can be seen in Box 16-1.

Box 16-1

Functions of the Skin

Protects against infection
Contains body fluids
Regulates body temperature
Produces vitamin D
Provides sensations of touch and temperature

The skin has three primary layers, the epidermis, dermis, and subcutaneous tissue. The epidermis is the thinnest layer, although it is thicker on some parts of the body where it is subjected to much "wear and tear," such as the soles of the feet and palms of the hands. The skin of men is generally thicker than that of women, and it becomes thinner with age.

The dermis contains the hair follicles, sweat glands, and sebaceous glands. There are also blood vessels, lymph vessels, and nerves in the dermis.

The subcutaneous tissue, or hypodermis, is mainly fat and provides heat, insulation, shock absorption, and a reserve of calories. It also has a nerve supply.

In addition to immune disorders, infectious diseases and cancer, disorders of the skin include those caused by injury, hormonal disorders, poor nutrition, impaired blood supply, and drug reactions.

Acne

Most adolescent boys and many adolescent girls experience acne vulgaris, which is the most common type of acne. It is a chronic disorder of the skin caused by inflammation of the hair follicles and sebaceous glands. It can appear as early as eight years of age but most often begins at puberty.

Predisposing Factors

Acne spots occur when a hair follicle becomes obstructed by **sebum.** The follicle becomes inflamed when the sebum is trapped because bacteria are able to multiply, producing the inflammatory response. No one is sure why this happens at puberty, but it seems to be linked to the release of hormones. There may be a hereditary factor too.

Other predisposing factors are drugs that increase oil production by the skin, barbiturates, isoniazid, **rifampin,** bromides, and iodides. Acne may also be caused by oil and grease, such as that at the hairline; regular contact with mineral or cooking oil as in restaurant kitchens may make the condition worse. Cosmetics with an oil base are another risk factor.

Symptoms

The places where acne occurs have a high concentration of sebaceous glands. They are found mainly in the face, center of the chest, upper back, shoulders, and around the neck. The most common acne spots are blackheads, whiteheads, pustules, nodules, and cysts. Some spots, particularly if squeezed or irritated, leave scars, and the cystic spots may leave scars even without being touched. The scars tend to be small, depressed pits.

Prevention

There is no known dietary substance that causes acne. However, each person may be sensitive to certain foods on an individual basis. Many myths have grown up around the disorder that is so disfiguring just when young people are becoming extremely sensitive about their appearance. No evidence shows that avoiding chocolate or any other dietary substance will help. Washing the affected areas twice daily will not prevent the disorder, but it may keep it from spreading. Washing simply removes surface oil.

Treatment

Many treatments are available for acne, but no cures. Topical treatments may relieve the condition by unblocking the pores and removing the sebum. They will also promote healing. If topical therapy is not effective, systemic drugs may be used. Antibiotics are sometimes used and can have a healing effect over a long period (up to 6 months). Recently, **retinoid** drugs have been prescribed to reduce oil secretions and facilitate

sebum	SE-bum
rifampin	RIF-am-pin
retinoid	RET-i-noyd

[Handwritten notes at top of page:]
Rosacea - not in book - redness / type of adult acne nose, cheeks, forehead, chin. cause unknown >female< males - worse in males who have it. avoid steroids ex hydrocortizone > oral treatment is better

drying on the skin, but they have dangerous side effects and cannot be used during pregnancy. Acne generally clears up by the end of the teenage years.

Dermatitis

Some forms of dermatitis are due to disorders of the immune system and were discussed in Chapter 2. Others have no known cause. **Seborrheic** dermatitis and contact dermatitis are two of the most common. Sometimes, dermatitis is known as eczema.

Seborrheic Dermatitis

A common site for seborrheic dermatitis is the eyebrows, although it may occur at many places on the body.

Predisposing Factors

The exact cause is unknown, but stress and neurologic conditions may be predisposing factors.

Symptoms

There is itching, redness, and inflammation in areas with many sebaceous glands, usually the scalp, face, and trunk, and in skin folds. The lesions may appear greasy. The victim also may have yellowish, scaly patches, and dandruff may be caused by a mild seborrheic dermatitis.

Prevention

No preventive measures are known.

Treatment

The basic treatment is frequent washing and shampooing with a medicated soap to remove the scales. Topical corticosteroids and/or antibiotics may also be used. Skin should be handled gently; scratching and irritating substances, such as detergents, should be avoided.

Contact Dermatitis

This kind of dermatitis is caused by something that has touched the skin.

Predisposing Factors

Contact dermatitis may be caused by an allergy to a substance such as poison ivy, or it may be due to a direct toxic effect of the substance. Common substances that cause the reaction are detergents, nickel, chemicals in rubber gloves and condoms, certain cosmetics, plants, and medications.

Symptoms

A rash occurs and varies considerably according to the substance that causes it. The skin is often itchy and may flake, or a blister may develop. The rash covers the area of skin that came in contact with the substance.

Prevention

Identification of the causative substance and avoidance in the future is the best means of prevention.

Treatment

Topical application of corticosteroids may be used for treatment of the rash.

Psoriasis

Psoriasis is a common skin disease characterized by thickened patches of inflamed, red skin that is often covered by silvery scaling. Close to two percent of the people in the United States and Europe are affected by the disease, which is not as common among blacks and Asians. The affected areas may be so extensive that the individual is embarrassed to go out in public, particularly if the patches are on exposed surfaces. Common sites of the patches are the knees, elbows, scalp, trunk, and back. The disorder occurs when new skin cells are produced at ten times the usual rate while the shedding of old cells does not change. The live cells accumulate, causing the thickened patches covered with dead, flaking skin. There are different forms of psoriasis; the most common form is discussed here.

Predisposing Factors

A number of possible causes are being investigated, and there may be a genetic basis. Psoriasis tends to recur in attacks that may be triggered by emotional stress, skin damage, and physical illness.

Symptoms

In addition to the red skin and silvery patches, the most common symptom is itching. Because the patches tend to be dry and become cracked and encrusted, there may also be pain. The disease usually begins with small red papules that enlarge and join into larger inflamed lesions. When they develop in skin folds, the lesions are smooth and have a deep red color. There may be small bleeding points if the scales are removed. Many individuals with psoriasis also have arthritic symptoms.

Prevention
No preventive measures are known.

Treatment
Treatment depends upon the severity of the attack and form of the disease. Sunlight or ultraviolet lamps in small doses can be helpful, along with an emollient to help soften the affected area. The same therapies are used in moderate attacks, with the addition of an ointment containing coal tar. More severe attacks are treated with corticosteroids and other drugs. A NSAID, antirheumatic drug, or **methotrexate** may be used to treat the arthritis that accompanies psoriasis.

DISORDERS OF THE MUSCULOSKELETAL SYSTEM

Without the muscles, bones and joints, and connective tissue, activity as we know it would not exist. Moreover, disease or disorder in the parts of the musculoskeletal system can cripple and incapacitate until a normal life is impossible. It is easy to think of a bone as something nonliving. Those we generally see from the human skeleton are dry and lifeless. But bones are living, productive parts of the body in addition to giving support. The center of each bone is a cavity in which blood cells are manufactured. And each bone is composed of a supply of minerals and fibrous tissue that are also active in various growth processes. Figure 16-1 shows the basic structure of a bone. In most

seborrheic	seb-o-RE-ik
psoriasis	so-RI-a-sis
methotrexate	meth-o-TREK-sat

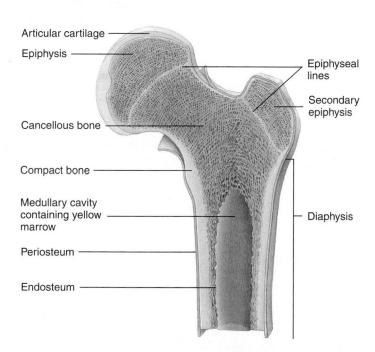

Articular cartilage

Epiphysis

Epiphyseal lines

Secondary epiphysis

Cancellous bone

Compact bone

Medullary cavity containing yellow marrow

Diaphysis

Periosteum

Endosteum

Figure 16-1
Structure of a bone.

chronic disorders of the musculoskeletal system, it is not the bone shafts that sustain injury, but the joints, which are susceptible throughout life to the stresses and strains of activity. One exception in the diseases that follow is osteoporosis, which is a metabolic bone disease affecting the integrity of the bone itself. Another exception is fibromyalgia, a disease of the muscles, tendons, and ligaments. Some of the other diseases affecting the musculoskeletal system are known to be neurologically or genetically oriented and will be dealt with in Chapters 17 and 18.

Disorders of the Joints
Osteoarthritis

Osteoarthritis is the most common form of arthritis and is present to some extent in everyone over sixty years of age. It is a chronic, progressive disorder causing deterioration of joint cartilage and bone. The body's response to this deterioration is to produce excess bone, which eventually makes joint movement painful and difficult, if not impossible.

Predisposing Factors

Continual exposure of the joint(s) to trauma such as in athletics or a professional trade, inherited predisposition, and normal aging processes all have been identified as predisposing factors.

Symptoms

In osteoarthritis, joint pain occurs, particularly after exercise or weight bearing, and is usually relieved by rest. There may also be stiffness in the morning, aching during changes in weather, limited movement, and fluid accumulation in the affected joint(s). Severity increases with poor posture, obesity, and occupational stress.

Prevention

Sensible exercise routines, but avoidance of athletic and occupational activities that cause constant stress to weight-bearing joints, may decrease the severity and deter the onset of osteoarthritis.

Treatment

The traditional treatment has been medication to relieve pain and surgery to replace joints that have been destroyed. Water exercise has been found to

be helpful for many. If analgesics no longer relieve the pain, three new treatments have been found to be effective in some patients with articular cartilage defects in the knee. The treatments involve cartilage transplants, bone grafts, or hyaluronic acid injected into the knee joint. They have helped alleviate pain in the short term (2 years) but more research is needed to determine long-term benefits.

Read the Did You Know? for information on pain relievers.

Gout

Gout is a painful arthritic disease that occurs most often in men. It involves a disruption of the body's control over uric acid production or excretion, resulting in high levels of uric acid in the blood. When the uric acid builds to a certain level in the blood, it crystallizes, and these crystals are deposited in connective tissue all over the body. When the crystals are deposited in the synovial fluid, they cause sudden sharp pain in the joint. Primary gout, which has a strong hereditary tendency, usually occurs in men over the age of thirty years and in postmenopausal women. Secondary gout, which arises as a result of another disorder, occurs in the elderly. The disease follows an intermittent course and may disappear for years and then return.

Predisposing Factors

Although excess use of alcohol may cause an exacerbation of the symptoms of gout, diet and "high living" are no longer considered the major factors. It is known that ingestion of excess amounts of protein can lead to high uric acid levels. Some evidence points to an inherited metabolic defect. Secondary gout may result from leukemia, chronic renal diseases, lead poisoning, and drugs such as chlorothiazide.

Symptoms

Primary gout is an interesting disease that may affect any joint at any time. The most frequent site, for some unknown reason, is the big toe. The victim may wake suddenly in the middle of the night with such excruciating pain that he or she cannot

For Osteoarthritis Pain Relief

Acetaminophen (Tylenol) was shown to be as effective as ibuprofen (Advil) in relieving some chronic pain caused by osteoarthritis. This surprising news was reported in *The New England Journal of Medicine* (July 1991). Acetaminophen had been known to be effective as an analgesic, but aspirin, ibuprofen, and other NSAIDs are usually prescribed first for arthritic conditions. Now it seems that acetaminophen, which has fewer side effects than NSAIDs, might be a better choice.

tolerate the touch of even a sheet. In fact, the uric acid level in the blood may have been increasing for some time. As the disease moves into a more advanced stage, hypertension and kidney stones with severe back pain may occur. When the first arthritic attack occurs, affected joints appear hot, tender, and inflamed. A low-grade fever may be present. A mild attack may subside quickly. In the final stages there is unremitting pain, and deposits of urate called **tophi** cause swollen and deformed joints at many sites, including fingers, hands, knees, and feet. The skin is drawn taut over these **tophaceous** deposits and may ulcerate, releasing a chalky white substance or pus. Gout can lead to chronic disability and crippling in addition to renal dysfunction.

Prevention
Decreasing the amount of protein in the diet could be of some help.

Treatment
Treatment for acute gout consists of bed rest, immobilization of the painful joints, local application of heat or cold, some dietary restrictions, and drugs to adjust the level of uric acid in the blood. **Colchicine,** a drug that was used 1500 years ago in the treatment of gout, is still the most effective drug in reducing pain and inflammation. It is used concomitantly with other analgesics. In severe cases that do not respond to other therapy, corticosteroids may be used.

Disorders of Muscle and Connective Tissue

Fibromyalgia
Fibromyalgia is a very common disease of the muscles, ligaments, and tendons that has only recently been recognized by medical science. According to the Arthritis Foundation, "There are, currently, millions of Americans who have been diagnosed with fibromyalgia."* In the past, it was called fibrositis, but because investigation has failed to show any inflammation in the muscles, the syndrome has been renamed. Fibromyalgia is more common in women than men, and those diagnosed with it are usually between the ages of twenty and fifty.

Predisposing Factors
The exact cause of fibromyalgia is not yet known, but a number of factors have been associated with the disease. Individuals with the syndrome have unfit or poorly developed muscles. It is not known whether the unfit muscles are the cause or the result of fibromyalgia. A second factor linked to the disease is sleep disturbances. In sleep laboratory studies, people with fibromyalgia show an interruption or disturbance of stage IV sleep. This is the deepest and most restful stage of sleep and the time when the body repairs tissue damage. There is also evidence to show that loss of stage IV sleep can lead to muscle pain. The combination of pain and fatigue that results leads to lack of physical exercise, which can contribute to the overall symptoms of the disease. Stress is a third factor linked to fibromyalgia. Although it is not thought that stress causes the syndrome, it is known that it can make the symptoms worse.

Symptoms
There are two major symptoms: pain and fatigue. Pain in fibromyalgia is felt as an aching, stiffness,

tophi	TO-fi
colchicine	KOL-chi-sin
fibromyalgia	FI-bro-mi-AL-jea
tophaceous	to-FA-shus

*Arthritis Foundation. Fibromyalgia Booklet. P.O. Box 1900, Atlanta, Georgia, 30326, 1991.

CASE STUDY

Fibromyalgia

The patient, a fifty-year-old woman, made an appointment with a family doctor because she couldn't work full time at her job. Her main complaints were "hurting all over" and extreme fatigue. The doctor examined her and ordered a blood test for rheumatoid arthritis (RA). When it came back negative, he suggested a new diet and some stress management techniques. The pain, swelling, stiffness, and fatigue remained but with visits to five other physicians over three years, she got essentially the same response as with the first one. Because more symptoms occurred, she made an appointment with a "new" doctor and told him of hurting "all over," a "clammy" feeling in her lower legs, periods of being suddenly too hot or cold, pain in the epigastric area, difficulty sleeping, fatigue, and depression. Her temperature and blood pressure were normal but when the RA test came back negative, she was referred to a rheumatologist. When this specialist checked her muscles for tender points, she found fourteen out of the eighteen used to diagnose another rheumatic disease. The diagnosis was fibromyalgia. The doctor prescribed medication to help the patient sleep at night, dietary restriction of caffeine and alcohol, and regular exercise. Within a few days, the treatment brought the symptoms under control and the woman was able to work full time again.

and tenderness around the joints. The pain may be general over much of the body or it may be localized. Extreme soreness is felt over points where muscles attach to bones (Figure 16-2). These sites are tender points or trigger points; they are the same for all people with fibromyalgia and are an important part of diagnosing the disease. The other major symptom, fatigue can be so severe that the individual must rest at one to two-2 hour intervals each day. People with fibromyalgia also have other symptoms that are confusing to doctors, such as **Raynaud's** phenomenon, tension headaches, migraine, dizziness, tingling and numbness, irritable bowel syndrome, muscle tremors, bladder spasms, and blurred vision.

Prevention
No preventive measures for fibromyalgia are known.

Treatment
The only treatment for fibromyalgia now is to help individuals increase their physical fitness, improve their sleep, and ease the pain and fatigue. Exercise is recommended to improve muscular and general physical fitness. An antidepressant is prescribed at bedtime to promote stage IV sleep. NSAIDs do

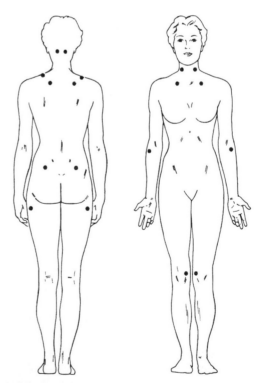

Figure 16-2
Tender points for fibromyalgia.

not seem to help the pain of fibromyalgia, which generally decreases as fitness and sleep improve. A hot bath may give temporary relief.

Carpal Tunnel Syndrome

This syndrome occurs when the median nerve that passes through the carpal tunnel at the wrist is compressed, cutting down the circulation and sensation in the thumb and fingers. It usually occurs in women between the ages of thirty and sixty. In recent years, the incidence has been increasing, possibly as a result of the computer age. Assembly line workers, packers, typists, guitar players, bakers, and computer operators are particularly susceptible.

Predisposing Factors   *Overuse*

There are many conditions that can cause swelling in the carpal tunnel and, subsequently, pressure on the nerve. Included in these are pregnancy, diabetes mellitus, menopause, rheumatoid arthritis, tuberculosis, and hypothyroidism. Dislocation or an acute sprain of the wrist may also cause the syndrome.

Symptoms

Carpal tunnel syndrome produces weakness, burning, tingling, numbness and/or pain in one or both hands. The sensations are usually felt in the thumb, forefinger, middle finger, and part of the fourth finger. Individuals may be unable to clench their fist; the fingernails may be smaller than normal, and the skin dry and shiny. Symptoms are often worse at night and in the morning. Shaking the hands vigorously or dangling them at the sides may relieve the symptoms temporarily.

Prevention

For people who perform repetitive tasks, regular breaks from their work may help. Correct posture, good chair level, and correct height for worktables are also important.

Treatment

The first step is to splint the wrist in a neutral position for one to two weeks. If symptoms persist, a small quantity of corticosteroid may be injected to reduce inflammation. If these measures do not

help, surgery is the only alternative. In some cases, it may be necessary to change occupations.

Tendinitis and Bursitis   *it's = inflammation*

Tendinitis and bursitis are two different disorders, but the predisposing factors, symptoms, prevention, and treatment are often the same. Tendinitis is a painful inflammation of tendons or tendon-muscle attachments. Bursitis is a painful inflammation of one or more of the bursae, the small, fluid-filled sacs that facilitate the movement of muscles and tendons over bony parts of joints. Figures 16-3 and 16-4 show common sites of tendinitis and bursitis.

Predisposing Factors   *overuse*

Strain during sports activity, repetitive movements, rheumatic diseases, congenital defects, postural misalignment, and gout are among the causes of both disorders. Infection of the bursae may also be a cause of bursitis.

Symptoms

Tendinitis often occurs in the shoulder, producing pain on movement and also localized pain, which is most severe at night and interferes with sleep. If

---

Raynaud's ra-NOZ

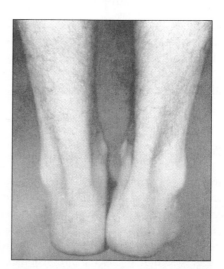

Figure 16-3
Common site of tendinitis.

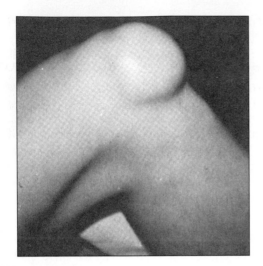

Figure 16-4
Common site of bursitis.

the tendinitis is due to calcium deposits, there may also be weakness. In bursitis, there are sudden or gradual pain and limitation of movement. Symptoms vary depending on the affected site.

Prevention
Maintaining adequate body strength and flexibility and avoiding stress and strain in sports activities are the principal preventive measures.

Treatment
Resting the joint, analgesics, and application of cold, heat, and ultrasound are helpful. In severe cases, an injection of an analgesic and cortico-steroids may be used to reduce inflammation.

Disorders of the Bone
Osteoporosis
Osteoporosis is a metabolic bone disorder resulting in resorption of calcium from the bone. More than one and a half million Americans have fractures related to osteoporosis each year. Because this dis-order affects so many of the elderly, Medicare pays the medical expenses, and the annual cost to the health care system is at least ten billion dollars.

Osteoporosis generally occurs after meno-pause and is linked to low levels of estrogen. It is estimated that half of the women over sixty years of age in North America have osteoporosis, and some elderly men also have it. Osteoporosis may also be secondary to another primary disease.

Osteoporosis is known to occur in women with anorexia nervosa. These women experience **amenorrhea,** low estrogen levels, and loss of bone mass, as do postmenopausal women. Highly trained women athletes also experience amenor-rhea and reduced bone mass. Studies have shown that women athletes who are deficient in estrogen regain their bone mass after treatment, as well as resumption of menses, whereas anorectics who are treated and regain at least eighty percent of their ideal weight do not regain their bone mass.

Predisposing Factors
Factors that have been linked to osteoporosis are race (white), smoking, alcohol consumption, European nationality or descent, sedentary living, and inadequate estrogen in women.

Symptoms
Osteoporosis is often discovered only after an elderly person breaks a bone. Although in the past, broken hips were attributed to falls, it is known now that the bone generally breaks first and causes the fall. (For research on hip replacement surgery, see the Did You Know? section that follows.) The most common symptom is backache pain that radiates around the trunk. This is due to broken vertebrae that snap easily when osteoporosis is present. Another common sign is kyphosis, a humped back condition that occurs because of crushed vertebrae. Breakage of a bone with no unusual stress having been placed upon it is a common occurrence in those with osteoporosis.

Primary Prevention
Individuals who get regular exercise and have a balanced diet with adequate calcium throughout life have less risk of developing osteoporosis.

Secondary Prevention
High calcium intake plus exercise involving active weight-bearing movement have been found to slow the loss of bone in some and increase bone mass in others.

DID YOU KNOW?

Meet Robodoc

Scientists have developed a robot to help surgeons in hip replacement. The robot named Robodoc, reams out the femur for placement of the prosthesis and does so with forty times more accuracy than the surgeon is capable of. The surgeon still must guide the robot, but it is hoped that the more precise dimensions of the hole, allowing ninety-five percent of the implant to contact the bone rather than only twenty percent by the current method, will lead to more comfortable, more stable, and longer lasting replacements. Expected to be approved soon by the FDA in America, it has been undergoing trials since the late 80's. Robodoc has been used in more than 2500 surgeries in Europe, many of these in Germany, with a high success rate.

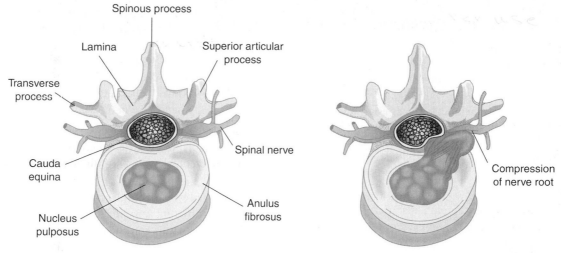

Figure 16-5
Herniated disk.

Treatment

A regular individualized activity program and increased dietary calcium are the best treatment. In severe cases, estrogen, fluoride, and supplemental calcium and vitamin D may be prescribed to decrease the rate of bone resorption.

Herniated Disk

Commonly called slipped disk, a herniated disk is the result when the soft central part of an intervertebral disk is forced through its outer covering (Figure 16-5). When this happens, the disk may press on a nerve, causing lower back pain. The

condition occurs more often in men, and usually in individuals under forty-five years of age.

Predisposing Factors

Although herniated disks usually occur in those under the age of forty-five, in elderly people they may occur because of degeneration of the joints. In younger men and women, the disk may herniate because of strain or trauma. Incorrect lifting and carrying procedures, especially if required

osteoporosis	os-te-o-por-O-sis
amenorrhea	a-men-o-RE-a

repeatedly because of occupation, can produce the condition. Some individuals may be more susceptible because of congenital spinal canal malformation.

Symptoms
Pain in the lower back and radiating down the sciatic nerve on one side to the buttocks, legs, and feet is the common sign of a herniated disk. Depending on the location of the hernia and nerves affected, there may be other symptoms.

Prevention
Good posture and proper lifting and carrying procedures can help prevent many back problems. Back exercises to strengthen those muscles that are subject to strain are very important.

Treatment
Instruction on proper care of the back along with rest, heat applications, and therapeutic exercises are the usual treatment. Analgesics and muscle relaxants may give relief from the pain. If the condition does not improve, surgery may be necessary.

Scoliosis
There are three common disorders having to do with the curve of the spine. Lordosis, commonly called swayback, is an accentuation of the normal curve that is present in the lower back and is generally the result of poor posture. **Kyphosis** is an exaggeration of the normal curve in the upper back and produces the disfigurement commonly called humpback or hunchback and will be discussed next. **Scoliosis** is a lateral curvature of the spine that generally affects the chest or lower back regions. It is often associated with lordosis and kyphosis. Scoliosis may begin in childhood or adolescence and progress until the age when growth stops, or it may begin in later life.

Predisposing Factors
Functional factors that lead to scoliosis are poor posture, a discrepancy in leg lengths, unfit muscles, and/or obesity. If it is structural, it may be congenital, caused by a disease that weakens muscles, such as polio; genes may also be a factor.

Symptoms
The most common curve is in an S shape. As the spine curves laterally, the body develops compensatory curves to maintain balance. Systemic symptoms do not occur until the curve becomes well established. When symptoms do occur, they include backache, fatigue, and dyspnea. If left untreated, there may be pulmonary insufficiency, back pain, degenerative arthritis of the spine, disk disease, and sciatica.

Prevention
Children, and particularly teenagers, are shy about their bodies and may not notice or allow anyone else to see whether there is a deformity. Doctors should check routinely during physicals, and teachers should know what to look for and screen students for signs of scoliosis or other back problems in each grade. Parents need to be educated about the possibility that scoliosis may develop, particularly if anyone else in the family has had it.

Treatment
Treatment depends upon the age of the individual and the severity of the deformity. It may include exercise, a brace, surgery, or a combination of these. If obesity is a factor, then dieting is necessary, and if different leg lengths is a factor, then orthopedic shoes are recommended also.

Kyphosis
Kyphosis is the medical term for excessive backward curvature of the spine. It usually affects the spine at the top of the back, resulting in either a hump or a more gradually rounded back.

Predisposing Factors
Kyphosis may be caused by a number of disorders affecting the spine. In adolescents, the disorder may result from growth retardation or congenital causes. In adults, it may be a result of aging, osteoporosis, endocrine disorders, steroid therapy, arthritis, polio, metastatic tumor, tuberculosis, and many other diseases.

Symptoms
In adolescents, there may be mild pain at the top of the curve, accompanied by fatigue, tenderness, or

stiffness in the involved area or along the entire spine. Symptoms for adults with kyphosis may be pain, weakness of the back, and generalized fatigue.

Prevention

Maintaining a correct posture, ideal weight, and good nutrition should help to reduce the risk factors.

Treatment

Treatment is rarely successful but is aimed at the underlying disorder.

scoliosis	sko-le-O-sis
kyphosis	ki-FO-sis

SUMMARY

Table 16-1 reviews the disorders of the skin and musculoskeletal system discussed in this chapter.

TABLE 16-1 Disorders of the Skin and Musculoskeletal System

Disease	Special Characteristics	Predisposing Factors	Common Symptoms	Prevention	Treatment
Acne	Experienced by most teenage boys and some teenage girls; inflammation of hair follicles and sebaceous glands	Obstruction of hair follicle by sebum leading to infection; linked to release of hormones; may be hereditary factor; may also be caused by drugs, oily skin, and cosmetics	Blackheads, whiteheads, pustules, nodules, and cysts on face and other parts of body with high concentration of sebaceous glands	None known; no dietary connection; washing affected area twice daily may keep it from spreading	Topical and systemic drugs; sometimes antibiotics; retinoid drugs to reduce oil secretions (cannot be used during pregnancy); no cure but generally clears up at end of teenage years
Seborrheic Dermatitis	Eyebrows are common site	Unknown; stress and neurologic conditions may have effect	Itching, redness and inflammation usually on scalp, face, trunk, and in skin folds; may appear greasy, yellowish and	None known	Frequent washing and shampooing with medicated soap; topical corticosteroids and/or antibiotics

Continued

TABLE 16-1	*Continued*				
Disease	**Special Characteristics**	**Predisposing Factors**	**Common Symptoms**	**Prevention**	**Treatment**
Seborrheic Dermatitis— Cont'd			scaly; may be cause of dandruff		
Contact Dermatitis	Caused by something that touches the skin	May be an allergic reaction or from a toxic substance	A rash that varies depending on cause; skin is itchy and may flake or blister; rash covers area that came in contact with substance	Identification of causative substance and avoidance in future	Topical application of corticosteroids
Psoriasis	Close to 2% affected in U.S. and Europe; not as common among blacks and Asians; may cause embarrassment; new skin cells produced at 10 times normal rate while shedding rate of old cells does not change	May be triggered by emotional stress, skin damage, physical illness; initial cause unknown	Thickened patches of inflamed skin often covered by silvery scaling; itching, pain; skin fold lesions smooth, deep red; bleeding if scales removed	None known	Sunlight or ultraviolet lamps, emollient, coal tar ointment, corticosteroids and other drugs depending on severity of attack
Osteoarthritis	Present to some extent in everyone over 60; deterioration of joint cartilage and bone; excess bone builds up, joint	Continual joint trauma and normal aging processes	Joint pain after exercise or weight bearing that is usually relieved by rest; stiffness in morning, aching during weather	Avoidance of athletic and occupational activities that place constant stress on joints and sensible exercise rou-	Medication for pain, surgery to replace joints, water exercise

TABLE 16-1	*Continued*				
Disease	**Special Characteristics**	**Predisposing Factors**	**Common Symptoms**	**Prevention**	**Treatment**
Osteoarthritis—Cont'd	movement difficult		changes, limited movement and fluid in joints; becomes worse with poor posture, obesity, and occupational stress	tines may help	
Gout	Occurs most in men over 40; secondary gout may occur in elderly; too much uric acid in blood	Inherited metabolic disorder	Most frequently strikes with severe pain in joints of big toe; sudden onset; hypertension, kidney stones, and back pain develop; affected joints are hot, tender and inflamed; may have a low-grade fever; tophi in final stages with unremitting pain; taut skin over tophi may ulcerate; chronic disability and renal dysfunction	None known; no connection with diet has been verified	Bed rest; immobilization of painful joints; local application of heat or cold; dietary restrictions; drugs (colchicine most effective); analgesics; corticosteroids
Fibromyalgia	Disease of muscles, ligaments, and	Unfit muscles, unrestorative sleep, stress	Pain and fatigue; tender points	Unknown	Exercise, antidepressant (to induce

TABLE 16-1	Continued				
Disease	**Special Characteristics**	**Predisposing Factors**	**Common Symptoms**	**Prevention**	**Treatment**
Fibromyalgia— Cont'd	tendons; much more in women than men, most ages 20–50	associated with disease; not known whether they are cause or result	where muscles attach to bones; other unexplained symptoms including Raynaud's phenomenon, tension headaches, migraine, dizziness, tingling and numbness, irritable bowel syndrome, muscle tremors, bladder spasms, and blurred vision		stage IV sleep), hot bath for temporary relief of pain
Carpal Tunnel Syndrome	Occurs when median nerve is compressed in carpal tunnel at wrist; usually in women age 30 to 60; occupational hazard	Anything that causes swelling in the carpal tunnel	Weakness, burning, tingling, numbness and/or pain in thumb and fingers; inability to clench fist; dry, shiny skin, fingernails smaller than usual	Splinting wrist for 1-2 weeks; corticosteroids, surgery only other choice	Wrist splint; corticosteroid injection; surgery; change of occupation
Tendinitis and Bursitis	Tendinitis is inflammation of tendons or tendon-muscle attachments; bursitis is	Strain during sports activity, repetitive movements, rheumatic diseases, congenital	Tendinitis often in shoulder, producing pain that may interrupt sleep; bursitis may be	Maintaining good body strength, posture, and flexibility, and avoiding physical	Resting joint; application of cold and heat; ultrasound; analgesic injection;

TABLE 16-1	*Continued*				
Disease	**Special Characteristics**	**Predisposing Factors**	**Common Symptoms**	**Prevention**	**Treatment**
Tendinitis and Bursitis—Cont'd	inflammation of bursae, fluid-filled sacs that help facilitate movement in joints	defects, postural misalign-ment, and gout all pos-sible causes; bursae may become infected	sudden with limitation of movement	stress, strain, and repetitive movements	cortico-steroids
Osteoporosis	Metabolic bone disorder resulting in resorption of calcium from bone; estimated over 50% of women over 60 have it in North America	White race, smoking, drinking, European descent, sedentary liv-ing have been linked to it	Easily broken bones, back-ache pain due to snapped vertibrae, kyphosis	Regular exercise, bal-anced diet, throughout life; secondary prevention: high calcium intake plus weight-bear-ing exercise	Individualized activity program; increased dietary cal-cium; estro-gen; fluoride; supplemental calcium; vitamin D
Herniated Disk	"Slipped disk" commonly; soft central part of inver-tebral disk is forced through outer covering; usually in people under 45 and more often in men	Strain, trauma, or, in elderly, degenerative joints	Pain in lower back, radiat-ing down sci-atic nerve to buttocks, legs, and feet on one side; other symp-toms depend-ing on loca-tion of hernia	Good posture, lifting, and carrying pro-cedures; exercises for muscles sub-ject to strain	Rest; heat; therapeutic exercises; analgesics; muscle relax-ants; surgery
Scoliosis	Lateral curva-ture of spine in chest and lower back regions; may begin in childhood, adolescence, or later life	Poor posture, different leg lengths, unfit muscles, obesity, mus-cle-weaken-ing disease; may also be genetic or congenital	Most common is an "S" shaped curve of spine; well established may lead to backache, fatigue, and dyspnea; if untreated,	Attention to underlying causes when possible, i.e., muscle fitness, posture	Exercise; a brace; surgery

TABLE 16-1	*Continued*				
Disease	**Special Characteristics**	**Predisposing Factors**	**Common Symptoms**	**Prevention**	**Treatment**
Scoliosis— Cont'd			pulmonary insufficiency, back pain, degenerative arthritis of the spine, disk disease, and sciatica		
Kyphosis	Excessive backward curvature of the spine; usually at top of back resulting in a hump or rounded back	Growth retardation, congenital defect, aging, osteoporosis, and many other diseases and disorders	Pain, fatigue, tenderness, stiffness along spine in children; pain, weakness of the back, generalized fatigue	Maintaining good posture, ideal weight, good nutrition, will help depending on cause	Aimed at underlying disorder

QUESTIONS FOR REVIEW

1. Describe the three layers of the skin.
2. What are the predisposing factors linked to acne?
3. What effect does diet have on acne?
4. What is the best treatment for acne?
5. What are the symptoms of seborrheic dermatitis?
6. What substances may cause contact dermatitis?
7. What process produces the symptoms of psoriasis?
8. What therapies are there for psoriasis?
9. How does osteoarthritis differ from rheumatoid arthritis?
10. What is the suspected cause of gout?
11. The symptoms of gout are a result of what process?
12. What predisposing factors have been linked to fibromyalgia?
13. How is fibromyalgia diagnosed?
14. What may be the cause of the recent increase of carpal tunnel syndrome?
15. What causes the symptoms of carpal tunnel syndrome?
16. Compare tendinitis and bursitis.
17. What is the cause of osteoporosis?
18. What is the best treatment for osteoporosis?
19. How can back problems be prevented?
20. How do lordosis, kyphosis, and scoliosis differ?

FURTHER READING

Aagaard, Eva M. Prevention of glucocorticoid induced osteoporosis: provider practice at an urban county hospital. *American Journal of Medicine* 107:456.

Aaron, Leslie A, and Mary M. Burke. 1999. Overlapping conditions among patients with chronic fatigue syndrome, fibromyalgia. *Archives of Internal Medicine* 160:221.

Adeyemi, E. O. 1999. Characterization of autonomic dysfunction in patients with irritable bowel syndrome by means of heart rate variablility studies. *American Journal of Gastroenterology* 94:816.

Affleck, G. 1999. Everyday life with osteoarthritis or rheumatoid arthritis: independent effects of disease and gender on daily pain, mood, and coping. *Pain* 83:601.

Alfonso, L. A. 1999. Contact dermatitis for primary care providers. *Nurse Practice Forum* 10:67.

Apgar, Barbara. 1999. Celecoxib for patients with arthritis and osteoarthritis. *American Family Physician* 60:296.

Apgar, Barbara. 1999. Comparing therapies for chronic plaque-like psoriasis. *American Family Physician* 60:1524.

Armamentarium against osteoporosis. *American Journal of Nursing* 99:14, 1999.

Arnold, Beth D. 1999. Hip fracture. *American Journal of Nursing* 99:36.

Atroshi, Isam, et al. 1999. Prevalence of carpal tunnel syndrome in a general population. *Journal of the American Medical Association* 282:153.

Azouriz, F. 1999. Dimensions of gut dysfunction in irritable bowel syndrome: altered sensory function. *Canadian Journal of Gastroenterology* 13:12A.

Beals, Katherine A., et al. 1999. Understanding the female athlete triad: eating disorders, amenorrhea, and osteoporosis. *Journal of School Health* 69:337.

Belsito, D. V. 1999. A sherlockian approach to contact dermatitis. *Dermatology Clinical* 17:705.

Berson, Diane, S., et al. 1999. Saving face: a treatment update for acne. *Patient Care* 33:257.

Blank, R. D. 1999. A genomic approach to scoliosis pathogenesis. *Lupus* 8:356.

Bohannon, A. D. 1999. Osteoporosis and African American women. *Journal of Women's Health and Gender Based Medicine* 8:609.

Bour, H., et al. 1999. T-cell repertoire analysis in chronic plaque psoriasis suggests an antigen specific immune response. *Human Immunology* 162:7480.

Boyd, A.S. 1999. Tamoxifen-induced remission of psoriasis. *Journal of the American Academy of Dermatology* 41:887.

Bradley, J. D. 1999. Comparison of an antiinflammatory dose of ibuprofen and analgesic dose of ibuprofen and acetaminophen in the treatment of patients with osteoarthritis of the knee. *New England Journal of Medicine* 325:87.

Briggs, A. 1999. Impact of osteoarthritis and analgesic treatment on quality of life of an elderly population. *Annal Pharmacotherapy* 33:1154.

Browning, S.A., et al. 1999. Constipation, diarrhea, and irritable bowel syndrome. *Primary Care* 26:113.

Caballero-Plasencia, A.M. 1999. Altered gastric emptying in patients with irritable bowel syndrome. *European Journal of Nuclear Medicine* 26:404.

Cerrato, Paul L. 2000. This osteoporosis drug prevents cancer. *RN* 63:86.

Chung, M.S. 1999. Prevalence of Raynaud's phenomenon in patients with idiopathic carpal tunnel syndrome. *Journal of Bone, Joint Surgery* 81:1017.

Claar, R.L. 1999. Functional disability in adolescents and young adults with symptoms of irritable bowel syndrome: the role of academic, social, and athletic competence. *Journal of Pediatric Psychology* 24:271.

Coward, Brandy L. 1999. Fibromyalgia. *American Journal of Nursing* 99:42.

Davis, J.C. 1999. A practical approach to gout. Current management of an "old" disease. *Postgraduate Medicine* 106:115.

Doube, Alan. 1999. Managing osteoporosis in older people with fractures. *British Medical Journal* 318:477.

Federman, Daniel G., Catherine W. Froelich, and Robert S. Kirsner. 1999. Topical psoriasis therapy. *American Family Physician* 59:957.

Fischer, T., et al. 1999. Clinical improvement of HIV associated psoriasis parallels a reduction of HIV viral load induced by effective antiretroviral therapy. *AIDS* 13:628.

Forseth, K.O. 1999. Prognostic factors for the development of fibromyalgia in women with self-reported musculoskeletal pain. A prospective study. *Journal of Rheumatology* 26:2458.

Franzblau, Alfred, and Robert A. Werner. 1999. What is carpal tunnel syndrome? *Journal of the American Medical Association* 282:186.

Gaby, A.R. 1999. Natural treatments for osteoarthritis. *Alternative Medicine Review* 4:330.

Goldenberg, Don L. 1999. Fibromyalgia syndrome a decade later. *Archives of Internal Medicine* 159:777.

Goulden, V. 1999. Prevalence of facial acne in adults. *Journal of American Academy of Dermatology* 37:273.

Gout and what to do about it. *American Family Physician* 59:1810, 1999.

Hackett, J.P. Allergic contact dermatitis in American aircraft manufacture. *American Journal of Contact Dermatitis* 10:169.

Harris, Mark D., Lori B. Siegel, and Jeffrey A. Alloway. 1999. Gout and hyperuricemia. *American Family Physician* 59:925.

Helwig, Amy L. 2000. Treating carpal tunnel syndrome. *Journal of Family Practice* 49:79.

Hormone therapy somewhat effective in elderly women with osteoarthritis. *Modern Medicine* 67:45, 1999.

Huffman, Grace Brooke. 2000. Reduction of fracture risk in women with osteoporosis. *American Family Physician* 61:859.

Huffman, Grace Brooke. 1998. Physical function, mobility and development of kyphosis. *American Family Physician* 57:1961.

Hurwitz, D. E. 1999. Effect of knee pain on joint loading in patients with osteoarthritis. *Current Opinion Rheumatology* 11:417.

Hwang, Mi Young, et al. 1999. Detecting carpal tunnel syndrome. *Journal of the American Medical Association* 282:206.

Increased osteoporosis risk in elderly hypertensive women. *American Family Physician* 61:1122, 2000.

Iqbal, Mohammad Masud. 2000. Osteoporosis: epidemiology, diagnosis, and treatment. *Southern Medical Journal* 93:2.

Isaksson, M. 1999. Occupational allergic contact dermatitis from olive oil in a massseur. *Journal of American Academy of Dermatology* 41:94.

Karachalios, T. 1999. Ten year follow up evaluation of a school screening program for scoliosis. *Spine* 24:2318.

Karakayli, Guliz, Grant Beckham, I. D. A. Orengo, et al. 1999. Exfoliative dermatitis. *American Family Physician* 59:625.

Karasek, M. A. 1999. Progress in our understanding of the biology of psoriasis. *Cutis* 64:319.

Kleinhenz, J. 1999. Randomized clinical trial comparing the effects of acupuncture and a newly designed placebo needle in rotator cuff tendinitis. *Pain* 83:235.

Koenig, Clint. 1999. Acupuncture in the treatment of fibromyalgia. *Journal of Family Practice* 48:497.

Koo, J. 1999. Systemic sequential therapy of psoriasis: a new paradigm for improved therapeutic results. *Journal of the American Academy of Dermatology* 41:S7.

Knee osteoarthritis stabilizes in some women on estrogen. *Geriatrics* 54:67, 1999.

Kripke, Clarissa C. 1999. Diuretics, NSAIDs and steroids for carpal tunnel syndrome. *American Family Physician* 59:166.

Kumar, A. 1999. Protein contact dermatitis in food workers. Case report of a meat sorter and summary of seven other cases. *Australas Journal of Dermatology* 40:138.

Lamberg, Lynn 1999. Patients in pain need round the clock care. *Journal of the American Medical Association* 281:689.

Lane, N. E. 1999. Exercise and osteoarthritis. *Current Opinion Rheumatology* 11:413.

Lazarov, A. 1999. Perianal contact dermatitis caused by nail lacquer allergy. *American Journal of Dermatology* 10:43.

Lee D. 1999. Diagnosis of carpal tunnel syndrome. Ultrasound versus electromyography. *Radiology Clinic of North America* 37:859.

Manente, G. 1999. A relief maneuver in carpal tunnel syndrome. *Muscle Nerve* 22:1587.

Martin, B. G. 1999. Contact dermatitis: evaluation and treatment. *Journal of American Osteopathy* 99:S11.

McCarthy, R.E. 1999. Management of neuromuscular scoliosis. *Ortho Clinic of North America* 30:435.

Meunier, P. J. 1999. Evidence based medicine and osteoporosis: a comparison of fracture risk reduction from osteoporosis randomized clinical trials. *International Journal of Clinical Practice* 53:122.

Miller, Karl E. 1999. Exercise can improve outcomes in osteoarthritis. *American Family Physician* 60:2659.

Miller, N. H. 1999. Cause and natural history of adolescent idiopathic scoliosis. *Orthop Clinic of North America* 30:342.

Mortz, C. G. 1999. Allergic contact dermatitis in children and adolescents. *Contact Dermatitis* 41:121.

Munger, Ronald G. 1999. Prospective study of dietary protein intake and risk of hip fracture in postmenopausal women. *American Journal of Clinical Nutrition* 69:147.

Nevitt, Michael, and Nancy Lane. 1999. Body weight and osteoarthritis. *American Journal of Medicine* 107:632.

Oestreich, A. E. 1999. Scoliosis circa 2000: radiologic imaging perspective. *Skeletal Radiology* 27:651.

Orfanos, C. E. 1999. Treatment of psoriasis with retinoids: present status. *Cutis* 64:335.

Osteoporosis among estrogen deficient women—United States, 1988-1994. *Journal of the American Medical Association* 281:224, 1999.

Osteoporosis guide provides specifics for prevention and treatment. *Modern Medicine* 67:36, 1999.

Papagrigoriadis, S. 1999. Smoking may be associated with complications in diverticular disease. *British Journal of Surgery* 86:923.

Pittman, Joel R., and Michael H. Bross. 1999. Diagnosis and management of gout. *American Family Physician* 59:1799.

Psoriasis affects quality of life in a manner similar to cancer or heart disease. *Geriatrics* 55:91, 2000.

Quintner, John L. 1999. Fibromyalgia falls foul of a fallacy. *The Lancet* 353:1092.

Rapp, S. R. 1999. Psoriasis causes as much disability as other major medical diseases. *Journal of the American Academy of Dermatology* 41:408.

Rayan, G. M. 1999. Carpal tunnel syndrome between two centuries. *Journal of Oklahoma State Medical Association* 92:493.

Rehman, Q. 1999. Getting control of osteoarthritis pain. An update on treatment options. *Postgraduate Medicine* 106:127.

Rganarsson, G. 1999. Abdominal symptoms are not related to anorectal function in the irritable bowel syndrome. *Scandinavian Journal of Gastroenterology* 34:250.

Richards, H.L. 1999. Patients with psoriasis and their compliance with medication. *Journal of the American Academy of Dermatology* 41:581.

Rothe, Marti Jill, and Jane M. Grant-Kels. 1999. Acne: update on therapeutic choices. *Consultant* 39:1061.

Rupp, John., et al. Psoriasis. *Consultant* 40:75.

Russell, John J. 1999. Topical therapy for acne. *American Family Physician* 61:357.

Saito, Naoto, et al. 1999. Natural history of scoliosis in spastic cerebral palsy. *The Lancet* 351:1687.

Sandor, T., et al. 1999. Comments on the hypotheses underlying fracture risk assessment in osteoporosis as proposed by the WHO. *Calcified Tissue International* 64:267.

Santori, N., and R. N. Villar. 1999. Arthroscopic findings in the initial stages of hip osteoarthritis. *Orthopedics* 22:405.

Saxon, L, et al. 1999. Sports participation, sports injuries and osteoarthritis: implications for prevention. *Sports Medicine* 28:123.

Schnirring, Lisa. 1999. Osteoporosis management: what's on the cutting edge. *Physician and Sports Medicine* 28:15.

Schnitzer, Thomas, and Verna Rose. 1999. Use of rofecoxib improves quality of life in osteoarthritis patients. *American Family Physician* 60:252.

Senior, Kathryn. 1999. Osteoarthritis research: on the verge of a revolution? *The Lancet* 355:208.

Sequeira, Winston. 1999. Yoga in treatment of carpal tunnel syndrome. *The Lancet* 353:689.

Sheppard, Robert. 1999. Mysterious malady: Doctors disagree on the causes of fibromyalgia. *Maclean's* 50.

Snaith, Michael. 1999. Gout through the ages. *The Lancet* 353:505.

So, J. B. 1999. Right-sided colonic diverticular disease as a source of lower gastrointestinal bleeding. *American Surgery* 65:299.

Sperber, A. D. 1999. Fibromyalgia in the irritable bowel syndrome, and Addison disease. *Archives of Internal Medicine* 159:2482.

Sperber, A.D. 1999. The sense of coherence index and the irritable bowel syndrome. A cross-sectional comparison among irritable bowel syndrome patients with and without coexisting fibromyalgia, irritable bowel syndrome non-patients, and controls. Scandinavian *Journal of Gastroenterology* 34:250.

Sternbach, G. 1999. The carpal tunnel syndrome from thrombosed persistent median artery. *Journal of Emergency Medicine* 17:437.

Stevens, J.C. 1999. Symptoms of 100 patients with electromyographically verified carpal tunnel syndrome. *Muscle Nerve* 22:1448.

Stitik, Todd P., and Patrick M. Foye. 1999. Osteoarthritis of the knee and hip: Part 2 keys to successful non-drug therapy. *Consultant* 24:38.

Stollerman, Gene H. 1999. Fibromyalgia after acute viral infection. *Hospital Practice* 43:24.

Stollman, N. H. 1999. Diverticular disease of the colon. *Journal of Clinical Gasteroentology* 29:241.

Therapeutic touch and osteoarthritis of the knee. *Journal of Family Practice* 48:11, 1999.

Thomas, Romano. 1999. Carpal tunnel syndrome in the workplace. *Archives of Internal Medicine* 59:1008.

Treating osteoporosis in men. *Amercian Journal of Nursing* 99:14, 2000.

Treatment of gout. *American Family Physician* 59:1624, 1999.

Trozak, D.J. 1999. Topical corticosteroid therapy in psoriasis vulgaris: update and new strategies. *Cutis* 64:315.

Vitamin D levels linked to incidence of hip osteoarthritis. *Geriatrics* 54:67, 1999.

Weinstein, James, N. 1999. A 45-year-old man with low back pain and a numb left foot. *Journal of the American Medical Association* 280:730.

Wever, D. J. 1999. A biomechanical analysis of the vertebral and rib deformities in structural scoliosis. *European Spine Journal* 8:252.

White, S. F. 1999. Patients' perceptions of overall function, pain, and appearance after primary posterior instrumentation and fusion for idiopathic scoliosis. *Spine* 24:1693.

Wilson, Emily J. 1999. Fibromyalgia at an educational facility. *Journal of Environmental Health* 61:20.

Wolf, William B. 1999. Calcific tendinitis of the shoulder. *Physician and Sports Medicine* 27:12.

Yawn, Barbara P., et al. 1999. A population based study of school scoliosis screening. *Journal of the American Medical Association* 282:1427.

Zhao, S. Z. 1999. Evaluation of the functional status of health-related quality of life of patients with osteoarthritis treated with celecoxib. *Pharmacotherapy* 19:1269.

SENSORY, NERVOUS, AND ENDOCRINE DISORDERS

O B J E C T I V E S

1. *Explain errors in refraction that make it necessary to wear glasses or contact lenses.*

2. *Describe the process that leads to a cataract.*

3. *Identify symptoms that may indicate the development of a cataract.*

4. *Explain why early detection of glaucoma is important.*

5. *Identify causes for hearing loss.*

6. *Compare the three types of cerebral palsy.*

7. *Describe the progression of symptoms for Parkinson's disease.*

8. *Explain the disease process in multiple sclerosis.*

9. *Identify the three stages of Alzheimer's disease.*

10. *Distinguish between Type I and Type II diabetes.*

11. *State characteristics, risk factors, symptoms, and prevention for the diseases in this chapter.*

EYE DISORDERS

Structure of the Eye

The eye is composed of four different layers; they are the sclera and cornea, the **uvea** (choroid, ciliary body, and iris) and the retina.

The sclera is a dense, white, and fibrous protective coat covered by a thin layer of fine elastic tissue. Continuous with the sclera is the cornea, which is the transparent, avascular, curved layer of the eye. Aqueous humor bathes the surface of the cornea, maintaining intraocular pressure. The sole function of the cornea is to refract light rays.

uvea	U-ve-a

The middle layer, or uvea, consisting of the iris, ciliary body, and choroid, is pigmented and vascular. The iris is suspended between the lens and cornea and perforated in the middle by the pupil. The ciliary body produces aqueous humor and controls the lens. The largest part of the uveal coat is the choroid, which is made up of blood vessels united by connective tissue containing pigmented cells.

The most essential structure of the eye is the retina, which receives the image formed by the lens. Light entering the eye passes through the cornea, then through the pupil, lens, and the jelly-like vitreous body behind the lens, to the retina. Through changes in the curvature of the lens brought about by its elasticity and contraction of the ciliary muscles, light rays are focused on the retina, where they stimulate the rods and cones, the sensory receptors. Sensory impulses are relayed via the optic nerve to the brain, where they register as visual sensations. (For an insight into treatment for corneal abrasion, see the Did You Know?)

Refractive Errors

When people have to wear glasses, it is generally for one or more refractive errors. The main types of refractive error are myopia (nearsightedness), hyperopia (farsightedness), presbyopia (difficulty in focusing), and astigmatism (unequal curvature of cornea and/or lens). Figure 17-1 shows how myopia and hyperopia are corrected with lenses. Refractive errors occur because of a genetic predisposition, and about one-third of the population wear glasses or contact lenses for them. Two other common disorders of the eye are cataract and glaucoma, which will be discussed next.

Cataract

There are a number of different types of cataract, but the most common are those that occur with aging. The lens gradually becomes opaque and the pupil turns white. Cataracts generally develop in both eyes at the same time but at different rates.

DID YOU KNOW?

To Patch or Not to Patch

If you have an eye injury, a patch can cause more pain while the eye is healing than if it were left uncovered. A study reported in *The Lancet* used thirty patients with corneal scratches. Half were asked to wear eye patches while the eye was healing, but the control half were not. In both groups the scratch healed in just two days. However, a day after the injury, three-quarters of the patients with a patch were experiencing pain, whereas only one-quarter of those in the control group had pain. The best treatment for a scratched cornea may be antibiotic drops alone.

From *The Lancet* 337:643, 1991. In *The Edell Health Letter* 10:4, 1991.

Predisposing Factors

Most cataracts develop in persons over seventy years of age and are considered to be a result of aging. Cataracts may be present in infants because of a genetic defect or because the mother contracted rubella during the first trimester of her pregnancy. Injury to the lens by a foreign body or toxic effects of drugs may also cause cataracts. Finally, cataracts may occur secondary to other disorders, such as glaucoma.

Symptoms

Blurring and loss of vision are generally the first signs of cataract. The patient may see halos around lights, and night driving may become more difficult because of the blinding glare of headlights. Sunlight may also cause an unpleasant glare and poor vision. Individuals with cataracts often see better in dim light.

Prevention

No means of prevention is known for senile cataracts. Prepubertal vaccination for rubella is recommended to reduce the incidence of congenital cataracts. Proper safety measures during involvement in activities that have a possibility of eye damage, as well as use of drugs only under

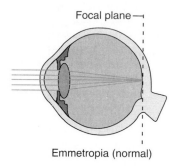

Emmetropia (normal)

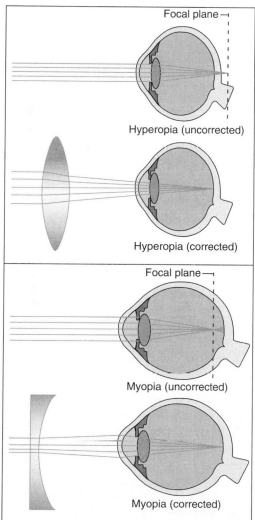

Figure 17-1

Visual disorders and their correction by various lenses.

medical supervision, might prevent other types of cataracts.

Treatment

Surgery to remove cataracts has improved steadily and can be performed on an outpatient basis. New and better techniques have led to a nincty-five percent effectiveness rate.

Glaucoma

Glaucoma is due to an increase in intraocular pressure leading to atrophy of the optic nerve and blindness (Figure 17-2). The disease occurs in women more than in men and accounts for fifteen percent of the blindness in the United States.

Predisposing Factors

Ninety percent of glaucoma cases result from an inherited predisposition to the disease, or it can occur as a result of other eye disease.

Symptoms

Generally there are no symptoms until the disease is advanced. Late symptoms include mild aching in the eyes, halos around lights, loss of peripheral vision, and reduced visual acuity that cannot be corrected with glasses.

Prevention

Everyone should have regular eye examinations. Individuals with a history of glaucoma should have yearly eye examinations, particularly after the age of forty. Screening for glaucoma is a routine practice in eye exams. Early detection can lead to good results with treatment.

Treatment

Treatment involves using drugs and eye drops to reduce the pressure in the eyes. If the disease has been detected early enough, it can be arrested.

EAR DISORDERS

Structure of the Ear

Hearing begins when sound waves in the air go through the auditory canal and reach the tympanic

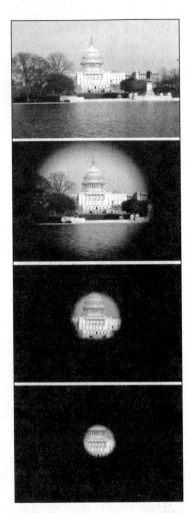

Figure 17-2
Progress in acute glaucoma.

membrane. The tympanic membrane vibrates the small bones in the middle ear (malleus, incus, and stapes), and the stapes sends these vibrations to the fluid in the inner ear by vibrating against the oval window. The fluid in the inner ear then conducts the sound across the hair cells of the organ of Corti (in the cochlea), which initiates auditory nerve impulses to the brain. An individual's balance is maintained by the fluid in the semicircular canals. Nerve cells line the canals and send messages to the brain by the acoustic nerve.

Hearing Loss

All hearing loss or deafness is either conductive or sensorineural. If the passage of sound from the external ear to the place where the stapes meets the oval window is blocked, then it is referred to as conductive loss of hearing. When the hearing loss occurs because there is no transmission of sound impulses from the inner ear to the brain, then it is called sensorineural loss of hearing. Both conditions may exist in the same person, and the hearing loss is then referred to as mixed. Total deafness is rare and is usually congenital. One in 1000 babies has sensorineural deafness at birth that is incurable. When deafness develops in young children, it is usually conductive and curable. Almost twenty-five percent of children starting school have some hearing loss from otitis media (middle ear infection). About twenty-five percent of people over sixty-five years of age need a hearing aid.

Predisposing Factors

The causes of hearing loss are many and different for conductive and sensorineural deafness. Common causes for conductive hearing loss are:

- Chronic middle ear infection (sticky fluid collects in the middle ear)
- **Cerumen** (earwax) blocking the outer ear canal
- Loss of mobility in stapes
- Damage to eardrum from sudden changes in air pressure, as in an airplane or underwater
- Perforated eardrum

Common causes for sensorineural hearing loss are:

- Birth injury or damage to developing fetus (measles, drugs, or other factors affecting the mother during pregnancy that can affect the fetus)
- Prolonged exposure to loud noise
- Ménière's disease
- Use of certain drugs, such as streptomycin
- Viral infections
- Degeneration of cochlea or labyrinth with old age
- Tumors on acoustic nerve

Symptoms

In young children, hearing loss may not become evident for a few days, when they do not turn their head at the sound of a voice. Although the hearing-compromised baby may cry as a hearing-normal child might, he or she will not make the babbling sounds that most children make preceding speech. Sometimes a child's seeming inattention to directions may be due to partial hearing loss. If the hearing loss is partial, there is generally difficulty in hearing very high or very low tones at first, which may not be noticed. This is the reason that early screening tests for hearing can be so beneficial. In older people whose hearing loss occurs because of a loss of hair cells in the organ of Corti, there may be **tinnitus,** or ringing in the ears; sounds become quieter, and some letter sounds (*s, f, z*) cannot be heard. Speech becomes harder to understand when there is background noise. When individuals are not aware that their hearing is impaired, they sometimes become paranoid, act confused, and have auditory hallucinations that can lead to withdrawal and depression if the problem is not diagnosed.

Prevention

Early treatment for diseases that may affect hearing, and avoidance of constant loud noise, will reduce the risk of hearing loss. Individuals who work in a noisy environment should wear protective mechanisms to guard their hearing. Children should not be exposed to music that is above a safe level. Prolonged exposure to loud noise (85 to 90 decibels) or brief exposure to noise greater than ninety decibels can cause hearing loss. Pregnant women should be educated about the dangers to the fetus if they are exposed to drugs, chemicals, or infection. The best secondary prevention is periodic hearing tests after the child enters school. If there is any suspicion of a hearing loss, in a child or adult, a doctor should be consulted immediately.

Treatment

In cases of hearing loss, the underlying cause must be identified first. Children who are born deaf must be taught sign language and speech. If a child becomes deaf from otitis media, then an operation is performed in which the eardrum is pierced in order to drain the fluid from the middle ear. If conductive hearing loss is caused by cerumen in the ear, a syringe is used to flush it out with warm water. A perforated eardrum will generally heal by itself. If it does not do so in two to three weeks, surgery may be necessary. The stapes can be replaced if conductive deafness occurs because of its lack of mobility. Hearing aids and training the individual to read lips are also part of treatment.

Ménière's Disease

Ménière's disease is a disorder of the inner ear. It occurs most often in adults between the ages of thirty and sixty and slightly more often in men. The symptoms are caused by an increase in the amount of fluid in the canals in the inner ear that control balance.

Predisposing Factors

The exact cause is not known. A number of theories have been set forth implicating one or more of the following: anatomic abnormality, heredity, immunologic, viral, vascular, metabolic, and/or psychologic factors.

Symptoms

Tinnitis and dizziness that may be severe enough to cause the individual to fall to the ground are symptoms of the disorder. Victims may also experience nausea, vomiting, sweating, jerky eye movements, and a feeling of pressure or pain in the affected ear. If the condition continues, sensorineural hearing loss occurs and finally deafness.

Prevention

No preventive measures are known.

Treatment

Atropine can stop an attack in twenty to thirty minutes. In a severe attack, other drugs may be

cerumen	se-ROO-men
tinnitus	tin-I-tus
Ménière's (disease)	MAN-e-arz

used. The victim is prescribed diuretics or a vasodilator, and salt intake is restricted. Antihistamines and mild sedatives may also help.

NERVOUS SYSTEM DISORDERS

Structure of the Nervous System

There are three main divisions to the nervous system, the central nervous system (CNS), which is composed of the brain and spinal cord, the peripheral nervous system, composed of the nerves that relay messages to and from all parts of the body to the CNS (Figure 17-3), and the autonomic nervous system, which regulates involuntary functioning of the internal organs (Figure 17-4).

The fundamental unit of the nervous system is the neuron, which consists of the cell body, axon, and dendrites (Figure 17-5). The axon carries messages away from the cell body, and the dendrites carry messages to the cell body. Thus, in the transmission of nerve impulses, the dendrites of one neuron receive a message from the axon of another neuron and transmit it through the cell body to another axon, which relays the message to other dendrites, and so on.

The minute space between the axon of one neuron and the dendrite of another neuron is called a synaptic gap. Special chemical substances called neurotransmitters diffuse across the gap and carry the message to the dendrites of the next neuron (Figure 17-6). A fatty substance called a myelin sheath envelops the axon and enables the impulse to pass at greater speed. Neurologic disorders occur when there is interference with the transmission of messages and can be crippling or life threatening, depending on what part of the system is involved.

Cerebral Palsy

In 1986 approximately one in every 200 children had cerebral palsy. The disorder can be very mild or severe enough to cause total disability. Cerebral palsy results from damage to the CNS that may occur before birth, at birth, or during infancy and childhood. The incidence is higher in whites and slightly higher in males. There are three forms of

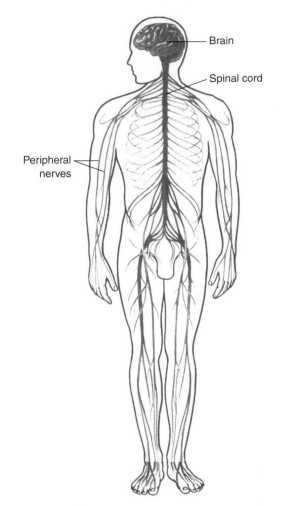

Figure 17-3
The central nervous system.

cerebral palsy: *spastic,* **athetoid,** and **ataxic.** Sometimes an individual has a mixture of the three. Many times other defects are present, such as mental retardation, disordered speech, and seizures.

Predisposing Factors
Any condition that results in damage to the brain may be a factor in cerebral palsy. During pregnancy, conditions in the mother such as German measles, diabetes, and malnutrition may be responsible. These

athetoid	ATH-e-toyd
ataxic	a-TAC-sic

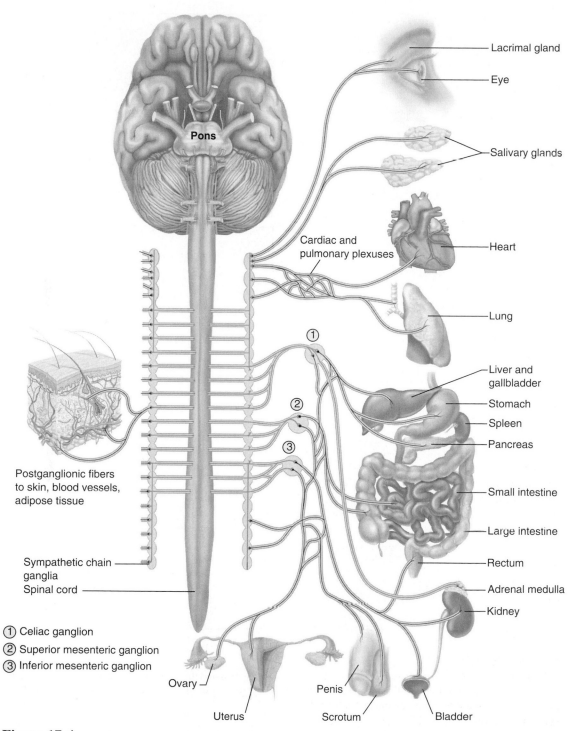

Lacrimal gland

Eye

Salivary glands

Pons

Cardiac and
pulmonary plexuses

Heart

Lung

①

Liver and
gallbladder

②

Stomach

③

Spleen

Pancreas

Small intestine

Postganglionic fibers
to skin, blood vessels,
adipose tissue

Large intestine

Rectum

Sympathetic chain
ganglia

Adrenal medulla

Spinal cord

Kidney

① Celiac ganglion
② Superior mesenteric ganglion
③ Inferior mesenteric ganglion

Ovary

Penis

Bladder

Uterus

Scrotum

Figure 17-4

The autonomic nervous system and organs affected.

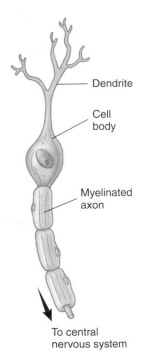

Dendrite

Cell
body

Myelinated
axon

To central
nervous system

Figure 17-5

The neuron, showing transmission of a message and
myelin sheath.

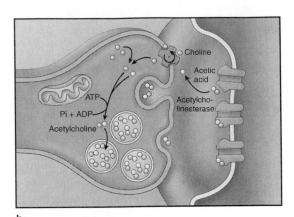

b

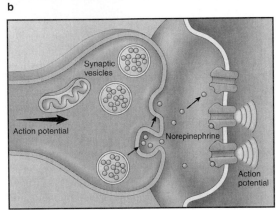

c

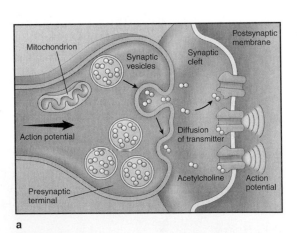

a

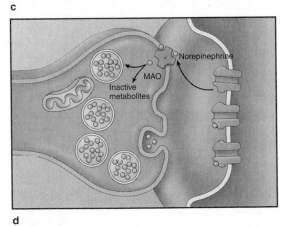

d

Figure 17-6

Synaptic Transmission. Acetylcholine (a) diffuses across the synaptic gap and (b) it is broken down into acetic acid and
choline. Choline is transported back to the presynaptic terminal where it is used to resynthesize acetylcholine. (c)
Norepinephrine diffuses across the synaptic gap and (d) is transported back into the presynaptic terminal and packaged
for reuse.

conditions are particularly dangerous to the fetus in the first trimester of pregnancy. Moreover, the earlier the condition occurs, the more severe the defect(s). In the birth process, a prolonged labor, forceps delivery, anesthetic, and other situations resulting in a reduced supply of oxygen to the baby could result in brain damage. Head trauma, brain infection, and brain tumor are also among the factors that might result in cerebral palsy for the infant or small child.

Symptoms

The spastic type of cerebral palsy is present in about seventy percent of the victims. Symptoms include excessive muscle contractions, muscle weakness, underdeveloped body parts (which are affected), and a tendency to walk on toes, with a scissorslike movement, crossing one foot in front of the other.

The athetoid form affects approximately twenty percent of the victims. These individuals have difficulty controlling the movements of their arms, legs, and/or facial muscles. The symptoms become more severe during stress, decrease when the individual is relaxed, and go away completely during sleep.

About ten percent of cerebral palsy victims have the ataxic type of the disorder. Their major problem is with balance, and they fall frequently.

Some children have a combination of these types. Individuals with cerebral palsy may be average or above average in intelligence, but as many as forty percent have mental retardation. About eighty percent have speech difficulties, and about twenty-five percent have seizure disorders.

Primary Prevention

Because the causative factors are linked to pregnancy and childbirth, there should be careful monitoring of the condition of the mother, particularly with respect to nutrition and drug use (including alcohol). Isolation from anyone who has rubella (vaccine should be given to girls before they reach puberty) is mandatory. Routine precautions must be taken in the use of forceps and anesthetic during childbirth. These procedures are all important in reducing the risk of cerebral palsy.

Secondary Prevention

Careful assessment and observation of infants for neurologic disorders by their doctor can lead to early

detection, which results in more effective treatment. If infants were premature or had a difficult birth, follow-up procedures to detect cerebral palsy or any other consequence of birth trauma are extremely important. A routine screening for cerebral palsy should be a part of every infant's six-month checkup.

Treatment

There is no cure for cerebral palsy, but with proper treatment and cooperation between all the child's care givers, children can be helped to reach their full potential within the limits set by their disorder. For very mild cases, this may be near normal. Treatment may include anticonvulsants, braces, exercises that involve range of motion, muscle relaxants, speech therapy, and other measures to control symptoms.

Epilepsy

Epilepsy is a seizure disorder related to disturbance of electrical patterns in the brain. Instead of firing in an ordered fashion, neurons discharge messages erratically, leading to an epileptic seizure. Epilepsy is in no way associated with lower intelligence or mental illness. One out of 200 in the population has the disorder. The seizures have different characteristics for different individuals and are identified by various terms.

Predisposing Factors

About half the cases of epilepsy are thought to be due to an abnormality in brain chemistry that is present at birth. Other factors include head injury, birth trauma, brain tumor, infectious diseases, and metabolic disorders.

Symptoms

Recurring seizures are the prevailing symptom in epilepsy. They range from mild to severe and may be partial or generalized.

Prevention

No preventive measures are known for epilepsy.

Treatment

With drug therapy, an individual with epilepsy can now be stabilized and remain seizure free. The epileptic has to be monitored for side effects and to maintain the proper dosage. If drug treatment fails, there are surgical techniques that may help in some cases.

Parkinson's Disease

Parkinson's disease is characterized by fine muscle, slowly spreading progressive tremors, muscular weakness and rigidity, and a peculiar gait. It was first described by Dr. James Parkinson in 1817. The deterioration continues for an average of ten years, at which time death usually occurs as a result of pneumonia or some other infection. The disease affects men more than women, with one in 100 over the age of sixty years becoming a victim. Over 60,000 cases are diagnosed annually in the United States, and with our aging population, this figure will rise.

Predisposing Factors
The cause is unknown, but individuals with Parkinson's have been shown to have a dopamine deficiency. Dopamine is known to have an inhibitory effect on nerve transmissions within the CNS.

Symptoms
Muscle rigidity, inability to control muscle movement, and an insidious tremor that begins in the fingers are the first symptoms of Parkinson's. The symptoms increase during stress or anxiety and decrease when moving purposefully and sleeping. There is no intellectual impairment from Parkinson's, although a concomitant disease such as arteriosclerosis may cause it. Lack of muscle control can lead to change of voice pitch, drooling, unusual gait, and strange cries, with upward or closed position of the eyes.

Prevention
No preventive measures are known.

Treatment
There is no cure for Parkinson's at present. The primary aim of treatment is to keep the patient as comfortable and as functional as possible. Drugs, physical therapy, and surgery (in extreme cases) are used.

Multiple Sclerosis

Multiple sclerosis (MS) is a chronic disease of the CNS that is a major cause of disability in young adults. Progressive demyelination of the nerve fibers of the brain and spinal cord leads to widely spread and varied neurologic dysfunction. It is a disease marked by remissions and exacerbations, and it may progress rapidly, causing death within months of the onset or, as in seventy percent of the cases, the patient may lead an active, productive life. The disease generally occurs between the ages of twenty and forty, with twenty-seven being the average. It affects more women than men (3:2) and more whites than blacks (5:1). Japan has a low incidence of the disease, and it occurs more often in cities and among upper income groups. In northern areas of the world, the incidence of the disease ranges from fifty to eighty per 100,000. It affects about 250,000 people in the United States.

Predisposing Factors
The exact cause of MS is unknown, but a family history of the disease and living in a cold, damp climate increase the risk. It is five times more common in temperate zones than in the tropics. There are many theories of causation, but one of the most widely held is that a slow-moving virus may be the disease agent. Other suspected factors include emotional stress, nutritional deficiencies, trauma, overwork, and acute respiratory infections.

Symptoms
For most patients, problems with the eyes and other sense organs are the first sign that anything is wrong. Numbness and tingling sensations, muscle weakness, urinary disturbances, and mood swings are included in the characteristic changes caused by the disease. Symptoms vary from being so mild that they are not noticed to being severe enough that the individual seems hysterical. Speech may be impaired also. As indicated before, remissions may occur and last for long periods, but then the disease may return with more severe symptoms than felt initially.

Prevention
No preventive measures are known.

Treatment
Various drugs are used to reduce the severity of the symptoms and the progression of the disease.

CASE STUDY

Multiple Sclerosis

A thirty-two year-old female instructor/coach at a large Midwestern university began having problems with her coordination. She noticed it particularly when she was coaching the softball team because she could not toss and hit the ball with her usual accuracy during practice. She also had some other signs that something was wrong including numbness, tingling, and some mood swings. When she went to her doctor, he examined her and immediately ordered a CAT scan. The diagnosis was multiple sclerosis. Not long after beginning drug therapy, she realized the symptoms were less and less pronounced until she had none. The doctor told her that the disease was in remission. She was able to continue teaching and coaching.

Among these are **adrenocorticotropic** hormone (ACTH) and prednisone to reduce edema, and ACTH and corticosteroids to relieve symptoms and speed up remission. There is no cure for the disease.

Alzheimer's Disease

This degenerative disease of the brain, Alzheimer's disease, which affects up to thirty percent of people over eighty-five years of age, is responsible for a great deal of suffering by the victims and their care givers. It is a progressive disease that rarely occurs in those under sixty years of age. There is no laboratory test to diagnose Alzheimer's disease, except an autopsy. If persons develop dementia (mental deterioration), and all other possible causes are ruled out, then they are diagnosed with Alzheimer's disease. For an idea of the chances of contracting Alzheimer's disease, see the Did You Know? section following.

Predisposing Factors

Even though our aging population and subsequent increased incidence of the disease have resulted in increased research efforts to find a cause, none has been identified to date. The latest research indicates that neurotransmitters and acetylcholine may play a part. Although no one cause has been identified, several factors are thought to be implicated including deficiencies in neurotransmitters, exposure to aluminum, slow viruses, trauma, and genetic immunologic factors.

Symptoms

There are generally three stages of the disease: (1) the individual is aware of increasing forgetfulness and attempts to compensate by writing lists or by asking others for help; (2) there is severe memory loss, particularly for recent events, accompanied by disorientation, difficulty in finding the right words when speaking, sudden and unpredictable mood changes, and personality changes; (3) all the symptoms of the second stage become more severe, and the victim may revert to childhood behaviors. The people who have the disease may become violent and difficult to control, or they may become quiet and withdrawn. They neglect habits of personal cleanliness, may be incontinent or wander aimlessly, not knowing where they are. At this stage, they require around-the-clock care and usually must be institutionalized. These symptoms range over a three- to ten-year period, and death is usually due to malnutrition or infection.

Prevention

No preventive measures are known.

---

adrenocorticotropic ad-re-no-KOR-ti-ko-trop-ik

Treatment

Tranquilizers and antidepressants can help control the behavior, but there is no real therapy available yet. Counseling the family to be sure they understand and can deal with the care of the person as long as possible is important. Adult day-care centers, home health aides, and extended-care facilities are all needed as the condition of the individual deteriorates.

ENDOCRINE DISORDERS

Disorders of Glands and Hormones

The endocrine glands include the pituitary gland, thyroid gland, parathyroid glands, adrenal glands, islets of Langerhans of the pancreas, and the ovaries and testes. These are ductless glands that produce an internal secretion that is discharged into the blood or lymph and circulated to all parts of the body. The hormones secreted by these glands may have a specific effect on an organ or tissue or a general effect on the entire body. The secretions of the endocrine glands may be under nervous control, under the control of chemical substances in the blood, or under the control of other hormones. If the glands do not function as they should, many disease conditions can occur. Diabetes mellitus will be discussed in this chapter.

Diabetes Mellitus

Diabetes mellitus is characterized by abnormal metabolism of carbohydrate, protein, and fat, resulting in increased levels of blood sugar. The adjective *mellitus* (for sweet) is used with diabetes to distinguish the disease from diabetes insipidus (tasteless), which is so rare that the word *diabetes* by itself generally refers to diabetes mellitus. The only thing that diabetes mellitus and diabetes insipidus have in common is polyuria, or frequent urination. There are two forms of diabetes mellitus: Type I, or insulin-dependent diabetes mellitus (IDDM), and Type II, or non-insulin-dependent diabetes (NIDDM).

Diabetes is one of the ten leading causes of death from disease in the United States. It is the result of an insufficient supply of insulin or an inadequate use of the insulin that is supplied from the islets of Langerhans in the pancreas. Diabetes contributes to fifty percent of myocardial infarctions and seventy-five percent of strokes. It is a contributing factor for renal disease, peripheral vascular disease, and blindness. Types I and II are the most common forms.

Type I

Type I was formerly known as "juvenile onset" diabetes, because it often begins in adolescence and usually before the age of thirty-five. Type I is a more severe form than Type II. It develops rapidly, the insulin-secreting cells in the pancreas are destroyed, and insulin production ceases almost completely. Without regular injections of insulin, the sufferer lapses into a coma and dies.

Predisposing Factors

Type I was thought to be hereditary. However, recent studies of identical twins indicate that there are other factors involved, because in almost half of the cases, only one twin developed the disease. No theory has yet been accepted that identifies the factors involved.

Symptoms

Type I has an abrupt onset, with dramatic weight loss, reversion to bedwetting, frequent urination, excessive thirst, and vaginal itching. It is often preceded by a flulike episode with slow recovery.

Prevention

No preventive measures are known.

Treatment

Diet, exercise, education, drugs (insulin), and self-testing are included in the treatment. Type I diabetes is not easily controlled, and because the victims are so young, it is difficult to keep them on a regular treatment schedule. Skipped insulin doses and neglect of self-testing can easily lead to diabetic coma and death.

Type II

Type II was formerly known as "adult onset," because it generally is not present until after the age of forty.

Predisposing Factors

Type II diabetes mellitus may also have a hereditary factor, but it is most often found in obese, sedentary adults. Other factors include physiologic or emotional stress, pregnancy, and oral contraceptives, and certain medications that are insulin antagonists. There is a high incidence among native Americans, blacks, and Hispanics.

Symptoms

Type II has a gradual onset, with frequent urination, fatigue, and blurred vision. Because it may also be asymptomatic, about half of those with Type II diabetes mellitus do not know they have it.

Prevention

Avoiding obesity, getting regular exercise, and learning to manage stress will reduce the risk.

Treatment

Type II may be managed by diet alone, which will mean a major change in eating habits. Exercise, education, a support group, and self-testing are also included. If the change in diet does not control the disease, then oral hypoglycemics (to stimulate insulin production) are used. It is not generally necessary for individuals with Type II to have injections.

A number of complications may occur in diabetes. If the blood glucose goes too low, *insulin shock* is the result. The improper metabolism of fatty acids, generally from carbohydrate deficiency, or inadequate utilization, results in too many ketone bodies in the blood, leading to ketosis. If the blood glucose becomes too high, the patient will go into *diabetic coma,* which is life threatening. Diabetics generally carry sugar in some form to alleviate the former.

Other problems for the diabetic include low resistance to infections, especially those involving the extremities, ulceration of lower extremities, increase in incidence of toxemia in pregnancy, cardiovascular and renal disorders, and eye disorders such as blindness. Diabetes is one of the contributing factors in fifty percent of heart attacks and also a contributing factor in about seventy-five percent of strokes.

SUMMARY

Table 17-1 summarizes relevant data on the sensory, nervous, and endocrine disorders discussed in this chapter.

TABLE 17-1	Disorders of the Senses, Nervous System, and Endocrine System			
Disorder	**Special Characteristics**	**Predisposing Factors**	**Common Symptoms**	**Prevention/ Treatment**
EYE				
Refractive Errors	Myopia (near-sighted), hyperopia (far-sighted), presbyopia (difficulty focusing), astigmatism (unequal curvature of cornea and/or lens)	Most often by inheritance	Difficulty in reading, recognizing people or objects at a distance, or very close; difficulty focusing; for astigmatism, variation in shades of print	None known; glasses, contact lenses
Cataract	Generally occur with aging; individual can often see better in dim light	Predisposition through inheritance most often; may also be secondary to glaucoma or may be present in a baby as a result of rubella in mother during pregnancy; abuse of drugs, eye injuries, can cause cataracts	Blurring of print and figures; halos around lights at night; headlights, sunlight, decrease vision	None for senile cataracts; pre-pubertal vaccination for rubella; protection of eyes in at-risk activities; medical supervision in use of drugs can prevent other kinds; laser surgery very successful
Glaucoma	Increase in intraocular pressure leading to atrophy of optic nerve and blindness; occurs in women more than men, accounts for 15% of blindness in U.S.	Inherited predis-position	None until disease is far advanced; mild aching in eyes, halos around lights, loss of peripheral vision and reduced visual acuity not corrected with glasses	Regular eye exams; yearly exams after age 40 if history of glaucoma in the family; eye drops used early in disease will control it

TABLE 17-1	*Continued*			
Disorder	**Special Characteristics**	**Predisposing Factors**	**Common Symptoms**	**Prevention/ Treatment**
EAR				
Hearing Loss	Almost 25% of children entering school have some hearing loss; about 25% of people over 65 need hearing aid		Baby doesn't "babble"; child doesn't turn head at sound of voice, inattention; tinnitus, loss of some letter sounds in older people; speech harder to understand with background noise; may become withdrawn or depressed if not aware of problem	Screening tests in school; protective equipment if exposed to long-term noise; education of pregnant women; treatment depends on cause; hearing aids help some, others may need to learn lip reading; some kinds may be cleared up by surgery or other medical treatment
Conductive	Passage of sound from the external ear to oval window blocked	Otitis media, earwax, immobile stapes, damaged eardrum, perforated eardrum		
Sensori neural	No transmission of sound from inner ear to brain; one in 1000 babies at birth have this type— incurable	Birth injury, fetus damage, loud noise, Ménière's, certain drugs, viral infections, degeneration of cochlea or labyrinth, tumors		
Ménière's Disease	Caused by increase in amount of fluid in inner ear;	Unknown	Tinnitus, dizziness, nausea, vomiting, sweating, jerky	Unknown; drugs used to stop an attack; vasodilators,

TABLE 17-1	*Continued*			
Disorder	**Special Characteristics**	**Predisposing Factors**	**Common Symptoms**	**Prevention/ Treatment**
Ménière's Disease— Cont'd	may lead to sensorineural hearing loss and deafness		eye movements, pressure or pain in ear	diuretics, anti-histamines and restricted salt intake may also be prescribed
NERVOUS SYSTEM				
Cerebral Palsy	Three kinds, spastic, athetoid, and ataxic; results from damage to CNS; about 70% are spastic	There are many, any condition during pregnancy, birth, or child-hood that results in dam-age to the brain; may be due to forceps delivery	Spastic: (70%) Excessive muscle contractions, muscle weak-ness, underde-veloped body parts, unusual walk. Athetoid: (20%) Difficulty con-trolling move-ment of body parts; more severe during stress, goes away completely during sleep Ataxic: (10%) Major problem is with balance—fall frequently	Monitoring of pregnant women, caution with forcep use in delivery, rou-tine screening at 6 months; treatment can help child to reach full potential— anti-convulsants, braces, exercises, mus-cle relaxants, speech therapy are among those used
Epilepsy	Seizure disorder related to dis-turbance of electrical pat-terns in the brain; not asso-ciated with lowered intelli-gence or men-tal illness; 1 out of 200 have the disorder	About half due to abnormality in brain chemistry pres-ent at birth; also due to head injury, birth trauma, brain tumor, infectious dis-ease, and meta-bolic disorders	Recurring seizures rang-ing from mild to severe	None known; individual can be free of seizures with drug therapy
Parkinson's Disease	Fine muscle, slowly	Unknown; may be due to	Muscle rigidity, inability to	None known; no cure; treatment

TABLE 17-1	*Continued*			
Disorder	**Special Characteristics**	**Predisposing Factors**	**Common Symptoms**	**Prevention/ Treatment**
Parkinson's Disease— Cont'd	spreading, progressive tremors, muscular weakness and rigidity; usually lasts about 10 years with death resulting from pneumonia or other infection; affects men (1 in 100 over age of 60) more than women; increasing with aging population	dopamine deficiency	control muscle movement, tremor beginning slowly in fingers; increase during stress, decrease during sleep; causes no intellectual impairment; may be change of voice pitch, drooling, unusual walk, strange cries with upward or closed position of eyes	to ease symptoms only
Multiple Sclerosis	Chronic disease of CNS— major cause of disability in young adults; progressive demyelination of nerve fibers; some may die in months, others (70%) lead an active, productive life; about 250,000 affected in U.S.	Unknown; family history of disease, cold, damp climate increase risk, may be slow-moving virus	Problems with eyes and other sense organs usually first sign; numbness, tingling, muscle weakness, urinary disturbances, and mood swings as disease advances; speech may be impaired and victim may seem hysterical at times; remissions have occurred for long periods but disease returns with more severe symptoms	Unknown; treatment for symptoms only
Alzheimer's Disease	Affects up to 30% of people over	No cause identified; three	Three stages:(1) increasing	None known

TABLE 17-1	*Continued*			
Disorder	**Special Characteristics**	**Predisposing Factors**	**Common Symptoms**	**Prevention/ Treatment**
Alzheimer's Disease— Cont'd	85; rarely occurs before age 60	major theories; aluminum; autoimmunity; slow viruses (most popular); 10%-30% have family history of disease	forgetfulness; (2) severe memory loss, disorientation, trouble finding right words when speaking, mood and per- sonality changes; (3) all symptoms become worse, childish behav- iors, wander aimlessly, incontinent neglect personal clean- liness, need round-the- clock care and usually institu- tionalized	
ENDOCRINE SYSTEM Diabetes Mellitus	Abnormal metabolism of carbohydrate, protein, and fat resulting in increased levels of blood sugar; a leading cause of death in U.S.; 5% of the population had diabetes in 1987; diabetics have low resis- tance to infec- tion, especially in extremities, increased incidence of			

TABLE 17-1	*Continued*			
Disorder	**Special Characteristics**	**Predisposing Factors**	**Common Symptoms**	**Prevention/ Treatment**
Diabetes Mellitus— Cont'd	toxemia in pregnancy, cardiovascular and renal disorders, and eye disorders many times leading to blindness; diabetes contributes to about 50% of myocardial infarctions and about 75% of strokes			
Type I	Insulin dependent; "juvenile onset" diabetes; usually begins before the age of 25	Unknown; may be hereditary factor	Abrupt onset, dramatic weight loss, bedwetting, frequent urination, vaginal itching, thirst; too much insulin can produce life-threatening insulin shock	Unknown; diet, exercise, education, drugs, and self-testing part of treatment; adolescents may not follow treatment guidelines resulting in diabetic coma and death from high blood sugar
Type II	"Adult onset," generally occurs after age 40	May also have hereditary factor but generally found in obese, sedentary adults; physiologic or emotional stress, pregnancy, oral contraceptives, certain drugs may all be predisposing factors	Gradual onset, frequent urination, fatigue, and blurred vision; may be asymptomatic	Avoiding obesity, regular exercise, stress management will reduce risk

QUESTIONS FOR REVIEW

1. What refractive errors are discussed in the text, and why do they occur?
2. What is a cataract?
3. What causes cataracts?
4. What symptoms may be due to a cataract?
5. What is the treatment for cataracts?
6. What causes glaucoma?
7. Why should glaucoma tests be performed regularly after the age of forty?
8. Name and describe the two kinds of hearing loss.
9. Identify risk factors for conductive and sensorineural hearing loss.
10. Why are hearing tests for children important?
11. What is otitis media?
12. What symptoms occur in Ménière's disease?
13. What types of treatment may be used for Ménière's disease?
14. What are the predisposing factors for cerebral palsy?
15. Name the three types of cerebral palsy and the symptoms for each.
16. What is epilepsy?
17. What is the treatment for epilepsy?
18. How prevalent is Parkinson's disease?
19. What are the symptoms of Parkinson's disease?
20. How effective is the treatment for Parkinson's disease?
21. What is the physiologic process leading to MS?
22. What can be said about the incidence of MS?
23. What are the symptoms of MS?
24. What is the treatment for MS?
25. How is Alzheimer's disease diagnosed?
26. Describe the three stages of Alzheimer's.
27. What treatment is available for Alzheimer's?
28. What are the differences between Type I and Type II diabetes mellitus?
29. What complications may occur in diabetes?
30. What measures can be taken to avoid Type II diabetes?

FURTHER READING

Aarsland, D. 1999. Mental symptoms in Parkinson's disease are important contributors to caregiver distress. *International Journal of Geriatric Psychiatry* 14:866.

Agnew, Christina M., Michael S. Nystul, and Mary C. Connor. 1998. Seizure disorders: An alternative explanation for students inattention. *Professional School Counselling* 2:54.

Ahmad, Khabir. 1999. Embryonic grafts have long term benefits in Parkinson's disease. *The Lancet* 354:1882.

Aikiya, M., et al. 1999. Predictors of seizure outcome in newly diagnosed partial epilepsy memory performance as a prognostic factor. *Epilepsy Res* 37:159.

Akiba, J. 1999. Retinal detachment associated with a macular hole in severely myopic eyes. *American Journal of Ophthalmology* 128:654.

Albereda, M. Merce, and Rosa Corcoy. 1998. Reversible impairment of renal function associated with enalapril in a diabetic patient. *Canadian Medical Association Journal* 59:1279.

Alendkamp, A. P., et al. 1999. An open nonrandomized clinical comparative study evaluating the effect of epilepsy on learning. *Journal of Child Neurology* 14:795.

Alevriadou, A., et al. 1999. Wisconsin card sorting test variables in relation to motor symptoms in Parkinson's disease. *Perceptual and Motor Skills* 89:824.

Al-Omaishi, J. 1999. The cellular immunology of multiple sclerosis. *Journal of Leukocyte Biology* 65:444.

Alzheimer's disease: Seeking new ways to preserve brain function. *Geriatrics* 54:42, 1999.

Andrews, D., et al. 1999. The assessment and treatment of concerns and anxiety in patients undergoing presurgical monitoring for epilepsy. *Epilepsia* 40:1535.

Arpino, C. 1999. Differing factors for cerebral palsy in the presence of mental retardation and epilepsy. *Journal of Child Neurology* 14:151.

Asita De Silva, H., Jeffrey K. Aronson, et al. 1998. Abnormal function of potassium channels in platelets of patients with Alzheimer's disease. *The Lancet* 352:1590.

Ault, Alicia. 1999. US FDA advisers back new myopia aid. *The Lancet* 353:300.

Bass, N. 1999. Cerebral palsy and neurodegenerative disease. *Current Opinion Pediatrics* 11:487.

Berg, A. T., et al. 1999. Childhood onset epilepsy with and without preceding febrile seizures. *Neurology* 53:1742.

Black, E. H. 1998. Corneal topography after cataract surgery using a clear corneal incision closed with one radial suture. *Ophthalmic Surgery and Lasers* 29:896.

Brown, C. J. 1998. Primary care physicians' knowledge and behavior related to Alzheimer's disease. *Journal of Applied Gerontology* 17:462.

Brown, Lisa., and Eric B. Rimm. 1999. A prospective study of carotenoid and vitamin A intakes and risk of cataract extraction in U.S. men. *American Journal of Clinical Nutrition* 70:517.

Budak, K. 1999. Preoperative screening of contact lens wearers before refractive surgery. *Journal of Cataract Refractory Surgery* 25:1080.

Budde, W.M. 1999. Family history of glaucoma in the primary and secondary open angle glaucomas. *Graefes Arh Clin Exp Ophthalmology* 237:554.

Burgess, I. A. 1998. Prenatal detection of congenital idiopathic cataracts. *Medical Journal of Australia* 169:385.

Burns, Alistari. 1999. Might olfactory dysfunction be a marker of early Alzheimer's disease? *The Lancet* 355:84.

Camras, C. B. 1999. Efficacy and adverse effects of medications used in the treatment of glaucoma. *Drugs and Aging* 15:377.

Chadwick, David. 1999. Seizures and epilepsy after traumatic brain injury. *The Lancet* 355:334.

Chasan-Taber, L. 1999. A prospective study of vitamin supplements intake and cataract extraction among U.S. women. *Epidemiology* 10:679.

Chrichton, Paul. 1999. No consolation for Alzheimer's disease. *The Lancet* 353:157.

Cohen, J. A., et al. 1999. Therapy of relapsing multiple sclerosis. *Journal of neuroimmunity* 98:29.

Coleman, Anne. 1999. Glaucoma. *The Lancet* 354:1803.

Colin, J. 1999. Retinal detachment after clear lens extraction for high myopia. *Ophthalmology* 106:2281.

Cortesi, R. 1999. Sleep problems and daytime behavior in childhood idiopathic epilepsy. *Epilepsia* 40:1557.

Craddock, Nick, and Corinne Lendon. 1998. New susceptibility gene for Alzheimer's disease on chromosome 12? *The Lancet* 352:1720.

Cross, T., and D. Rintell. 1999. Children's perceptions of parental multiple sclerosis. *Psychology, Health and Medicine* 4:355.

Davison, Steven P., and Mitchell S. Marion. 1998. Sensorineural hearing loss caused by NASAID-induced, aseptic meningitis. *Ear Nose and Throat Journal* 68:820.

Delagaza, Vincent W. 1998. New drugs for Alzheimer's disease. *American Family Physician* 58:1175.

Deuschle, Michael, and Liv Bode, et al. 1998. Borna disease virus proteins in cerebrospinal fluid of patients with recurrent depression and multiple sclerosis. *The Lancet* 352:1828.

Devinsky, O. 1999. Risk factors for poor health-related quality of life in adolescents with epilepsy. *Epilepsia* 40:1715.

Dillon, James, Roy C. Milton, Sheila K. West, et al. 1999. Sunlight exposure and cataract. *Journal of the American Medical Association* 281:229.

Do I have diabetes? *American Family Physician* 58:1371, 1998.

Doraiswamy, P. Murali, Cecil H. Charles, et al. 1998. Prediction of cognitive decline in early Alzheimer's disease. *The Lancet* 352:1678.

Douglas, Carolinda, and Patrick J. Fox. 1999. Health care utilization among clients with Alzheimer's disease: Public implications from the California Alzheimer disease diagnostic and treatment center program. *Journal of Applied Gerontology* 18:99.

Dunnett, S. B., and A. Bjoerklund. Prospects for new restorative and neuroprotective treatments in Parkinson's disease. *Nature* 399:A23.

Ebers, G. C., G. Rice, et al. 1998. Randomized double blind placebo-controlled study of interferon beta-la in relapsing/remitting multiple sclerosis. *The Lancet* 352:1498.

Egge, K. 1999. Survival of glaucoma patients. *Acta Ophthalmology Scandi* 77:397.

Eggink, C.A. 1999. Photorefractive keratectomy with an ablatable mask for myopic astigmatism. *Journal of Refractory Surgery* 15:550.

Emara, B. 1998. Correlation of intraocular pressure and central corneal thickness in normal myopic eyes and after laser in situ keratomileusis. Journal of Cataract and Refractive Surgery, 24:1320.

Ewbank, Douglas C. 1999. Deaths attributable to Alzheimer's disease in the United States. *American Journal of Public Health* 89:90.

Feely, Morgan. 1999. Drug treatment for epilepsy. *British Medical Journal* 318:106.

Feldman, Howard. 2000. Causes of Alzheimer's disease. *Canadian Medical Journal* 162:65.

Finucane, Alexandra K. 1999. Epilepsy, driving and the law. *American Family Physician* 59:199.

Fiscella, R.G. 1999. Cost considerations of medical therapy for glaucoma. *American Journal of Ophthalmology* 128:426.

Foley, Daniel. 1999. Sorting out sleep in patients with Alzheimer's disease. *The Lancet* 354:2098.

Fransen, E., et al. 1999. High prevalence of symptoms of Ménière's disease in three families with a mutation in the coch gene. *Human Molecular Genetics* 8:1425.

Fritch, C. D. 1998. Risk of retinal detachment in myopic eyes after intraocular lens implantation: A 7-year study. *Journal of Cataract and Refractive Surgery* 24:1357.

Gabrieli, C.B. 1999. Excimer laser photorefractive keratectomy for high myopia and myopic astigmatism. *Ophthalmic Surgery Lasers* 30:442.

Gale, Catherine A., et al. 1999. Mortality from Parkinson's disease and other causes in men who were prisoners of war in the Far East. *The Lancet* 354:2116.

Garrett, S. K. 19 99. Methodology of the VECAT study. *Ophthalmic Epidemiology* 6:181.

Gelisse, P., et al. 1999. Is schizophrenia a risk factor of epilepsy or acute symptomatic seizures? *Epilepsia* 40:1566.

Gentilucci, M., and A. Negrotti. 1999. The control of an action in Parkinson's disease. *Experimental Brain Research* 129:269.

George, S. P. 1999. Photorefractive keratectomy retreatments: comparison of two methods of excimer laser epithelium removal. *Ophthalmology* 106:1481.

Goodkin, Donald E. 1998. Interferon beta therapy for multiple sclerosis. *The Lancet* 352:1486.

Goodrich, M.E. 1999. Plasma fibrinogen and other cardiovascular disease risk factors and cataracts. *Ophthalmic Epidemiology* 6:279.

Gordon, J. 1999. Improving outcome of cataract surgery in developing countries. *The Lancet* 355:158.

Gorell, J. M. 1999. Occupational exposure to manganese, copper, lead, irons, mercury and zinc, and the risk of Parkinson's disease. *Neurotoxicology* 20:239.

Green, Keith. 1999. Marijuana smoking vs. cannabinoids for glaucoma therapy. *Journal of the American Medical Association* 281:402.

Grether, J.K. 1999. Interferons and cerebral palsy. *Journal of Pediatrics* 134:324.

Haberkamp, T. J. 1999. Management of idiopathic sudden sensorineural hearing loss. *American Journal of Otology* 20:1435.

Hagnebo, C., L. Melin, and G. Andersson. 1999. Coping strategies and anxiety sensitivity in Ménière's disease. *Psychology, Health and Medicine* 4:10.

Hall, K.S. Low education and childhood rural residence: risk of Alzheimer's disease in African Americans. *Neurology* 54:95

Haraguchi, H. 1999. Progressive sensorineural hearing impairment in professional fishery divers. *Annal Otology Rhinology Larngology* 108:1165.

Harper, R.A. 1999. Glaucoma screening: the importance of combining test data. *Optom Vis Sci* 76:537.

Harris, Stewart B., Sara J. Meltzer, et al. 1998. New guidelines, for the management of diabetes: A physician's guide. *Canadian Medical Association Journal* 159:973.

Hearing aids underused; patient support, education needed. *Modern Medicine* 66:10, 1998.

Heller, T. 1999. Residential transitions from nursing homes for adults with cerebral palsy. *Disabil Rehability* 318:1021.

Ho, W. K. 1999. Long term sensorineural hearing deficit following radiotherapy in patients suffering from nasopharyngeal carcinoma: a prospective study. *Head Neck* 21:547.

Hollis, L. 1999. Ménière's disease. *Hospital Medicine* 60: 574.

Holmes, Gregory L. 1999. Buccal route for benzodiazepines in treatment of seizures? *The Lancet* 353:608.

Hopkins, K. D. 1998. More benefits attributed to good glycaemic control in type II diabetes. *The Lancet* 352:1528.

Horner, D. G. 1999. Myopia progression in adolescent wearers of soft contact lenses and spectacles. *Optom Vis Sci* 76:474.

Hourihan, Fleur, and Paul Mitchell. 1999. Possible associations between computed tomography scan and cataract. *American Journal of Public Health* 89:1864.

Huang, T.S. 1999. Three new surgeries for treatment of intractable Ménière's disease. *American Journal of Otology* 20:233.

Hung, G. K. 1999. Model of human refractive error development. *Current Eye Res* 19:41.

Iviere, Stephanie, et al. 1999. Nutrition and Alzheimer's disease. *Nutrition Reviews* 57:363.

Jain, S. 1999. Phototherapeutic keratectomy for treatment of recurrent corneal erosion. *Journal of Cataract Refractory Surgery* 25:1610.

Jankovic, J. 1999. Reemergenet tremor of Parkinson's disease. *Journal of Neurology Neurosurgery Psychiatry* 67:404.

Jimyenez-Alfaro, I. 1998. Clear lens extraction and implantation of negative power posterior chamber intraocular lenses to correct extreme myopia. *Journal of Cataract and Refractive Surgery* 24:1310.

Job, Agnes, Marc Raynal, et al. 1999. Hearing loss and use of personal stereos in young adults with antecedents of otitis media. *The Lancet* 353:35.

Jones, N.S. 1999. A prospective case controlled study of patients presenting with idiopathic sensorineural hearing loss to examine the relationship between hyperlipidaiemia and sensorineural hearing loss. *Clinical Otolaryngology* 24:531.

Jones, N.S. 1999. A prospective case controlled study of 197 men, 50-60 years old selected at random from a population at risk from hyperlipidaemia to examine the relationship between hyperlipidaemia and sensorineural hearing loss. *Clinical Otolaryngology* 24:449.

Julius, M.C. 1999. The prevention of type I diabetes mellitus. *Pediatric Annual* 28:585.

Kane, Michael N. 1999. Factors affecting social work students' willingness to work with elders with Alzheimer's disease. *Journal of Social Work Education* 35:71.

Kaplan, Sheldon L. 1999. Prevention of hearing loss from meningitis. *The Lancet* 350:158.

Kessel, L. 1999. Diabetic versus non-diabetic color vision after cataract surgery. *British Journal of Ophthalmology* 83:1042.

Kirchner, Jeffrey T. 1997. Inhaled corticosteroids and risk of cataract formation. *American Family Physician* 56:2333.

Klein, B. E. 1998. Diabetes, cardiovascular disease, selected cardiovascular disease risk factors, and the 5-year incidence of age-related cataract and progression of lens opacities: The Beaver Dam eye study. *American Journal of Ophthalmology* 126:782.

Knoblock, Mary Jo, and Steven K. Broste. 1998. A hearing conservation program for Wisconsin youth working in agriculture. *Journal of School Health* 68:313.

Kolahdouz-Isfahani, A. H. 1999. Clear lens extraction with intraocular lens implantation for hyperopia. *Journal of Refractive Surgery* 15:316.

Kraft, George. 1999. Rehabilitation still the only way to improve function in multiple sclerosis. *Multiple Sclerosis* 354:2016.

Kroencke, D.C., and D.R. Denney. 1999. Stress and coping in multiple sclerosis: exacerbation, remission and chronic subgroups. *Multiple Sclerosis* 5:89.

Kuopio, A. M. 1999. Environmental risk factors in Parkinson's disease. *Mov Diord* 14:928.

Kwan, Patrick, and Martin J. Brodie. 1999. Early identification of refractory epilepsy. *New England Journal of Medicine* 342:314.

Lampe, John B., and John B. Bodensteiner. 1998. Life expectancy of children with cerebral palsy. *Clinical Pediatrics* 37:578.

Langdon, D. W. 1999. Multiple sclerosis: a preliminary study of selected variables affecting rehabilitation outcome. *Multiple Sclerosis* 5:94.

Lee, K.E. 1999. Changes in refractive error over a 5 year interval in the Beaver Dam Eye study. *Invest Ophthalmology Vis Sci* 40:1645.

Lenarz, T. 1999. Sensorineural hearing loss in children. *Int Journal of Otorhinolaryngology* 49:S179.

Lerman-Sagie, T., and P. Lerman. 1999. Phenobarbital still has a role in epilepsy treatment. *Journal of Child Neurology* 14:820.

Lieu, A. S., and S.L. Howng. 2000. Intracranial meningiomas and epilepsy: incidence, prognosis and influencing factors. *Epilepsy Resident* 38:45.

Lim, R. 1999. Refractive associations with cataract. *Invest Ophthalmology Visual Science* 40:3021.

Lipton, G. E. 1999. Factors predicting postoperative complications following spinal fusions in children with cerebral palsy. *Journal of Spinal Disorders* 12:197.

Liu, X. 1999. Effects of visual feedback on manual tracking and action tremor in Parkinson's disease. *Exp Brain Res* 129:477.

MacAndie, C. 1999. Sensorineural hearing loss in chronic otitis media. *Clinical Otolaryngology* 24:220.

Macdougall, C. F., T. Cheetham, and M. Craig. 1998. Minerva. *British Medical Journal* 317:1668.

Marosn, D.C. 1999. Error behaviors associated with loss of competency in Alzheimer's disease. *Neurology* 53:1983.

Mason, J. 1999. A systematic review of foot ulcer in patient with type 2 diabetes mellitus. *Diabetes Medicine* 16:801.

Massaro, Dominic W., and Michael M. Cohen. 1999. Speech perception in perceivers with hearing loss: Synergy of multiple modalities. *Journal of Speech, Language, and Hearing Research* 42:21.

Mathern, G. W., et al. 1999. Postoperative seizure control and antiepileptic drug use in pediatric epilepsy surgery patients: the UCLA experience. *Epilepsia* 40:1740.

Mathews, S. 1999. Sclera expansion surgery does not restore accommodation in human presbyopia. *Ophthalmology* 106:873.

McAllister, Carol L., and Myrna A. Silverman. 1999. Community formation and community roles among persons with Alzheimer's disease: A comparative study of experiences in a residential Alzheimer's facility and a traditional nursing home. *Qualitative Health Research* 9:65.

McDonald M.B. 1999. Photorefractive keratectomy for low to moderate myopia and astigmatism with a small beam tracker directed excimer laser. *Ophthalmology* 106:1481.

McNamara, J.O. 1999. Emerging insights into the genesis of epilepsy. 399:A15.

Menegon, Alessandra, and Philip G. Board. 1998. Parkinson's disease, pesticides, and glutathione transferase polymorphisms. *The Lancet* 352:1344.

Mesec, A. 1999. The deterioration of cardiovascular reflexes in Parkinson's disease. *Acta Neurolo Scan* 100:296.

Miller, Karl. 1998. Exercise and weight training in adolescents with type I diabetes. *American Family Physician* 58:1655.

Mitchell, P. 1999. The relationship between glaucoma in myopia. *Ophthalmology* 106:2010.

Mitchell, P. 1999. Inhaled corticosteroids, family history, and risk of glaucoma. *Ophthalmology* 106:2301.

Mitchell, P. 1999. The relationship between glaucoma and myopia: the Blue Mountains eye study. *Ophthalmology* 106:2010.

Mittendorf, Robert, et al. 1999. Association between cerebral palsy and coagulase-negative staphylococci. *The Lancet* 354:1875.

Mohr, D.C., et al. 1999. Treatment adherence and patient retention the first year of a phase III clinical trial for the treatment of multiple sclerosis. *Multiple Sclerosis* 5:192.

Moore, B. 1999. A clinical review of hyperopia in young children. *Journal of the American Ophthalmology Association* 70:215.

Murer, M.G. 1999. Levodopa in Parkinson's disease: neurotoxicity issue laid to rest? *Drug Saf* 21:339

Newborn and infant hearing loss: Detection in the nursery. *Pediatrics* 103:527, 1999.

Nickells, R. W. 1999. Apoptosis of retinal ganglion cells in glaucoma: an update of the molecular pathways involved in cell death. *Surv Ophthalmology* 43:S151.

Noseworthy, J. H. 1999. Progress in determining the causes and treatment of multiple sclerosis. *Nature* 399:A40.

O'Connor, Paul W. 1999. Reason for hope: the advent of disease modifying therapies in multiple sclerosis. *Canadian Medical Association* 162:83.

O'Hara, Ruth, 2000. Update on Alzheimer's disease: recent findings and treatments. *Western Journal of Medicine* 172:115.

Osher, R. H.1999. Cataract surgery combined with implantation of an artificial iris. *Journal of Cataract Refractory Surgery* 25:1540.

Palacios, Entrique, and Galdino Valvassori. 1999. Vestibular aqueduct syndrome. *ENT: Ear, Nose and Throat Journal* 78:676.

...epilepsy
...gs. *Pediatrics*

Pellock, John M. 199... syndromes with...ed atmospheric
104:1106. ...y. *Journal of Cataract*

Peters, N.T. 199...20.
pressure o... 999. Multiple sclerosis and
*Refracto...*em demyelination. *Journal of*
Pouly, S., ...:297.
centr...99. Progress in functional
Au...ery for Parkinson's disease. *The Lancet*
Quin... ...8.

...ant, A. D., et al. 1999. Sensory symptoms of
...ultiple sclerosis: a hidden reservoir of morbidity.
Multiple Sclerosis 5:179.

Ramsay, A. L. 1999. Simultaneous bilateral cataract
extraction. *Journal of Cataract Refractory Surgery*
25:753.

Ravalico, G. 1999. Effect of astigmatism on multifocal
intraocular lenses. *Journal of Cataract Refractive
Surgery* 25:804.

Rose, Verna L. 1999. Near sightedness and light exposure
during sleep. *American Family Physician* 60:328.

Rose, Verna L., and Paul R. Solomon. 1998. Study
evaluates for screening test for Alzheimer's disease.
American Family Physician 58:2099.

Rosenberg, Seth I. 1999. Vestibular surgery for Ménière's
disease in the elderly: a review of techniques and
indications. *Ear, Nose and Throat Journal* 78:443.

Rowsey, J. J. 1998. Surgical correction of moderate
myopia: Which method should you choose? I.
Radial keratotomy will always have a place. *Survey
of Ophthalmology* 43:147.

Rubinstein, J. T. 1999. How do cochlear prostheses
work? *Current Opinion Neurobiology* 9:399.

S disease. *Geriatrics* 55:26, 2000.

Sadovnick, A., et al. 1999. School based hepatitis B
vaccination program and adolescent multiple
sclerosis. *The Lancet* 355:549.

Sadovsky, Richard. 1998. Enalapril for attenuating renal
function decline in diabetes. *American Family
Physician* 58:1884.

Saw, S.M. 1999. Estimating the magnitude of close up
working school age children: a comparison of
questionnaire and diary instruments. *Ophthalmic
Epidemiology* 6:291.

Schapira, A. H. V. 1999. Parkinson's disease. *British
Medical Journal* 318:311.

Schein, Oliver D., et al. 2000. The value of routine
preoperative medical testing before cataract surgery.
New England Journal of Medicine 342:168.

Schwartz, Lisa B. 1998. Infertility and pregnancy in
epileptic women. *The Lancet* 352:1952.

Selai, C.E., et al. 2000. Quality of life pre and post
epilepsy surgery. *Epilepsy Resident* 38:67.

Senior, Kathryn. 1999. Inpatient rehabilitation helps
patients with multiple sclerosis. *The Lancet* 353:301.

Sharma, N. 1999. Complications of pediatric cataract
surgery and intraocular lens implantation. *Journal of
Cataract and Refractory Surgery* 25:1585.

Shinzato, M. 1999. Eye disease in a patient with
rheumatoid arthritis. *Postgraduate Medicine Journal*
75:676.

Shulan Hsieh, Lee Shia-Ying. 1998. Source memory in
Parkinson's disease. *Perceptual and Motor Skills*
89:355.

Shu-Li, Lin. 2000. Coping and adaptation in families of
children with cerebral palsy. *Exceptional Children*
66:201.

Skyler, Jay S. 1998. Simplifying the diagnosis of diabetes
mellitus. *American Family Physician* 58:1290.

Sloane, Philip D. 1998. Advances in the treatment of
Alzheimer's disease. *American Family Physician*
58:1577.

Smith, Philip E. M. 1998. The teenager with epilepsy.
British Medical Journal 317:960.

Smith, P.M., and C.L. Darlington. 1999. Recent
developments in drug therapy for multiple sclerosis.
Multiple Sclerosis 5:110.

Sperling, N.M.1999. A patient benefit evaluation of
unilateral congenital conductive hearing loss
presenting in adulthood: should it be repaired?
Laryngoscope 109:1386.

Spierer, A. 1999. Changes in astigmatism after cataract
extraction and intraocular lens implantation in
children. *Eye* 13:360.

Stacy, Mark. 1999. Parkinson's disease: therapeutic
choices and timing decision in patient management.
Geriatrics 54:44.

Steenerson, R.L. 1999. Treatment of tinnitus with
electrical stimulation. *Otolaryngology Head Neck
Surgery* 121:511.

Stern, C. 1999. New refractive surgery procedures in
ophthalmology and the influence on pilot's fitness
for flying. *European Journal of Medical Res*
4:382.

Storr-Paulsen, A. 1999. Possible factors modifying the surgically induced astigmatism in cataract surgery. *ACTA Ophthalmology Scand* 77:548.

Stuckey, B. 1999. Health promotion for cataract day case patients. *Professional Nurse* 14:638.

Sundaram, M., et al. 1999. EEG in epilepsy: current perspectives. *Canadian Journal of Neurology* 26:255.

Tandberg, E. 1999. Excessive daytime sleepiness and sleep benefit in Parkinson's disease: a community based study. *Mov Disord* 14:922.

Taniguchi, H. 1999. Cataract and retinal detachment in patients with severe atopic dermatitis who were withdrawn from the use of topical corticosteriod. *Journal of Dermatology* 26:658.

Thorne, Barbara. 1999. Living with diabetes as a transformational experience. *Qualitative Health Research* 9:786.

Tikellis G. 1999. The VECAT study: methodology and statistical power for measurement of age-related macular features. *Ophthalmic Epidemiology* 6:181.

Vittoria, Anne K. 1999. Our own little language: Naming and social construction of Alzheimer's disease. *Symbolic Interaction* 22:361.

Wallace, H., S. Shorvon, et al. 1998. Age specific incidence and prevalence rates of treated epilepsy in an unselected population of 2,052,922 and age specific fertility rates of women with epilepsy. *The Lancet* 352:1970.

Wallace, L. M. Alward. 1998. Medical management of glaucoma. *The New England Journal of Medicine* 339:1298.

When the diagnosis is Alzheimer's disease. *American Family Physician* 58:1589, 1998.

Wang, J. J. 1999. Cataract and age-related maculopathy: the Blue Mountain study. *Ophthalmic Epidemiology* 6:317.

Whitehead, E. 1999. Sudden sensorineural hearing loss with fracture of the stapes footplate following sneezing and parturition. *Clinical Otolaryngology* 24:462.

Wiebe, S., et al. 1999. Bu Health study. *Canadian 26:263.

Wiebe, Samuel. 2000. Managing the Ontario *British Medical Journal* 7226:

Wissel, J. 1999. Botulism toxin A of spastic gait disorders in childre adults with cerebral palsy. *Neurope 30:120

Wittink, Harriet, 2000. Pain in persons with ce palsy. *Physical Therapy* 80:199.

Woods, C. 1999. Clinical performance of an innova back surface multifocal contact lens in correcting presbyopia. *CLAO* 25:176.

Woolf, Steven H., and Stephen F. Rothemich. 1998. New diabetes guidelines: A closer look at the evidence. *American Family Physician* 58:1287.

Woolley, A. L. 1999. Risk factors for hearing loss from meningitis in children: the Children's Hospital experience. *Arch Otolaryngology Head Neck Surgery* 125:509.

Wunsch, Hannah. 1998. Abnormality in blood cytokines may cause cerebral palsy. *The Lancet* 352:1199.

Yamamoto, T. A patient with cerebral palsy whose mother had a traffic accident during pregnancy: a diffuse axonal injury? *Brain Development* 21:334.

Zadnik, K. 1999. Ocular predictors of the onset of juvenile myopia. *Invest Ophthalmol Vis Science* 40:1912.

Zafeirious, D.I. 1999. Characteristics and prognosis of epilepsy in children with cerebral palsy. *Journal of Child Neurology* 14:289.

Zenner, H. Peter, and Hans Leysieffer. 1998. Totally implantable hearing device for sensorineural hearing loss. *The Lancet* 352:1751.

GENETIC AND PEDIATRIC DISORDERS

O B J E C T I V E S

1. *Distinguish between the terms* **congenital** *and* **genetic.**

2. *Explain how genetic disorders may occur.*

3. *State characteristics of at least one disease that occurs because of (1) a chromosome abnormality, (2) a unifactorial defect, and (3) a multifactorial defect.*

4. *Tell what is meant by autosomal dominant, autosomal recessive, and X-linked recessive.*

5. *Explain why a chorionic villus biopsy may be preferred over amniocentesis.*

6. *Explain why the transmission of Huntington's chorea may be difficult to prevent.*

7. *Distinguish between sickle cell trait and sickle cell anemia.*

8. *Identify a common risk factor for having a child with Down syndrome and other genetic diseases.*

9. *Explain when and why drinking alcohol is a high risk for a pregnant woman.*

10. *Compare respiratory distress syndrome and sudden infant death syndrome.*

GENES AND GENETIC DISORDERS

Many theories have been developed over the years to explain how humans develop and why behavior differs from person to person. Early theorists believed the transmission of hereditary traits to be much simpler than we know it to be today. Knowledge in the field of genetics has grown at such a rapid pace that new findings outdate books on the subject before they are off the press.

In the last ten years, one of the most exciting occurrences in science has been the on-going project of the U.S. federal government—deciphering the human **genome.** The human genome is the totality of the hereditary

genome	JE-nom

information encoded in our genes. The Human Genome Project began in the late 1980s. The initial goals were: to construct a genetic map of the 100,000 or so genes that make up the human genome; produce a variety of physical maps that make DNA accessible to scientists for further research and, determine the complete sequence of human DNA. The original target date to complete the project was 2005 but, spurred on by competition from the private sector and faster progress than anticipated, completion of a "working draft" is scheduled for 2001 with completion of the full sequence by 2003. Once the project is completed, researchers will be able to determine how each gene functions—or malfunctions, to trigger illnesses. For some time it has been known that specific genes are a factor in some of the congenital disorders but this project has identified many more genes that play a role in human disease. Some of these can be seen in Table 18-1.

TABLE 18-1	Some of the Diseases Identified in the Human Genome Project	
Disorder	**System**	**Comments**
Alzheimer's Disease	CNS	Fourth leading cause of death in adults; incidence rises sharply with age; mutations in four genes are believed to play a role
Amyotrophic Lateral Sclerosis (ALS)	CNS	Also known as "Lou Gehrig's disease" after a famous baseball player who developed the disease; a gene has been identified as being associated with many cases of ALS; it is thought that anti-oxidants might help
Asthma	Respiratory	Affects more than 5% of the population in the United States; a number of genes contribute to a person's susceptibility to the disease; research on-going to identify specific genes
Atherosclerosis	Cardiovascular	A protein coded for by a gene found on chromosome 19 is important for removing excess cholesterol from the blood; many of the treatments proposed for this condition are in the experimental phase
Breast Cancer	Reproductive	Second major cause of cancer death in American women; two breast cancer susceptibility genes have been identified; general screening of the population for these genes could reduce mortality but is not recommended yet
Colon Cancer	Digestive	One of the most common inherited cancer syndromes; two key genes have been found to help repair mistakes in DNA replication; if they are mutated, mistakes aren't repaired, leading to damaged DNA and colon cancer
Cystic Fibrosis	Respiratory	Most common fatal genetic disease in the U.S. today; caused by a defective gene; several hundred mutations of the gene have been found; severity of disease related to particular mutations; the normal gene was cloned but treatment with it was not as successful as hoped; further research will be necessary before this "gene therapy" is useful in combating CF
Duchenne Muscular Dystrophy	Muscular	Most prevalent type of muscular dystrophy; all are X-linked, affecting many males
Diabetes Type I (Juvenile Onset)	Endocrine	Chronic metabolic disorder; greatly increases risk of blindness, heart disease, kidney failure, neurologic disease and other conditions; complex trait, mutations in several genes contribute to the disease; one identified on chromosome 6

TABLE 18-1	*Continued*	
Disorder	**System**	**Comments**
Glaucoma	CNS (Extension)	A group of diseases that can lead to damage to the eye and result in blindness; affects over 3 million Americans; asymptomatic at first; one gene identified related to nearly 100,000 cases; efforts to clone the gene are underway
Huntington's Disease	CNS	HD gene was identified in 1983 and cloned in 1993; a predictive test was developed enabling those at risk to find out if they will develop the disease
Lung Cancer	Respiratory	Most common cause of cancer deaths among both men and women; a deletion of part of chromosome 3 was first observed in 1982 but, like other cancers, mutations in a variety of genes have been observed; no one mutation is likely to result in cancerous growth
Malignant Melanoma	Integumentary (Skin)	Most aggressive kind of skin cancer; a mutation of a tumor suppressor gene on chromosome 9 has been identified; sun protection and early detection are still the best prevention
Obesity	Total body effect	Probably more than one cause genetic, environmental, psychological, and others; hormone leptin discovered about 3 years ago in mice; one related gene has been mapped to chromosome 7; much research needed to identify all the factors in obesity
Pancreatic Cancer	Endocrine	About 90% of pancreatic cancer shows a loss of part of chromosome 18; in 1996, a possible tumor suppressor gene was discovered from the section that is lost in pancreatic cancer; other tumor suppressor genes, if mutated or absent, can contribute to cancerous growth in a variety of tissue
Parkinson's Disease	CNS	Gene mapped in 1997 to chromosome 4; mutations of this gene have been linked to Parkinson's disease families; further research is needed to understand the exact function of the gene
Phenylketonuria (PKU)	Digestive	Caused by mutations in both alleles of a gene found on chromosome 12; with careful dietary supervision, children born with PKU can lead normal lives and mothers who have the disease can produce healthy children
Prostate Cancer	Reproductive	Second leading cause of cancer death in American men; susceptibility locus discovered on chromosome 1, may account for 1 in 500 cases; next step is to clone the gene

In October 1997, the CDC's Office of Genetics and Disease Prevention was established to coordinate the projects dealing with genetics in the CDC. The Human Genome Project is considered the most ambitious scientific investigation ever. With its completion, a valuable resource will be available for scientists in their unending search for the causes and subsequent cures for disease. However, with all the good it will do, this tremendous undertaking has already presented us with many difficult questions.

The U.S. Department of Energy (DOE) and the National Institutes of Health (NIH), co-sponsors of the project, were aware of the ethical, legal, and social issues related to gene mapping and allotted three percent to five percent of their annual Human Genome Project budgets toward studying these issues. ELSI (ethical, legal, and social issues) represents the largest bioethics program in the world and has become a model for other "ELSIs." Some of the issues that have been identified are:

- Fairness in the use of genetic information by insurers, employers, courts, schools, adoption agencies, and military, among others.
  - Who should have access and how will it be used?
- Privacy and confidentiality of genetic information.
  - Who owns and controls it?
- Psychologic impact and stigmatization caused by an individual's genetic differences.
  - How does the information affect an individual and society's perceptions of that individual?
- Genetic testing of an individual for a specific condition because of family history (prenatal, carrier, and presymptomatic testing) and population screening (newborn, premarital, and occupational).
  - Should testing be performed when no treatment is available?
  - Should parents have the right to have their minor children tested for adult-onset diseases?
  - Are genetic tests reliable and interpretable by the medical community?
- Reproductive issues including informed consent for procedures, use of genetic information in decision making, and reproductive rights.
- Clinical issues including education of health service providers, patients, and the general public; and implementation of standards and quality control measures in testing procedures.
- Commercialization of products: issues include property rights (patents, copyrights, and trade secrets) and accessibility of data and materials.
- Conceptual and philosophical implications regarding human responsibility, free will versus genetic determinism, and concepts of disease and health.*

*Adapted from "Human Genome Project Information: Ethical, Legal, and Social Issues," [www.ornl.gov/hgmis/resource/elsi.htm]

From great discoveries come great responsibility. This generation needs to become knowledgeable about the Human Genome Project and become involved so that the power of this information can be used humanely for all humanity.

Genetics now has three main branches: (1) **Mendelian** genetics, the study of the transmission of traits from one generation to the next; (2) molecular genetics, the study of the chemical structure of genes and how they operate at the molecular level; and (3) population genetics, the study of the variation of genes among and within populations. In this chapter, we will be most concerned with Mendelian and molecular genetics. The treatment will be necessarily brief, and students are urged to follow the literature in the field to increase their knowledge of genetics and keep up with new developments.

Genes

The essential ingredient of heredity is **deoxyribonucleic** acid (DNA). Along with some associated protein, DNA makes up the twenty-three pairs of chromosomes in the nuclei of all human cells. A gene corresponds to a small section of DNA on a chromosome. Each gene has the responsibility for directing the creation of a specific human trait, such as hair color or the lining of the stomach. It is estimated that each human cell holds more than 50,000 genes within its nucleus. These genes direct the development and functioning of every organ and system within the body.

With the exception of the egg and sperm cells, each cell in a person's body contains an identical set of genes. However, in different locations in the body, some genes are active and others are idle, depending upon the location. (For example, different genes are active in stomach cells than in liver cells.) We know that our genes have an important role in the structure and function of the body, but their role in personality, behavior, and mental ability is not as clear.

Each body cell has forty-six chromosomes (23 pairs), including two sex chromosomes. Females have a matched (**homologous**) pair, XX, whereas males have an unmatched (**heterologous**)

DID YOU KNOW?

A Wider Perspective

Marfan's syndrome is a rare disease, but famous people have been afflicted with the disorder. The sports world was shocked when Flo Hyman, a famous volleyball player, suddenly slipped off the bench on the sidelines of a game in Japan and was pronounced dead. Doctors suspected a heart attack, but an autopsy revealed that she had died of a ruptured aorta caused by Marfan's syndrome. People with the disorder are often taller than other family members and have arms that are disproportionately long. Defective genes are responsible for the syndrome, causing critical changes in the protein that gives connective tissue its strength. Marfan's syndrome victims also tend to have long fingers, deformities of the breastbone, and nearsightedness. Some experts believe that Abraham Lincoln may have had Marfan's syndrome because of his long fingers and great height. It is a difficult disease to diagnose and many times remains hidden until sudden death occurs as it did with Hyman. Even with all the physical examinations that athletes are exposed to, a hint of Marfan's syndrome was not detected by physicians. Flo Hyman was considered to be in excellent health.

pair, XY. Each gene occupies a specific place or locus on the chromosome. There are different loci for different traits, such as hair color, eye color, and so on. Genes are able to fulfill their function by directing the manufacture of proteins. The directions for making the necessary body proteins are encoded within the sequence of DNA that makes up the gene.

Whenever a cell divides, the DNA is first copied. This is an extremely complicated process and sometimes mistakes are made, resulting in mutant or defective genes that can lead to genetic disorders.

Genetic Disorders

A genetic disorder is any disorder caused by a defect or defects in the inherited genetic material. A genetic disorder may be congenital (with birth) or it may not appear for many years. There are many congenital disorders that are not genetic, and some of these will be discussed in this chapter also. See the Did You Know in this section.

With the exception of identical twins, every human being has a unique genetic makeup. Some of us have inherited a predisposition or susceptibility to certain diseases. If we do not come in contact with an initiating factor for a disease for which we are susceptible, we will never have it.

For example, if a man has a genetic makeup that makes him susceptible to lung cancer, but never smokes and never is exposed to smoke or other carcinogenic substances in the air, lung cancer is not likely to develop. Or consider a woman who has inherited a tendency for skin cancer but spends most of her time indoors and little time in the sun—she is not likely to get skin cancer.

For persons to have a genetic disorder, the genetic material that is abnormal must usually be present in each of their cells. For this to happen, the defect must be present in the egg or sperm cell (or both) from which the individuals were formed. This abnormal genetic material may have been present in the parent(s) at birth, or a mutation may have occurred during the formation of the egg or sperm cell. Because of mutations, a child with a genetic disorder may be born into a family that does not have a history of a known disorder. Figure 18-1 shows the pedigree of such a mutation in the royal family of England. One-third of the cases of hemophilia, which will be discussed later, are due to new mutations.

Mendelian	MEN-del-ean
deoxyribonucleic	de-OK-se-ri-bo-nu-kle-ik
homologous	ho-MOL-o-gus
heterologous	HET-er-ol-o-gus

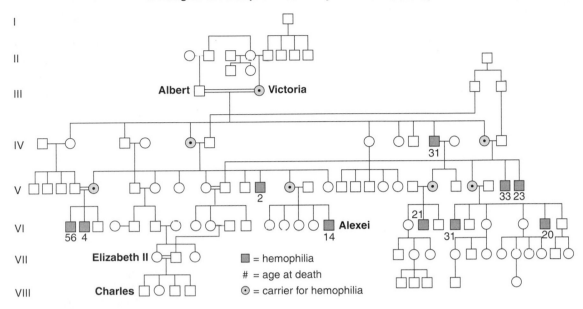

A Pedigree of Hemophilia in the Royal Families of Europe

Selected members of the pedigree
- I-1 = King George III
- III-1 and III-2= Prince Albert and Queen Victoria
- IV-5 and IV-6= Alice of Hesse and Ludwig IV of Hesse
- V-13 V-14= Alix and Nicholas II (Tsar of Russia)
- VI-16 = Alexei
- VIII-1 = Prince Charles

Figure 18-1

Partial pedigree for descendants of Queen Victoria showing the appearance of hemophilia A in one of her sons and his descendants and the descendants of her daughters and granddaughters. Black squares indicate hemophiliacs; black spots indicate carriers.

Classifications of Genetic Disease

Genetic diseases can be broadly classified as caused by chromosome abnormalities, unifactorial defects, and multifactorial defects. Down syndrome is the best known example of a chromosome abnormality. Children born with this disorder have an extra chromosome. Unifactorial disorders occur rarely, but there are many of them. They are caused by a single defective gene or pair of genes. Unifactorial disorders can be divided into three groups:

Autosomal dominant disorders occur when a person carries only one defective gene, but because it is dominant, it overrides the normal gene and the individual can get the disease. Examples include Huntington's chorea and Marfan's syndrome.

Autosomal recessive disorders occur when a recessive defective gene is acquired from both parents who are carriers and have no apparent disease. With two recessive genes for the same disease, the child will get the disease. Examples of such disorders are cystic fibrosis and sickle cell anemia.

X-linked recessive disorders occur when the defective gene is on the X chromosome. As has been stated earlier, women have two X chromosomes and men have one X and one Y. Men get the X chromosome from their mothers and pass it on to their daughters. When a woman inherits a defective single sex gene, it is masked by the gene on her other X chromosome, and she has no apparent disease. When a man inherits the defective gene, he has no normal X gene on another chromosome, and he will get the disease.

Examples are color blindness, hemophilia, and muscular dystrophy.

There are many disorders that fall into the category of multifactorial disorders. These disorders are thought to be determined by a number of different genes plus environmental influences. Examples of multifactorial disorders can be seen in Table 18-2.

TABLE 18-2	Noninfectious Diseases Thought to Have Genetic Predispositions	
Disease	**Associated Pathophysiology or Hypothesis**	**Environmental Factors**
Coronary heart disease (especially early disease) (several different syndromes)	Familial hypercholesterolemia	Dietary fat, saturated fat, polyunsaturated fat, total fat intake
	LDL recetor defects	
	Other high cholesterol?	Exercise, alcohol, diet
	Low HDL	Smoking
	Endothelial factors?	
	Diabetes I and II	
	Hypertension (especially early onset)	
	Multiplicative interactions of history and risk factors	
Stroke	Hypertension and diabetes	
Hypertension	Age at onset?	Salt, stress, obesity
	Severity? Etiology?	Polyunsaturated fat, calcium, exercise
Type I diabetes	Islet cell destruction	Viral infection
	Immunologic cause	Seasonal variation
		Complications a function of blood sugar control for years
Type II diabetes	Insulin resistance or decreased production	Obesity
		Dietary sugar and fiber
		Exercise protective
		Complications a function of blood sugar control and function
Breast cancer	Possibly estrogen related	Age at first birth
	Certain benign tumor precursors	Alcohol?
		Female hormones
Colon cancer	Several different types of syndromes	Fiber intake
	Often benign polyps are precursors	Dietary fat? (converted by bacteria to carcinogens)

| | TABLE 18-2   *Continued* | |

Disease	Associated Pathophysiology or Hypothesis	Environmental Factors
Lung cancer	Chemical carcinogens from environment encounter enzymatically susceptible subjects	Cigarette smoke Environmental pollutants Radiation exposure
Rheumatic heart disease	Immunologic cross-reactivity to bacteria and heart valves	Strep bacterial infection
Asthma and other allergies	Immunologically reactive	Many possible allergens—fur, dust, pollen, mold, etc.
Autoimmune disorders	Autoantibodies to thyroid, adrenal, synovium, platelets	Viral infections trigger immune responses
Psychiatric disorders: manic-depressive, depression, schizophrenia	Neurochemical disorders in brain tissue	Uncertain influence Dramatic success with drug treatment for first two
Kidney stones	Mineral-acid-base imbalance	Milk? Soda pop? Other fluids?
Gallstones	Fat, cholesterol, bilirubin balance	Dietary fat Obesity?
Obesity	Less energy wasted? Decreased thermogenesis in brown fat?	Dietary fat, sugar, and total calories Stress, etc., affecting appetite Exercise level Cultural perceptions attractive to be fat or thin
Gout	Several different enzyme defects found	Dietary intake of meat, etc.
Multiple sclerosis	Autoimmune demyelination of nerve fibers	Slow virus? Climate dependent
Peptic ulcer disease	Excess acid production and/or decreased mucosal resistance	Stress Diet Dramatic drug Rx
Lactose intolerance	Deficiency of lactase enzyme in intestinal mucosa	Milk products
Alcoholism	Possible neurochemical origin? Associated with other psychiatric disorders	Ethyl alcohol intake Social factors

Research in and Determination of Genetic Disease Prevention

Scientists have developed the capability of manipulating some genes before birth to prevent genetic diseases or provide each of us with the defenses to ward off disease. The procedures are still in the experimental stage for the most part, and there are hard ethical problems to be solved before these procedures can be used on humans. Tests have been used for some time that can detect genetic defects in the unborn fetus. Figure 18-2 shows one of these tests, **amniocentesis.** Another test used to identify genetic defects in the fetus is **chorionic villus** biopsy. This technique can be done earlier in the pregnancy (2 months) than amniocentesis (5 months), resulting in earlier diagnosis. However, there is more chance of miscarriage with chorionic villus biopsy. Both procedures have advantages and disadvantages.

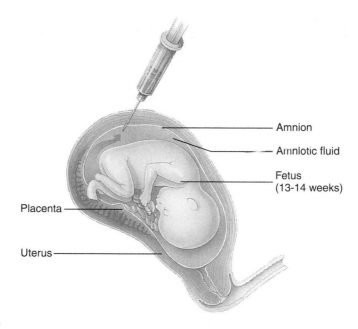

Figure 18-2
Amniocentesis.

AUTOSOMAL DOMINANT DISORDER

Huntington's Chorea

Huntington's chorea is an inherited disease of the central nervous system that usually has its onset between the ages of thirty and fifty. Patients gradually lose their mental capabilities and musculoskeletal control. Death usually results ten to fifteen years after onset of the disease, from suicide, congestive heart failure, or pneumonia.

Because of the late onset of Huntington's, the victim has often had children before the disease becomes apparent. Because many families tend not to talk about any relative who has a neurologic disorder, there may be no record or recollection of anyone in the family having Huntington's. The stigma of "mental" disease has not yet been overcome, even with our increased understanding of the cause of these disorders. Therefore, this disease, which results in so much suffering and an early death, is unknowingly passed on from generation to generation.

Predisposing Factors
If a parent has had the disease, each child has a fifty percent chance of inheriting it.

Symptoms
The disease begins slowly with momentary loss of balance. Gradually, symptoms become more pronounced, with progressively severe uncontrolled movements. In the beginning, these movements are unilateral and occur more in the legs, arms, and face. As the chorea becomes more violent, the patient also loses mental competence, and personality changes such as obstinacy, untidiness, apathy, and paranoia take place.

Prevention
No preventive measures are known.

Treatment
There is no known cure for Huntington's, and treatment is aimed at relieving symptoms and

amniocentesis	AM-ne-o-sen-TE-sis
chorionic villus	ko-re-ON-ik VIL-us

CASE STUDY

Huntington's Disease

Ted M. was a married man with two daughters and a son. He was in the army, exercised regularly, and was well liked by friends and family. Ted was thirty-five years old when he became depressed and complained of fatigue after physical effort. He was transferred to work in the office and discharged with honor. In the next few years his symptoms became worse as he started to have difficulty with his balance, had several accidents and had trouble concentrating. Ted went to see his doctor and after a routine physical, was referred to a neurologist. He was diagnosed with Huntington's disease. He had not known that anyone in the family had had it but realized his father had some of the same symptoms. Ted's condition gradually deteriorated until he could no longer be managed at home and spent the last few years of his life in an extended-care facility.

---

providing support. Drugs can help control the involuntary movements and alleviate depression and discomfort. Emotional support and genetic counseling are needed for patient and family to help them understand the disease.

AUTOSOMAL RECESSIVE DISORDERS

Cystic Fibrosis

Cystic fibrosis is an inherited disease of the exocrine glands, affecting the pancreas, respiratory system, and sweat glands. One gene for cystic fibrosis, located on the long arm of chromosome 7, must be inherited from each parent. Cystic fibrosis kills more children than any other genetic disease. The average life span has improved from age sixteen to age twenty-eight or older.

Predisposing Factors

The disease is more common in children of Central European ancestry and rare in blacks. In a family in which both parents carry the defective gene, there is a twenty-five percent chance in every pregnancy that the baby will develop the disease.

Symptoms

In the newborn, intestinal mucus may be so sticky that it blocks the bowel, which leads to obstruction, rupture, and even death. The child does not gain weight, although a good appetite is present. The air passages in the lungs become blocked with mucus, leading to collapsed lungs and emphysema. Chronic respiratory infection and heat intolerance are also symptoms of the disease. If the child lives long enough, the bile ducts may become obstructed, leading to cirrhosis with portal hypertension. Many children with cystic fibrosis also have diabetes mellitus.

Prevention

No preventive measures are known.

Treatment

Because there is no cure at present, the goal of treatment is to help the child live as normal a life as possible. Breathing exercises, physical therapy, and postural drainage help to manage the lung problems, and antibiotics can be used to hold off the threat of staphylococcal pneumonia. Oral pancreatic enzymes are used to offset the enzyme deficiencies. Extra salt on food and salt tablets in hot weather are used to combat electrolyte loss through sweating. Air conditioners and humidifiers help to decrease vulnerability to respiratory infections, and oxygen therapy is used as needed. The patient and the family need education about the disease and emotional support throughout the illness. Heart and/or lung transplants may be performed if the patient lives long enough.

Phenylketonuria

Phenylketonuria, or PKU, is an inherited disorder in which an enzyme that converts phenylalanine (an amino acid) into tyrosine (another amino acid) is defective. When phenylalanine builds up in the body, it causes severe mental retardation. About one baby in 14,000 is born with PKU in the United States.

Predisposing Factors
PKU is transmitted by a recessive gene. The incidence is higher among those of Celtic origin and Central Europeans.

Symptoms
Babies generally show no signs of PKU at birth, but by four months of age, neurologic disturbances, including epilepsy, become evident. PKU babies have an unpleasant musty, mousy smell about them caused by a breakdown product of phenylalanine excreted in their sweat and urine. Most of these children (90%) have blond hair and blue eyes that are effects of the condition. They may also have eczema, an abnormally large head, and a steep decline in IQ during the first year. They may be hyperactive, irritable, and display purposeless, repetitive motions.

Prevention
Early screening for PKU (by blood test) is now mandatory in most states and is the best means of prevention. Early detection and treatment of the disorder can minimize the damage to the central nervous system.

Treatment
PKU is treated with a diet free of phenylalanine, which is a natural constituent of most protein foods. Milk substitutes are given to babies, and after weaning they are given a very low protein diet that is mainly vegetarian. Some physicians believe this diet should be followed throughout life, but others believe it can be discontinued by the age of twelve years.

Sickle Cell Anemia

Individuals with sickle cell anemia have blood cells that are abnormal and become sickle shaped and thus unable to carry sufficient oxygen. The genetic defect is largely confined to blacks and is transmitted as a dominant characteristic by either sex. If both parents carry the defective gene, the child will have sickle cell anemia. If only one parent carries the gene, the child will have *sickle cell trait,* which means being a carrier of the disease. Approximately two out of every twenty-five black people carry the disease. The sickle cell trait may provide protection from malaria.

Predisposing Factors
Most of those with sickle cell anemia are members of the black race.

Symptoms
The symptoms, which usually do not occur until after six months of age, include heart problems, fatigue, breathlessness on exertion, joint swelling, and leg ulcers, especially around the ankles. Upon getting older, the child has acute crises when the anemia is intensified and suffers from severe abdominal pain and other symptoms, depending on the type of crisis.

Prevention
No preventive measures are known.

Treatment
When an acute crisis occurs, the child is hospitalized for transfusions. At other times, the patient can stay at home and be treated for the symptoms.

X-LINKED RECESSIVE DISORDER

Hemophilia A

Hemophilia is an inherited bleeding disorder that occurs because of a deficiency of certain clotting factors. There are several different forms of hemophilia, but A is the most common. Most hemophiliacs are male, because it is an X-linked recessive trait. Women who are carriers have a fifty percent chance of passing the disease on to their sons but transmit only the gene to their daughters (50% chance also). About one male in 10,000 is born with hemophilia. Affected males pass the gene on

---

Phenylketonuria   FEN-il-KE-to-NU-re-a

to none of their sons but to all of their daughters, who become carriers of the condition. In about one third of the cases, there is no family history of hemophilia. Since the advent of AIDS, the problems of hemophiliacs have increased because of the chance of transmission of AIDS through blood transfusions, which hemophiliacs must have to treat their condition (Figure 18-3). Blood screening has reduced the risk of transmission by transfusion until it is now estimated that chances of getting HIV in this way are one in several million.

Predisposing Factors

Hemophilia is passed on from mothers who are carriers to half of their sons, who are born with the condition, or to half of their daughters, who become carriers. All daughters of hemophiliac fathers are carriers. Rarely, the daughter of a father with hemophilia and a mother who is a carrier may have hemophilia.

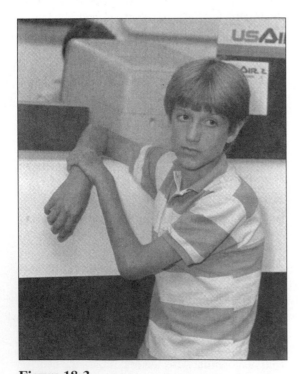

Figure 18-3

Ryan White, hemophiliac who contracted AIDS because of blood transfusions.

Symptoms

There is great variation in symptoms among those who have hemophilia. Most bleeding episodes involve hemorrhage into joints and muscles. They often begin when an affected child begins to walk and becomes susceptible to falls. Pain accompanies the bleeding episodes, and if they are not treated, there may be crippling of the joints involved. If it is a mild case, it may not be diagnosed until surgery or some other major trauma causes bleeding. In addition to the pain, there may be other symptoms, depending upon the location of the bleeding, which may be internal as well as external.

Prevention

Children who have hemophilia need to avoid activities that expose them to risk of injury, such as contact sports. If a person who has hemophilia must have surgery, careful management is needed by a physician who has expertise in hemophilia care.

Treatment

Fifty years ago, most hemophiliacs did not survive to adulthood. Today, bleeding episodes can be controlled by a transfusion. Infusions of the missing clotting factor should be given as quickly as possible after the start of bleeding. Because of the threat of HIV in the blood supply, efforts are under way to develop a synthetic replacement for the clotting factor that hemophiliacs need.

CHROMOSOMAL ABNORMALITIES

Down Syndrome

Down syndrome occurs in one per 650 births overall. A child with Down syndrome has forty-seven chromosomes instead of forty-six. This genetic disorder may be inherited from either of the two parents, who may have no physical or mental abnormalities themselves. Life expectancy for individuals with Down syndrome is short, with up to one-third dying before ten years of age.

Predisposing Factors

The age of the mother at the time of birth seems to be a significant factor in the development of Down syndrome, because the incidence increases with mothers older than thirty-five.

Symptoms

Some typical signs and symptoms of the disorder are mental retardation; slanting, almond-shaped eyes; protruding tongue, small skull, abnormal dental development, small ears, and short neck (Figure 18-4). These persons often have heart disease, pelvic bone abnormalities, poorly developed genitalia, and delayed puberty. They are especially susceptible to leukemia and chronic infections.

Prevention

No preventive measures are known.

Treatment

Surgery to correct heart defects and antibiotics for chronic infections have helped to extend life for these individuals. They can be cared for at home or may be institutionalized. There is no cure.

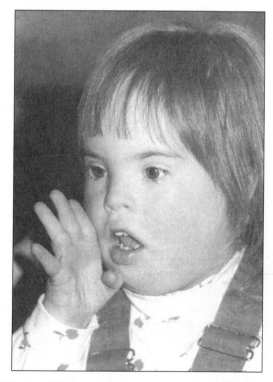

Figure 18-4
A child with Down syndrome.

Klinefelter's Syndrome

One in every 600 males has Klinefelter's syndrome, a genetic abnormality resulting from one or more extra X chromosomes. This disease is usually not apparent until puberty, when the secondary sex characteristics develop. Although this genetic disorder occurs only in males, Turner's syndrome is a similar disorder in females. Both syndromes result in sterility. However, Turner's syndrome occurs in only one out of 10,000 live female births.

Predisposing Factors

The disorder usually results from one extra chromosome. The possibility of this occurrence increases with the age of the mother, as with many other genetic disorders.

Symptoms

Mild cases may not have any apparent symptoms. The inability of a couple to conceive may be the first indication of the infertility of the male. Some of the characteristic features are a small penis and prostate; small, firm testicles; sparse facial and abdominal hair; impotence, and **gynecomastia.** The syndrome is also associated with mental retardation, osteoporosis, alcoholism, antisocial behavior, increased incidence of pulmonary disease, and breast cancer.

Prevention

No preventive measures are known.

Treatment

Hormonal treatment and psychotherapy to treat emotional problems, with acceptance of the disorder, are the best treatment, sometimes mastectomy in extreme cases. Nothing can be done to deter the changes that lead to infertility.

COMMON DISORDERS IN INFANTS AND CHILDREN

A number of disorders are present at birth that are not due to genetic abnormalities, but rather to unfavorable environmental factors for the fetus, or to lack of sufficient developmental time in the womb.

gynecomastia ji-ne-ko-MAS-te-a

The damage that can be caused to the baby by disease agents such as syphilis, gonorrhea, and rubella when they infect the mother during pregnancy has already been mentioned. In addition, some congenital disorders have been associated with the use of cocaine and other illegal drugs. Disorders that may occur because of prenatal drug use are spontaneous abortion, detached placentas, premature deliveries, sudden infant deaths, fetal urogenital tract malformations, and low birth weight. Women who smoke regularly during pregnancy also tend to have low-birth-weight babies, and those who drink may deliver a baby with fetal alcohol syndrome. Three of the most common of these disorders are discussed in the rest of this chapter.

Fetal Alcohol Syndrome

Fetal alcohol syndrome (FAS) is a combination of birth defects found in a baby at birth. Alcohol and tobacco both interfere with the growth of the fetus. Alcohol crosses the placenta in an amount equal to that in the mother's bloodstream. The fetal liver is underdeveloped and cannot oxidize the alcohol, and as a result the fetal brain is soaked in alcohol until the mother's blood alcohol count drops.

Almost twenty percent of these babies die during the first few weeks of life.

Predisposing Factors

FAS results when a pregnant woman consumes alcohol. It is now thought that any amount of alcohol can cause difficulties for the fetus, but most cases of FAS occur in babies whose mothers were heavy drinkers during pregnancy. Alcohol consumed during the first three months is especially damaging to the fetus. Binge drinking is thought to be particularly harmful, because it produces high blood alcohol levels.

Symptoms

Low birth weight, small head, mental retardation, learning disabilities, joint problems, and heart abnormalities are included in the signs and symptoms of FAS. FAS babies also tend to have distinctive facial features: small eyes that have vertical skin folds extending from the upper eyelid to the side of the nose, and a small jaw (Figure 18-5). The baby may also have a small brain, cleft palate, heart defects, a dislocated hip, and other joint deformities. As a newborn, the baby sleeps badly, sucks poorly, and is irritable because of alcohol withdrawal.

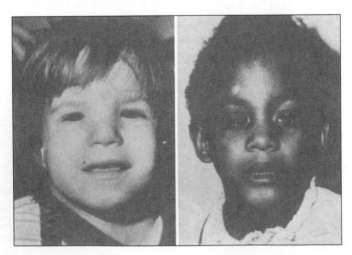

Figure 18-5
Children with fetal alcohol syndrome.

Prevention

Most experts now believe that a woman should abstain from drinking if there is a chance she could be pregnant. Because the worst damage can occur in the first few months, any woman who has unprotected intercourse should not drink until she knows she did not conceive.

Treatment

Treatment depends upon the type and extent of defects. Some defects can be corrected, but the mental and physical retardation will last for life.

Respiratory Distress Syndrome

The most common cause of death of newborn babies, respiratory distress syndrome (RDS), results in 40,000 deaths every year. This lung disorder causes increasing difficulty in breathing, resulting in insufficient oxygen in the blood.

Predisposing Factors

A deficiency of **surfactant,** a chemical that keeps the alveoli open, is the cause of the syndrome in babies. It occurs most often in premature babies. About three percent of newborn babies die of RDS.

Symptoms

Babies make grunting noises and draw in the chest wall when they breathe. The baby will eventually turn blue as the condition worsens, and death may result if treatment is not given.

Prevention

Prenatal care to help the woman carry her baby to full term could reduce the risk of RDS in newborns.

Treatment

Babies who have the disorder are kept in an intensive care unit, where they can be given oxygen. If the condition worsens, they may need an endotracheal tube inserted through the nose or mouth, or a tracheostomy.

Sudden Infant Death Syndrome

When a baby is found dead in its crib and there is no known reason for its death, sudden infant death syndrome (SIDS) is suspected. SIDS is the most common cause of death for infants one month to one year old in the United States and other developed countries. Three quarters of the time the baby is under six months of age. SIDS occurs slightly more frequently in boys, among second children, and in cold weather. For reasons unknown, more of these deaths occur between midnight and 9 a.m. and on weekends. Most experts believe there is no single cause of SIDS and that most deaths are caused by a respiratory or cardiac abnormality.

Predisposing Factors

Risk factors include prematurity, low birth weight, bottle feeding, and cold weather; young, single mothers; smoking, drug addiction, or anemia in the mother; poor socioeconomic background; the death of a brother or sister as a result of SIDS; and infants who have been discovered near death and were revived.

Symptoms

No symptoms have been identified for certain, but it is known that some of the babies have mild cold symptoms for several days previous to the death, and some have shown unexplained loss of weight.

Prevention

When the cause of a death cannot be identified, there is no way of being positive about preventive measures. It is possible that good prenatal care, avoidance of smoking, alcohol, and drugs during pregnancy, good obstetric care, breast-feeding, and close observation of any baby who has symptoms of being sick, no matter how minor, could help. Recently, studies have shown that infants who sleep on their backs are less likely to have SIDS. There is an alarm that can be used to detect if a baby stops breathing, but there is no evidence that use of this will prevent the disease.

Treatment

There is obviously no treatment for SIDS. However, it is such a shock to the family that it is important that they have help in working through their grief and probable feelings of guilt.

surfactant	sur-FAK-tant

SUMMARY

Genetics is one of the most rapidly developing fields in science. Transmission of the genetic code is complicated, but scientists have deciphered much of it and are on the verge of being able to correct genetic defects before birth. Ethical problems will need to be addressed.

Genes direct the development and functioning of every organ and organ system in the body. We are not sure how much genes have to do with personality characteristics, but everyone inherits characteristics that might protect them from certain diseases, as well as predispositions to certain diseases that may be triggered by an initiating factor.

Genetic diseases may be caused by chromosome abnormalities, unifactorial defects, or multifactorial defects. Unifactorial disorders may be autosomal dominant, autosomal recessive, or X- linked recessive. There are many multifactorial disorders, and some believe that a genetic factor may be present in every disease. If all goes according to schedule, by 2003 all human genes will be identified and located as a result of the Human Genome Project.

Tests have been used for some time to detect defects in the fetus. If defects are found, parents must make a difficult choice. It is hoped that genetic engineering may eventually make the choice unnecessary.

Table 18-3 summarizes relevant data on genetic and pediatric disorders.

TABLE 18-3	Genetic and Pediatric Disorders			
Disorder	**Special Characteristics**	**Predisposing Factors**	**Common Symptoms**	**Prevention/ Treatment**
Huntington's Disease	Onset between 30 and 50; death 10-15 years after onset from suicide, heart failure, or pneumonia	Parent with disease—50% chance	Begin slowly, become more pronounced gradually; loss of mental capabilities and musculoskeletal control; personality changes—apathy and paranoia	No known prevention; cannot be cured; treatment to ease symptoms only
Cystic Fibrosis	Disease of the exocrine glands; half die by age of 16, rest by age of 30	Genetic	Sticky mucus blocks bowel in newborn—may lead to rupture and death; child does not gain weight; air passages become blocked with mucus leading to emphysema; respiratory infection, heat	No prevention or cure, treatment is palliative

TABLE 18-3	*Continued*			
Disorder	**Special Characteristics**	**Predisposing Factors**	**Common Symptoms**	**Prevention/ Treatment**
Cystic Fibrosis— Cont'd			intolerance, eventually cirrhosis with portal hypertension	
Sickle Cell Anemia	Red blood cells sickle shaped; mostly in black race; carriers have sickle cell trait	Parents with disorder; member of black race	Heart problems, fatigue, joint swelling, leg ulcers, breathlessness on exertion; later, acute crises: anemia intensified	No prevention, no cure, hospitalized during acute crises
Down Syndrome	1 per 650 births, short life expectancy; child has an extra chromosome; may be inherited from either parent	Mother past 35 at time of birth	Typical symptoms include: mental retardation, slanting almond-shaped eyes, protruding tongue, small skull, abnormal dental development, small ears, short neck; often have heart disease, and puberty is delayed; especially susceptible to leukemia and chronic infections	No prevention and no cure; treatment for defects when possible
Klinefelter's Syndrome	One in 600 males; have 1 or more extra X chromosomes; usually not apparent until puberty; Turner's syndrome in	Possibility increases with age of mother	Penis and testicles fail to develop; infertility; mental deficiency and gynecomastia tendency; also associated with some chronic	No prevention; can be treated with hormones and psychotherapy; changes leading to infertility cannot be deterred

TABLE 18-3	*Continued*			
Disorder	**Special Characteristics**	**Predisposing Factors**	**Common Symptoms**	**Prevention/ Treatment**
Klinefelter's Syndrome— Cont'd	women is similar but occurs in only 1 in 10,000 live female births		diseases; may be no apparent symptoms	
Hemophilia A	Several kinds, "A" is most common; deficiency in clotting factor; passed from mother to sons; gene only passed on to daughters, disease passed on to sons; 1/3 of cases have no family history of disorder; some have become infected with HIV from transfusions	Fifty percent of sons of mother who is a carrier are born hemophiliacs	Main symptom is uncontrollable bleeding accompanied by pain; degree varies; sometimes not diagnosed until surgery or other major trauma causes bleeding	Children need to avoid activities that may cause injury; there must be careful management of any surgery; treatment is by transfusion; synthetic clotting factor may be developed
Phenylketonuria	Child is born without an enzyme necessary for amino acid conversion; one in 12,000 born with PKU in the U.S.	Recessive gene; Celtic or Central European origin	Neurologic disturbances, musty, mousy smell; blond hair, blue eyes caused by condition; eczema, large head, steep decline in IQ; may be hyperactive, irritable, display repetitive motions	Early detection and treatment are best prevention; diet controlled to be free of phenylalanine, milk substitutes and very low protein diet; some doctors believe the diet can be discontinued
Fetal Alcohol Syndrome	Alcohol crosses placental membrane, underdeveloped fetal liver cannot	Alcohol in any amount during first 3 months of pregnancy can produce	Low birth weight, small head, mental retardation, joint problems, heart	Any woman who has a chance of becoming pregnant should not

TABLE 18-3	*Continued*			
Disorder	**Special Characteristics**	**Predisposing Factors**	**Common Symptoms**	**Prevention/ Treatment**
Fetal Alcohol Syndrome— Cont'd	oxidize it; baby's brain soaked in alcohol until mother's blood alcohol drops; almost 20% die within first few weeks of life	damage; binge drinking any time dangerous to fetus	abnormalities; tend to have distinctive facial features; any other defects possible	drink any beverage containing alcohol; some defects can be corrected but mental and physical retardation last for life
Respiratory Distress Syndrome	Most common cause of death in newborn babies	Deficiency of surfactant that is necessary to keep alveoli open; occurs mostly in premature babies	Grunting noises and chest wall drawn in when breathing; baby will turn blue and die without treatment	Good prenatal care to produce full term babies; treatment is in an intensive care unit where oxygen can be given and a tracheostomy performed if necessary
Sudden Infant Death Syndrome	Baby found dead in crib for no apparent reason; most common cause of infant death in 1 month to 1 year olds; most of time, baby is under 6 months; more on weekends and between midnight and 9 a.m.	Prematurity, low birth weight; bottle feeding; cold weather; young, single mother; smoking, drug addiction, or anemia in the mother; poor socioeconomic background; death of sibling from SIDS; infant discovered near death and revived	May be mild cold symptoms, and/or unexplained weight loss; none identified for sure	Placing baby on back to sleep may help; family needs help with grief and possible guilt feelings

QUESTIONS FOR REVIEW

1. What is the Human Genome Project?
2. For what are genes responsible?
3. How do genes fulfill their function?
4. What is DNA?
5. What does an initiating factor have to do with disease?
6. How does a genetic disorder occur?
7. Define and give examples of the following: chromosome abnormality, unifactorial defect, multifactorial defect, autosomal dominant, autosomal recessive, X-linked recessive.
8. What is the difference between amniocentesis and chorionic villus biopsy?
9. What is genetic engineering?
10. Why is it difficult to keep the genetic defect that causes Huntington's chorea from being transmitted?
11. What is the progression of the symptoms for Huntington's chorea?
12. Why is cystic fibrosis such a devastating disease?
13. What physiologic problems can a child with cystic fibrosis have?
14. What are some of the therapies that may be used for cystic fibrosis?
15. What is the difference between sickle cell anemia and sickle cell trait?
16. Why can some individuals who are not black develop sickle cell anemia?
17. What are the symptoms of sickle cell anemia in the beginning stages and as the child gets older?
18. How often does Down syndrome occur?
19. What are the risk factors for Down syndrome?
20. What are the symptoms of Down syndrome?
21. What causes Klinefelter's syndrome?
22. What is the predisposing factor for Klinefelter's syndrome?
23. What are the chances that a baby will be born with hemophilia?
24. What are the chances of being infected with HIV through a blood transfusion?
25. What can be said about the symptoms of hemophilia?
26. How may it be possible for the person with hemophilia to avoid blood transfusions in the future?
27. What causes phenylketonuria?
28. What are the symptoms of PKU?
29. What is the best prevention for PKU?
30. How is PKU treated?
31. Why may one alcoholic drink be dangerous for the fetus?
32. What are the symptoms of fetal alcohol syndrome?
33. How can fetal alcohol syndrome be prevented?
34. What causes respiratory distress syndrome in babies?
35. What are the symptoms of RDS?
36. How is RDS treated?
37. What is the most common cause of death in infants in the United States?
38. What is thought to be the cause of sudden infant death syndrome?
39. What symptoms have been identified for SIDS?
40. What can be said about prevention and treatment for SIDS?

FURTHER READING

Acosta, P. B. "Nutrient intake and growth of infants with phenylketonuria." *J Pediatr Gatroenterol Nutr,* Sep. '98, 27(3):287–91.

Andrews, T. C., et al. 1999. Huntington's disease progression. *PET and clinical observations* 122:842.

"A new gene map of the human genome." The International RH Mapping Consortium, GeneMap '98, National Center for Biotechnology Information, National Library of Medicine, National Institute of Health. www.ncbi.nlm.nih.gov/genemap98.

Arnold, G. L. "Factors affecting cognitive, motor, behavioral, and executive functioning in children with phenylketonuria." *Acta Pediatr* 87:565.

Aurora, P., et al. 1999. Lung transplantation and life extension in children with cystic fibrosis. *The Lancet* 354:1591.

Bagasra, O. 1998. Viral burden and disease progression in HIV-1- infected patients with sickle cell anemia. *American Journal of Hematology* 59:199.

Barr-Agholme, M. 1998. Periodontal conditions and salivary immunoglobulins in individuals with Down syndrome. *Journal of Periodontology* 69:1119.

Bilenker, J. H. 1998. The costs of children with sickle cell anemia: Preparing for managed care. *Journal of Pediatric Hematology Oncology* 20:528.

Blair, Peter. 1999. Babies sleeping with parents: case control study of factors influencing the risk of the sudden infant death syndrome. *British Medical Journal* 319:7223.

Bonelli, Raphael, Peter Koltringer, et al. 1998. Reversible Huntingdon's disease? *The Lancet* 352:1520.

Bosch, Xavier. 1998. Geneticists discuss ethics of human genome project. *The Lancet* 352:1448.

Centerwall, Siegried, A., and Willard R. Centerwall. 2000. The discovery of phenylketonuria: The story of a young couple, two retarded children. *Pediatrics* 105:17.

Chan, D. Q. 1999. Fetal alcohol syndrome. *Optom Vis Sci* 76:678.

Collins, Francis S., Ari Patrinos, Elke Jordan, et al. 1998. New goals for the US human genome project: 1998-2003. *Science* 282:682.

Collins, Marietta, Nadine Kaslow, Karla Doepke, et al. 1998. Psychosocial interventions for children and adolescents with sickle cell disease. *Journal of Black Psychology* 24:432.

Cusick, W. 1999. Fetal Down syndrome screening: A cost effectiveness analysis of alternative screening programs. *Journal of Maternal Fetal Medicine* 8:243.

Decrutenaere, M. 1999. Psychological functioning before predictive testing for Huntington's disease: The role of the parental disease, risk perception, and subjective proximity of the disease. *Journal of Medical Genetics* 36:897.

Development of guidelines for treatment of children with phenylketonuria. *Pediatrics* 104:1376, 1999.

Dwyer, Terence, Anne-Louise Ponsonby, et al. 1999. Tobacco smoking exposure at one month of age and subsequent risk of SIDS a prospective study. *American Journal of Epidemiology* 149:593.

Emery, J.L., et al. 1999. Debate on cot death. *British Medical Journal* 320:310.

Feigin, A. Advances in Huntington's disease: implications for experimental therapeutics. *Curr Opin Neurol,* Aug. '98, 11:357.

Foca, M., et al. 1999. Rational treatment of pulmonary infections in patients with cystic fibrosis. *Current Opinion in Infectious Diseases* 12:257.

Glass, Richard. 1999. Facts about sickle cell anemia. *Journal of the American Medical Association* 281:36.

Guggino, W. B. 1999. Cystic fibrosis and the salt controversy. *Cell* 96:607.

Halvorson, D.J. 1998. Management of chronic sinusitis in the adult cystic fibrosis patient. *Annals of Otology, Rhinology and Laryngology* 107:946.

Hardin, D.S. 1999. Diabetes mellitus in cystic fibrosis. *Endocrinology Metabolism Clinic of North America* 28:787.

Hasleton, P.S. 1999. Adult respiratory distress syndrome. *Histopathology* 34:285.

Haworth, Charles S., Peter L. Selby, et al. 1998. Severe bone pain after intravenous pamidronate in adult patients with cystic fibrosis. *The Lancet* 352:1753.

Hoffmann, N. 1999. Understanding the neuropsychiatric symptoms of Huntington's disease. *Journal of Neuroscience Nursing* 31:309.

Hudson, Thomas J. 1998. The human genome project: Tools for the identification of disease genes. *Clinical and Investigative Medicine* 21:267.

Ievers, C. E. 1998. Family functioning and social support in the adaptation of caregivers of children with sickle cell syndromes. *Journal of Pediatric Psychology* 23:377.

Isaacson, Glenn. 1998. Cystic fibrosis and sinusitis. *Ear, Nose and Throat Journal* 77:886.

Japan study of cot death. *Pediatrics* 103:A64, 1999.

Jeffery, Heather. 1999. Why the prone position is a risk factor for sudden infant death syndrome. *Pediatrics* 104:263.

Jensen, P. 1998. Crime in Huntington's disease: A study of registered offences among patients, relatives, and controls. *Journal of Neurology, Neurosurgery and Psychiatry* 65:467.

Johnson-Robbins, Lauren A., Joanne C. Porter, and Michael J. Horgan. 1999. Splenic rupture in a newborn with hemophilia A: A case report and review of the literature. *Clinical Pediatrics* 38:117.

Kinney, Thomas R. 1999. Silent cerebral infarcts in sickle cell anemia: A risk factor. *Pediatrics* 103:640.

Koch, Richard K. 1999. Issues in newborn screening for phenylketonuria. *American Family Physician* 60:1462.

Kuppermann, Miriam, James D. Goldberg, Robert F. Nease Jr., et al. 1999. Who should be offered pre-natal diagnosis? The 35-year-old question. *American Journal of Public Health* 89:160.

Lander, Eric S. 1998. Scientific commentary: The scientific foundations and medical and social prospects of the Human Genome Project. *Journal of Law, Medicine and Ethics* 26:184.

Leonard, S. 1999. Medical aspects of school aged children with Down syndrome. *Dev Med Child Neurol* 41:683.

Levy, H.L. 1999. Phenylketonuria: Old disease, new approach to treatment. *National Academy of Science* 96:2339.

Lewis, Jeffery. 1999. The performance of a lifetime: a metaphor for the phenotype. *Perspectives in Biology and Medicine* 43:112.

Mapping the human genome: The genetics revolution. *British Medical Journal* 319:1282, 1999.

Marshall, Bruce C. 1999. The information explosion in cystic fibrosis. *The Lancet* 353:333.

McCarthy, Michael. 1999. Inhaled antibiotics effective for cystic fibrosis. *The Lancet* 353:215.

Messmore, Jr., and L. Harry. 1999. Hemophilia. *Journal of the American Medical Association* 283:124.

Mitchell, Edwin. 1999. Changing infants sleep position increases risk of sudden infant death syndrome. *The Journal of American Medical Association* 283:986.

Murphy-Brennan, Majella, et al. 1999. Is there evidence to show that fetal alcohol syndrome can be prevented? *Journal of Drug Education* 29:5.

Mutton, David, and Roy G. Ide. 1998. Trends in pre-natal screening for and diagnosis of Down's syndrome: England and Wales. *British Medical Journal* 317:922.

Myers, L. B. 1999. The relationship between control beliefs and self-reported adherence in adults with cystic fibrosis. *Psychology, Health and Medicine* 4:387.

Nunley, D. R. 1998. Pulmonary aspergillosis in cystic fibrosis lung transplant recipients. *Chest* 114:1321.

Percivial, S. S. 1999. Altered copper status in adult men with cystic fibrosis. *Journal of Am. Coll Nutrition* 18:614.

Pietz, J. 1998. Neurological outcome in adult patients with early treated phenylketonuria. *European Journal of Pediatrics* 157:824.

Pitulle, C. 1999. Novel bacterium isolated from a lung transplant patient with cystic fibrosis. *Journal of Clinical Microbiology* 37:3851.

Price, D. L. 1998. Genetic neurodegenerative diseases: The human illness and transgenic models. *Science* 282:1079.

Private venture to sequence human genome launched. *Issues in Science and Technology* 15:28, 1998.

Quinn, N. 1998. Huntington's disease and other choreas. *Journal of Neurology* 245:709.

Reddy, P. H., et al. 1999. Recent advances in understanding the pathogenesis of Huntington's disease. *Trends in Neurosciences* 22:248.

Reilly, Philip R. 1998. Introduction: Reading the human genome: Gothic tale or happy ending? *Journal of Law, Medicine and Ethics* 26:181.

Roach, M.A. 1999. Mothers and fathers of children with Down syndrome: Parental stress and involvement in childcare. *American Journal of Mental Retardation* 104:422.

Russell, D. 1998. Evaluating motor function in children with Down's syndrome: Validity of the GMFM. *Developmental Medicine and Child Neurology* 40:693.

Saenz, Rebecca B. 1999. Primary care of infants and young children with Down syndrome. *American Family Physician* 59:381.

Schechter, Alan. 2000. Sickle cell anemia therapy. *Science* 287:592.

Schlaud, M., et al. 1999. Prevalence and determinants of prone sleeping position in infants: Results from two cross sectional studies on risk factors for SIDS in Germany. *American Journal of Epidemiology* 150:51.

Shreve, M.R., et al. 1999. Impact of microbiology practice on cumulative prevalence of respiratory tract bacteria in patients with cystic fibrosis. *Journal of Clinical Microbiology* 37:753.

Smith, Maurice A., et al. 1999. Motor disorder in Huntington's disease begins as a dysfunction in error feedback control. *Nature* 403:544.

Soubani, A. O. 1999. Acute respiratory distress syndrome. *South Medical Journal* 92:450

Soucie, J. M. 1998. Occurrence of hemophilia in the United States. The hemophilia surveillance system project investigators. *American Journal of Hematology* 59:288.

Sullivan, J. E. 1999. Review emotional and behavioral functioning in phenylketonuria. *Journal of Pediatric Psychology* 24:281.

Takeuchi, Y. 1999. Klinefelter's syndrome accompanied by mixed connective tissue disease and diabetes mellitus. *Internal Medicine* 38:875.

Tolstoi, Linda, G., et al. 1999. Human genome project and cystic fibrosis: A symbiotic relationship. *Journal of the American Dietetic Association* 99:1421.

Tuemmler, B., and C. Kiewitz. 1999. Cystic fibrosis: an inherited susceptibility to bacterial respiratory infections. *Molecular Medicine Today* 5:351.

Usner, D. W. 1998. Hemophilia morbidity, cognitive functioning and academic achievement. *Journal of Pediatrics* 133:782.

Valta, P. 1999. Acute respiratory distress syndrome. *Critical Care Medicine* 27:2367.

Wappner, R. 1999. Management of phenylketonuria of optimal outcome: a review of guidelines for phenylketonuria management and a report of surveys of parents, patients, and clinic directors. *Pediatrics* 104:d68.

Welch, Gilbert H., and Wylie Burke. 1998. Uncertainties in genetic testing for chronic disease. *Journal of the American Medical Association* 280:1525.

White, D. A. 1998. Cognitive and behavioral function of children with sickle cell disease: A review and discussion of methodological issues. *Journal of Pediatric Hematology/Oncology* 20:458.

Wilschanski, Michael, Joseph Rivlin, Solomon Cohen, et al. 1999. Clinical and genetic risk factors for cystic fibrosis—related liver disease. *Pediatrics* 103:52.

Wyllie, Robert. 1999. Gastrointestinal manifestations of cystic fibrosis. *Clinical Pediatrics* 38:735.

Wyncoll, Duncan, et al. 1999. Acute respiratory distress syndrome. *The Lancet* 354:497.

Xiang, F. 1998. A Huntington's disease-like neurodegenerative disorder maps to chromosome 20p. *American Journal of Human Genetics* 63:1431.

Zimmermann, S. A. 1998. Inherited DNA mutations contributing to thrombotic complications in patients with sickle cell disease. *American Journal of Hematology* 59:267.

Zuckerman, J.B. 1999. A phase I study of adenovirus mediated transfer of the human cystic fibrosis transmembrane conductance regulator gene to a lung segment of individuals with cystic fibrosis. *Human Gene Therapy* 1461:731.

GLOSSARY

A

ACE inhibitor   Drug used to treat hypertension and heart failure

acetylcholine   Type of neurotransmitter

acromegaly   Rare disease characterized by abnormal enlargement of bone; caused by a benign tumor of the pituitary gland in an adult

ACTH   Adrenocorticotropic hormone that stimulates the adrenal cortex to release other hormones (corticosteroids)

active artificial immunity   Acquired through vaccination with a weakened form of an active or disease-causing microorganism

active natural immunity   Acquired through exposure to a disease-causing microorganism

acyclovir   Antiviral drug used to treat herpes simplex infection

adenocarcinoma   A malignant adenoma arising from a glandular organ

adenovirus   One of a group of closely related viruses that can cause infections of the upper respiratory tract

adrenocorticotropic   Having a stimulating effect on the adrenal cortex

AIDS   acquired immunodeficiency syndrome

alimentary   Referring to parts of the digestive system

allergen   Agent that causes an allergic reaction

alpha antitrypsin   An inhibitor of trypsin that may be deficient in patients who have emphysema

alveolar sacs   Small saclike structures at the end of the bronchioles that contain the alveoli

alveoli   Terminal saccules of the alveolar ducts where gases are exchanged in respiration

amantadine   An antiviral agent; also used to treat Parkinson's disease

amebiasis   Infection with amebas

amenorrhea   The absence or suppression of menstruation; it occurs normally before puberty, after menopause, and during pregnancy and lactation

amniocentesis   Test to identify genetic defects in a fetus as young as five months of age

anaerobic   Lacking oxygen—some organisms multiply in anaerobic conditions

analgesic   Agent that relieves pain without causing loss of consciousness

anaphylactic shock   Rare, severe, life-threatening reaction to an allergen

aneurysm   Weakened area of a blood vessel, usually an artery, which dilates (expands) with the pressure of blood flowing through it. May be caused by disease, injury, or a congenital defect. Usually results in severe pain; may rupture

angina pectoris   Squeezing or crushing tightness in the chest; a symptom of coronary artery disease

angioplasty   Insertion of a balloon into an artery; the balloon is inflated to widen the lumen, which has been narrowed by atherosclerotic plaques

angiotensin   Vasopressant involved in regulating blood pressure

Anopheles   A genus of mosquitoes belonging to the family Culicidae, order Diptera; a vector of *Plasmodium,* the causative agent of malaria, and may be involved in transmitting the causative agent of dengue, filariasis, and possibly other diseases

antibody-mediated immunity   *See* humoral immunity

antiemetic   Drug used to treat nausea and vomiting

antigen   Any substance that can trigger the immune response resulting in the body's production of antibodies

antipyretic   Relieving fever; agent that relieves or reduces fever

antisera   *See* antitoxin

antitoxin   Antibody produced in response to and capable of neutralizing a toxin

antrum   Lower part of the stomach; churns food with enzymes and acids to produce chyme

apoptosis   Cell deletion by fragmentation into membrane-bound particles that are phagocytosed by other cells

aqueous humor   Transparent liquid contained in the anterior and posterior chambers of the eye

arsphenamine   Also called *606*, first drug used to treat syphilis

arteriosclerosis   Hardening of and loss of elasticity in the arteries

arthralgia   Pain in a joint

arthropod vector   Organism that transports a disease agent from infected to noninfected individuals

ascariasis   Condition resulting from infestation by *Ascaris lumbricoides* (pin worm)

ascites   Excess of fluid in the peritoneal cavity—the space between the two layers of membrane that line the inside of the abdominal wall and the outside of the abdominal organs

asymptomatic   Without any apparent symptoms

ataxic   Defective muscular coordination, especially that manifested when voluntary muscular movements are attempted

atherogenesis   Formation of masses of plaque in the arteries

atheroma   Mass of plaque, formed of cholesterol and cellular debris

atherosclerosis   Deposits of plaque formed within the arteries; a form of arteriosclerosis

athetoid   Resembling or affected with athetosis

atrioventricular   Pertaining to both the atrium and the ventricle

atrophy   Shrinkage or wasting away of a tissue or organ; a reduction in the number or size of cells

atropine   Drug sometimes used to treat Ménière's disease and other disorders

autoimmune disorder   Misdirected immune response wherein the body's immune system attacks the body's own tissues

autoinfection   Infection by an agent already present in or on the body

autolysis   Enzymatic digestion of cells (especially dead or degenerate) by enzymes present within them (autogenous); occurs after death and in some pathological conditions

autonomic process   Process controlled by the part of the nervous system that regulates the motor functions of body organs

avenue of escape   *See* portal of exit

avian   Pertaining to birds

axon   Part of a neuron that carries messages away from the cell body

azidothymidine (AZT)   Drug that inhibits the human immunodeficiency virus that causes AIDS

B

bacilli   Rod-shaped bacteria; tuberculosis is caused by bacilli

bacteremia   Presence of bacteria in the blood

bacteria   Single-celled, plantlike organisms, some are harmless, some beneficial, and a minority cause disease; common groups of bacteria are bacilli, cocci, and spirilla

BCG   Vaccination that provides immunity to tuberculosis

benign   Noncancerous, as a growth or tumor

beta blockers   Drugs prescribed mainly for heart disease

bile   Liquid secreted by liver that carries away waste products of the liver and helps break down fat in the small intestine

bilirubin   Bile pigment that, along with cholesterol and calcium, forms gallstones

biofeedback   Technique of furnishing an individual with auditory or sensory information that enables the individual to gain control over autonomic processes such as blood pressure or heart rate

bolus   Mass of chewed food that is ready to be swallowed

Borrelia   A genus of spirochetes, some of which are causative agents for relapsing fevers and Lyme disease in humans; though classed as bacteria, spirochetes differ in physical appearance from most bacteria in that they have a spiral shape

bradycardia   Slowness of the heartbeat, as evidenced by slowing of the pulse rate to less than 60

bradykinin   Normally present in blood in an inactive form and similar to trypsin in action; one of a number of the plasma kinins, a potent vasodilator, and one of the physiologic mediators of anaphylaxis released from cytotropic antibody-coated mast cells following reaction with antigen (allergen) specific for the antibody

bronchial tubes   Larger air passageways of the lungs

bronchiole   One of the finer subdivisions of the branched bronchial tree

bronchodilator   Drug used to relieve breathing difficulties such as those occurring in asthma

bubo   Tender, enlarged, and inflamed lymph node, particularly in the axilla or groin and present in infections such as bubonic plague

bursa   Small, fluid-filled sac that facilitates the movement of muscles and tendons over body parts or joints

C

calcium channel blocker   Used in the treatment of angina pectoris, hypertension, and certain types of dysrhythmia

calculus   A hard, crystalline mass formed from precipitates of body fluids, most often found in biliary or urinary tract

Candida albicans   Thrush fungus; a species that is ordinarily a part of normal human gastrointestinal flora, but which becomes pathogenic when there is a disturbance in the balance of flora or in debilitation of the host from other causes; resulting disease states may vary from limited to generalized cutaneous or mucocutaneous infections, to severe and fatal systemic disease including endocarditis, septicemia, and meningitis

candidiasis   Infection with, or disease caused by, *Candida,* especially *C. albicans*

carcinogen   Cancer-causing substance

cardiac catheterization   Diagnostic test wherein a fine tube (catheter) is introduced into the heart, through a blood vessel, to investigate its condition

cardiovascular system   Composed of heart, blood vessels, and lymphatics

carrier   Individual who, although infected with a disease, has no discernible symptoms, and is capable of spreading the disease to others

catarrhal stage   Stage of whooping cough marked by inflammation of the mucous membrane in the air passages of the head and throat

cell-mediated immunity   Involves the production of lymphocytes (T cells) in response to exposure to an antigen

cerebrovascular accident   Stroke

cerumen   A substance secreted by glands at the outer third of the ear canal

chancre   Characteristic sore and first apparent symptom of syphilis

chemotaxis   Movement of an organism or cells in response to a chemical attractant; in the inflammatory reaction, chemicals called mediators lure leukocytes to travel toward the site of an injury

chemotherapy   Use of drugs (chemicals) to treat disease

chest physiotherapy   Process of massaging and pressure applied to the chest

cholecystectomy   Surgery to remove the gallbladder

cholesterol   Lipid that plays an important part in the formation of atheromas in the arteries; also important in normal body processes

chorea   Involuntary muscular twitching of face or limbs

chorionic villus biopsy   Test to identify genetic defects in a fetus as young as two months of age

choroid   Layer of blood vessels that lies at the back of the eye behind the retina

chylomicron   Lipoprotein composed primarily of triglycerides

chyme   Liquid produced in the antrum of the stomach during the digestive process and released gradually to the duodenum

cilia   Fine hairlike projections in the respiratory passages; also found in other parts of the body

ciliary body   Membrane of the eye between the iris and front of the choroid

claw hand   Flexion and atrophy of the hand and fingers occurring in leprosy and other disorders

clinical   Stage of a disease when the characteristic symptoms appear

Clostridium tetani   The causative organism of tetanus or lockjaw; it produces a powerful exotoxin, one portion of which affects nerve tissue and the other of which is hemolytic

Coccidioides immitis   A genus of fungi found in the soil of the semiarid areas of the southwestern United States and small areas throughout Central and South America, but has not been found elsewhere; causes coccidioidomycosis

coccidioidomycosis   An inapparent, benign, severe, or fatal systemic mycosis caused by inhalation of dust particles containing arthrospores of *Coccidioides immitis;* in benign forms of the infection the lesions are limited to the upper respiratory tract and lungs; in a low percentage of cases the disease disseminates to other visceral organs, bones, joints, and skin and subcutaneous tissues

colchicine   Drug used 1500 years ago and still used today in the treatment of gout

COLD   Chronic obstructive lung disease (*see* COPD)

collateral circulation   Side branches of blood vessels

colostomy   The opening of a portion of the colon through the abdominal wall to its outside surface

complement   Contained in the plasma secreted by capillaries during the body's immune response; enhances the phagocytosis of the antigen by causing the destruction of its cell membrane

completed stroke   Maximal damage in the beginning

computed axial tomography (CAT scan)   Diagnostic technique using X rays and a computer to produce clear, cross-sectional images of the tissue being examined

congenital disorder   Disorder present at birth

contact inhibition   Pertaining to the cancer cell's inability to know when to stop reproducing

contact investigation   Finding those known to have been exposed to a disease agent

convalescence   Recovery stage of a disease

COPD   Chronic obstructive pulmonary disease— often a combination of chronic bronchitis and emphysema; chronic asthma may also be present

cornea   Part of the eye that refracts light rays

cor pulmonale   Failure of right ventricle caused by disorders of the lungs, pulmonary vessels, or chest wall

corticosteroids   Drugs similar to the natural hormones produced by the adrenal glands, which are prescribed in hormone replacement therapy

cruciferous vegetable   Vegetable such as cauliflower, broccoli, or brussels sprouts that contains nutrients and nonnutrients that protect against cancer

cryosurgery   Tissue destruction by freezing

cyanosis   Blueness caused by reduced oxygen in general circulation

cystectomy   Bladder removal

cystoscope   Tube with a light and various attachments; used to examine and treat diseases of the bladder and urethra

D

debilitated   Weakened by some disease process

debridement   Removal of foreign material and dead, damaged, or infected tissue from a wound or burn until surrounding healthy tissue is exposed

decline   Stage of a disease when the symptoms begin to fade

defecation   Expulsion of feces via the anus

dementia   Mental deterioration

demyelination   Destruction or removal of myelin sheath of nerve tissue

dendrite   Part of neuron that carries messages to the cell body

deoxyribonucleic acid (DNA)   Principal carrier of genetic information in almost all organisms

dermis   Layer of skin containing hair follicles, sweat glands, sebaceous glands, blood vessels, lymph vessels, and nerves

desquamation   Shedding of epithelial elements, chiefly of the skin, in scales or small sheets

diabetic coma   Life-threatening condition in diabetics, occurring if blood glucose becomes too high

diapedesis   The passage of blood, or any of its formed elements, through the intact walls of blood vessels

diastolic pressure   Resting period of the heart muscle; the second reading when blood pressure is measured

diethylstilbestrol (DES)   Synthetic estrogen used therapeutically to treat menopause and as a "morning after" pill until it was discovered that daughters of women who were given the drug during pregnancy developed vaginal cancer later in life

differentiation   Term used in classifying cancer cells

dopamine   Neurotransmitter that is deficient in individuals with Parkinson's disease

duodenum   First section of the small intestine

dysentery   Diarrhea

dyspepsia   Indigestion

dyspnea   Difficult or labored breathing

dysrhythmia   Abnormal, disordered, or disturbed rhythm

E

ectopic pregnancy   Pregnancy that develops outside the womb, usually in a fallopian tube

edema   Presence of abnormally large amounts of fluid in the intercellular tissue spaces of the body

Ehrlichia   A genus of small, often pleomorphic coccoid to ellipsoidal, nonmotile gram-negative bacteria that occur either singly or in compact inclusions in circulating mammalian leukocytes

electrodesiccation   Tissue destruction by heat

electrolyte   Substance that plays an important part in regulation of heartbeat

embolism   Obstruction of a blood vessel by foreign substances or a blood clot

embolus   Moving blood clot

emigration   During the inflammatory response, leukocyte movement along the endothelium and escape through the walls of blood vessels

emollient   Agent that softens skin or soothes irritated skin or mucous membrane

encapsulated   Enclosed in a sheath not normal to the part as in a benign tumor

encephalitides   Inflammation of the brain

endemic   Constantly present in a particular area or specific population

endocardium   Internal lining of the heart

endocrine gland   Ductless gland that discharges its secretions directly into the bloodstream

endogenous   Arising from causes on or within the organism

endometritis   Inflammation of the inner mucous membrane of the uterus

endometrium   Lining of the uterus

endothelium   Lining of the blood vessels and other body parts

Entamoeba histolytica   A pathogenic species of ameba, the cause of amebic dysentery and tropical liver abscess

enteritis   Inflammation of the intestine, applied chiefly to the small intestine

Enterovirus   Genus of virus that includes the polio virus

eosinophilia   Pulmonary infiltrates seen as transient migratory shadows on the chest X-ray film, accompanied by blood

epidemic   Disease occurring suddenly in numbers clearly in excess of normal expectancy

epidemiologic theory   Whether anyone gets a disease depends on the relationship among three factors: the disease, the host, and the environment

epidemiology   Science of studying the factors that determine and influence the frequency and distribution of disease

epidermis   Outermost and thinnest layer of the skin

epididymitis   Inflammation of the epididymis

erythema   Redness of the skin produced by congestion of the capillaries

erythema chronicum migrans (ECM)   Characteristic rash resulting from the bite of a tick carrying Lyme disease; the rash is a red spot that expands gradually, leaving a clear area in the middle

erythematous   Relating or marked by erythema

erythromycin   Drug used to treat infections of the skin, chest, throat, and ears

esophageal   Pertaining to the esophagus

esophageal varices   Dilated, incompetent veins in the esophagus that are a result of liver disease

etiology   Study of the factors that cause disease

excise   To cut out diseased tissue

exocrine gland   Gland that discharges its secretions through a duct opening on an internal or external surface of the body

exogenous   Originating outside the organism

exotoxin   Toxic substance formed by species of certain bacteria that is found outside the bacterial cell

external barrier   Body's first line of defense against invaders

exudate   Material escaping from blood vessels that have increased permeability during the inflammatory responses

F

familial hyperlipoproteinemia   Increase in three fatty substances in the blood: cholesterol, phospholipid, and triglyceride (lipoproteins) more common in some families

feces   Waste material of digestive tract, expelled through the anus; consists of indigestible food residue (fiber), dead bacteria, dead cells shed from intestinal lining, secretions from intestines such as mucus, bile from the liver, and water

fibrinous   Pertaining to an exudate containing fibrin, an aid to formation of a clot in the healing process; produced in a moderately severe wound

fibromyalgia   Chronic pain in muscle and soft tissues surrounding joints

fibrotic regeneration   Repair of a wound with fibrous tissue

foamy macrophage   Macrophage containing lipids

fomite   Inanimate object capable of harboring pathogenic organisms and thus conveying an infection from one person to another; respiratory infections such as colds and influenza are most commonly transmitted this way

fontanelle   One of two soft areas on a baby's scalp; a gap between the bones of the skull covered by a membrane

food poisoning   Term commonly used to denote any illness that seems to be the result of ingesting food

Franciscella   A genus of nonmotile nonsporeforming aerobic bacteria that contains small gram-negative cocci and rods; capsules are rarely produced and the cells may show bipolar staining

fundus   Upper part of the stomach that holds food as it is gradually delivered to the lower part

fungi   Single- or multicelled plantlike organisms that release enzymes that digest cells

G

gangrene   Death of tissue, usually because of inadequate oxygen supply to the area

gastrin   Hormone secreted mainly by cells in the stomach to aid in digestion

gastroenterologist   Specialist in treating disorders of the digestive tract

gastroesophageal   Concerning the stomach and esophagus

genome   The complete set of chromosomes, and thus the entire genetic information present in a cell

giardiasis   Infection with the flagellate protozoan

glomerulonephritis   A form of nephritis in which the lesions involve primarily the glomeruli

glomerulus   Element in the nephron of the kidney that filters the blood

glucocorticoids   Any steroidlike compound capable of significantly influencing intermediary metabolism such as promotion of hepatic glycogen deposition, and of exerting a clinically useful anti-inflammatory effect; cortisol is the most potent of the naturally occurring glucocorticoids; most semisynthetic glucocorticoids are cortisol derivatives

gold salts   Sometimes used to treat arthritis

grading   Classification of tumor cells by grades (I to IV) depending on their degree of difference from normal cells and their growth rate

griseofulvin   Drug prescribed to treat fungi orally when creams and lotions have not been effective

gumma   Advanced lesion of syphilis

gynecomastia   Excessive development of the male mammary glands

H

hajj   Pilgrimage to Mecca

heartburn   Burning pain in center of chest that may travel from tip of breastbone to throat; generally a result of overeating, eating spicy foods, or drinking alcohol

Helicobacter pylori   A motile, gram-negative bacterium that causes some peptic ulcers, which are treated with combined antibiotics and agents to block gastric acid secretions

helminth   A wormlike animal

hemangioma   Birthmark caused by abnormal distribution or excess of blood vessels

hematuria   Blood in the urine

hemoccult test   Test to detect blood in the stool, a sign of colorectal cancer

hemorrhagic exudate   Exudate that appears in a severe injury, when a lesion is deep enough to penetrate blood vessels and allow red blood cells to escape

hemorrhoids   Varicose veins in the anal area

hepatomegaly   An enlargement of the liver

hepatorenal   Relating to the liver and the kidney

hepatosplenomegaly   An enlargement of the liver and spleen

herpetic whitlow   Painful herpes simplex virus infection of a finger, often accompanied by lymphangitis and regional adenopathy, lasting up to several weeks; most common in physicians, dentists, and nurses as a result of exposure to the virus in a patient's mouth

heterologous   Made up of cell tissue not normal to the part

hiatal hernia   The protrusion of the stomach upward into the mediastinal cavity through the esophageal hiatus of the diaphragm

high-density lipoprotein (HDL)　Removes cholesterol from the blood and sends it to the liver to be processed and excreted (good cholesterol)

histamine　Substance released in an allergic reaction or as part of the inflammation response

Histoplasma capsulatum　A dimorphic fungus species of worldwide distribution that causes histoplasmosis in man and other mammals; the organism's natural habit is soil fertilized with bird and bat droppings, where it grows as a mold, fragments of which, following inhalation, produce the primary pulmonary infection

homologous　Similar in fundamental structure and in origin but not necessarily in function

human immunodeficiency virus (HIV)　Virus that causes AIDS

human T-cell lymphotrophic virus (HTLV)　Name once used for the virus that causes AIDS

humoral immunity　Protection against disease through B lymphocytes, or B cells, which produce antibodies in the blood; also called antibody-mediated immunity

hydrocephalus　An increased amount of fluid, usually under increased pressure within the skull

hypercalcemia　Abnormally high level of calcium in the blood

hypercholesterolemia　Excess of cholesterol in the blood

hyperesthesia　Increased sensitivity to sensory stimuli such as pain and touch

hyperlipidemia　Excess of fats in the blood

hyperplasia　Excessive proliferation of normal cells in the normal tissue arrangement of an organ

hypersecretion　An abnormal amount of secretion

hypersensitivity disorder　Also called allergy, an inappropriate reaction of the immune system, e.g., allergic rhinitis, urticaria, angioedema, asthma

hypertension　High blood pressure

hypertrophy　Enlargement of an organ or tissue caused by increase in size, rather than number, of its cells

hyperuricemia　Excess uric acid in the blood

hypochondriac　Individual with an unreasonable belief or fear that he or she has a serious illness despite medical reassurance

hypodermis　Layer of skin consisting mainly of fat, which provides heat, insulation, shock absorption, and a reserve of calories; also has a nerve supply

hypothermia　Significant loss of body heat

hypoxemia　Too little oxygen in the blood

I

I.M.　Intramuscular administration of a liquid form of a drug

I.V.　Intravenous administration of a liquid form of a drug

idiopathic hypertension　*See* primary hypertension

immunology　Branch of biomedical science concerned with the response of the organism to antigenic challenge, the recognition of self and not-self, and all aspects of immune phenomena

incidence rate　Number of new cases of a disease occurring during a specified time

incubation　Period from the time when the agent enters the body to the appearance of the first symptoms

inflammation　First response of the body when pathogenic agents penetrate external barriers

insidious　Indicating the occurrence of a disease that comes on in such a way (no symptoms) that the individual is unaware of the onset

in situ　Localized

insulin shock　State occurring in diabetics if blood glucose becomes too low

interferon　Protein that protects the body against viral infection; released during the inflammatory response if the cell injury is due to a viral infection

intermediate-density lipoprotein (IDL)　Lipid quickly removed from plasma or converted to LDL

ischemia　Deficiency of blood in an area caused by constriction or obstruction of a blood vessel

islets of Langerhans　Areas in the pancreas containing the beta cells that produce insulin

Ixodes scapularis　The black-legged or shoulder tick, a species found on animals in the southern and eastern United States; capable of inflicting a painful bite to humans

J

jaundice　Yellowing of the skin and whites of the eyes; indicative of a liver and/or biliary system disorder

K

Kaposi's sarcoma　A multifocal malignant neoplasm of primitive vasoformative tissue occurring in the skin and sometimes in lymph nodes or viscera, consisting of spindle cells and irregular small vascular spaces frequently infiltrated by hemosiderin-pigmented macrophages and extravasated red cells

ketosis   Potentially serious condition when chemical substances called ketones accumulate in the blood if there is not enough sugar available to use as energy; may be a result of untreated or inadequately controlled diabetes

Koplik's spots   Small irregular, bright red spots on the inside of the mouth with a minute bluish-white speck in the center of each; seen in the prodromal stage of measles (rubeola)

kyphosis   An exaggeration or angulation of the normal posterior curve of the spine, giving rise to the condition commonly known as humpback, hunchback, or Pott's curvature; it may be due to congenital anomaly, disease, malignancy, or compression fracture

L

laparoscopy   Means of examining the abdominal cavity by means of a laparoscope (viewing tube)

laryngoscopy   Means of examining the larynx with a laryngoscope (viewing tube)

leproma   Superficial granulomatous nodule characteristic of lepromatous leprosy

Leptospira   A genus of aerobic bacteria containing thin, tightly coiled organisms six to twenty micrometers in length; they possess an axial filament, and one or both ends may be bent into a semicircular hook

leptospirosis   Infection with species of *Leptospira*

leukotrienes   Products of arachidonic acid metabolism with postulated physiologic activity such as mediators of inflammation and roles in allergic reactions; differ from the related prostaglandins and thromboxanes by not having a central ring; they are so named because they were discovered in association with leukocytes and because of three double bonds in the first leukotriene discovered (most have four); letters *A* through *E* identify the five metabolites thus far isolated, with subscript numbers to indicate the number of double bonds

lindane   Drug used for infestation with scabies or lice

lipid   Fatty substance; includes triglycerides, phospholipids, and sterols such as cholesterol

lipoprotein   Lipids in the plasma; they circulate attached to protein

lithotripsy   The application of physical force to crush a calculus in the bladder or urethra

lordosis   Commonly called *swayback,* an accentuation of the normal curve of the spine

low-density lipoprotein (LDL)   Lipid strongly correlated with atherosclerosis

lumen   Space in a tubular organ such as an artery

lymphadenopathy   Swollen lymph glands

lymphadenopathy-associated virus (LAV)   Name once used for the virus that causes AIDS

lymphokine   Substance released by lymphocytes that have come in contact with an antigen; helps produce cellular immunity by stimulating macrophages and monocytes

lymphotrophy   Nourishment of the tissues by lymph in parts devoid of blood vessels

lysosome   A cytoplasmic membrane-bound vesicle measuring five to eight nanometers (primary lysosome) and containing a wide variety of glycoprotein hydrolytic enzymes active at an acid pH; serves to digest exogenous material, such as bacteria, and effete organelles of the cells

M

macrophage   Large cell that performs the final function of the body's immune response; i.e., "cleanups" by killing and digesting antigens

macule   Discolored spot on the skin that is not elevated above the surface

magnetic resonance imaging (MRI)   Provides high quality cross-sectional images of organs and structures within the body without the use of X rays or other radiation

malaise   Vague feeling of bodily discomfort

malignant   Cancerous; used to describe neoplasm or tumor

malignant hypertension   Severe form of high blood pressure in which blood pressure rises rapidly with possible injury to the arterioles

mastectomy   Excision of the breast

mediators   Chemicals that lure leukocytes to an inflammatory site

Mendelian genetics   Study of the transmission of traits from one generation to the next

Ménière's disease   A recurrent and usually progressive group of symptoms including progressive deafness, ringing in the ears, dizziness, and a sensation of fullness or pressure in the ears

menopause   Time during which menstruation ceases and changes occur in a woman's body because of reduced hormone production

metastasize   To spread, as a tumor, through the circulatory and lymphatic systems and to invade surrounding tissue

metazoon   Multicellular parasitic animal (worm) that can cause disease

methotrexate   Drug originally used in cancer chemotherapy

metronidazole   An antibiotic effective against infections caused by anaerobic bacteria; also used to treat protozoan infections

miasma theory   Theory that attributed disease to bad odors or emanations from the earth

mitral stenosis   Narrowing of the mitral valve opening

mode of conveyance   Means by which disease organisms pass from one host to another

molecular genetics   Study of the chemical structure of genes and how they operate at the molecular level

moniliasis   Candidiasis

monoclonal antibody therapy   Experimental treatment for cancer whereby "clones" of antibodies carry substances to cancer cells and destroy them

mucolytic   Pertaining to a class of agents that liquefy sputum or reduce its viscosity

mucolytic agent   Drug that makes mucus less sticky and easier to cough up

mucous membrane   Soft, pink layer that lines many cavities and tubes of the body and secretes a fluid containing mucus to keep structures moist

myalgia   Muscle pain

myocardial infarct (MI)   Heart attack

myocarditis   Inflammation of the myocardium, the muscular walls of the heart

N

nebulizer   Device used to administer a drug in aerosol form through a face mask; often used for asthma attacks

necrosis   Death of tissue

neoplasm   New or abnormal growth

nephron   Anatomical and functional unit of the kidney providing the filtering, reabsorption, and excretion functions

neuroblastoma   A malignant hemorrhagic tumor composed principally of cells resembling neuroblasts that give rise to cells of the sympathetic system, especially adrenal medulla

neuron   Fundamental unit of the nervous system consisting of the cell body, axon, and dendrites

neurotransmitter   Chemical substance that diffuses across the synaptic gap and carries a message from the axon of one neuron to the dendrite of another

nocturia   Increased urination at night

nodule   Small lump of tissue—hard or soft—usually more than one quarter of an inch in diameter

nonsteroidal anti-inflammatory drug (NSAID)   One of a number of drugs used to reduce inflammation and pain

O

occlusion   Blockage of any canal, opening, or vessel of the body

oncogene   Gene in tumor cells whose activation is associated with the conversion of normal cells into cancer cells

oncogenesis   Tumor formation and development

oncologist   Physician who specializes in treating cancer

oral hypoglycemic   Drug used to stimulate insulin production

orchitis   Inflammation of the testes

osteoporosis   A general term describing any disease process that results in reduction in the mass of bone per unit of volume. The reduction is sufficient to interfere with the mechanical support function of bone.

otitis   Inflammation of the ear

P

palliative   Affording relief but not cure

pallor   Paleness; absence of normal skin coloration

pandemic   Widespread epidemic of a disease

papilloma   A circumscribed benign epithelial tumor projecting from the surrounding surface

Papillomavirus Any of a group of viruses that cause papillomas or warts in humans and animals

Pap smear Test for cancer of the cervix

papule Small circumscribed, superficial, solid elevation of the skin

Paramyxovirus A genus of viruses that includes Newcastle disease, mumps, and parainfluenza viruses

parasitic Pertaining to or caused by a parasite, a plant or animal that lives upon or within another living organism at whose expense it obtains some advantage

paresthesia Abnormal sensation, as burning or prickling

parotid glands Salivary glands located on either side of the face, above the jaw and in front of the ear

paroxysmal Recurring sudden intensification of symptoms or spasms

passive artificial immunity Acquired through inoculation with antibodies

passive natural immunity Acquired through the transfer of antibodies from a mother to her baby through the placenta and, later, through breast milk

patent ductus arteriosus Persistence of a communication between the main pulmonary artery and the aorta, after birth. The condition of patent and persistent ductus arteriosus in preterm infants has been treated successfully by using drugs that inhibit prostaglandin synthesis.

pathogenic Disease-causing

pavementing Adherence of leukocytes to the endothelium of venules after the immediate inflammatory response

pediculous Infested with lice

Pediculus capitis The head louse that lives in the fine hair of the head, although the beard and eyebrows may also be infested. Its eggs, commonly called *nits,* are glued to hairs and frequently form nests in the vicinity of the ears. This organism is the cause of pediculosis capitis.

pepsin Chief digestive enzyme in the stomach

perianal Around the anus

pericarditis Inflammation of the membrane that surrounds the heart

peripheral neuritis Inflammation of nerves in peripheral nervous system

peristalsis Wave of contraction propelling contents through a tubular organ

permeability The property of being permeable

phagocytes Cells that attack and are capable of ingesting antigens that enter the body

phagocytosis The process of ingestion and digestion by cells of solid substances, for example, other cells, bacteria, bits of necrosed tissue, or foreign particles

pharyngeal Relating to the pharynx

phenylketonuria Phenylpyruvic acid in the urine

phospholipid Lipid that contains phosphorus

photophobia Sensitivity to light

Phthirus pubis The crab louse; infests primarily the pubic region but it may also be found in armpits, beard, eyebrows, and eyelashes

plaque In the arteries, deposits containing cholesterol, foamy macrophages, smooth muscle cells, and cellular debris

Pneumocystis carinii A minute lung-infecting protozoan characterized by cysts that develop into intracystic organisms

poliomyelitis Inflammation of the gray matter of the spinal cord

polyuria Frequent urination

population genetics Study of the variation of genes among and within populations

portal of entry Avenue through which a pathogenic organism gets into a new host

portal of exit Way for a pathogenic organism to leave the host

positron emission tomography (PET) Produces three-dimensional images that reflect the metabolic and chemical activity of tissues being studied

PPNG Penicillinase-producing *Neisseria gonorrhoeae*

predisposing factor *See* risk factor

prednisone Corticosteroid drug used to reduce inflammation and pain

prevalence rate Number of cases of a particular disease in a community at a specified time

primary healing *See* resolution

primary hypertension Another name for essential hypertension, the most common form of high blood pressure

primary prevention Measures taken before disease occurs to reduce susceptibility, such as a vaccination

proctosigmoidoscopy Visual examination of the rectum and sigmoid colon by use of a sigmoidoscope

prodromal Second stage of a disease when nonspecific symptoms appear

progressive stroke   Stroke that starts with slight neurologic impairment that worsens in twenty-four to forty-eight hours

prophylactic   Drug, procedure, or equipment used to prevent disease

prostaglandin   Any of a class of physiologically active substances present in many tissues, with effects such as vasodilation, vasoconstriction, stimulation of intestinal or bronchial smooth muscle, uterine stimulation, and antagonism to hormones influencing lipid metabolism; prostaglandins are prostanoic acids with ortho sidechains of varying degrees of unsaturation and varying degrees of oxidation; often abbreviated PGA, PGB, PGC, PGD, etc., with numerical subscripts, according to structure

proteinuria   Passage of increased amounts of protein in the urine

protooncogene   Normal gene that with alteration becomes an oncogene

protozoon   Single-celled parasitic animal that may release toxins and enzymes that destroy cells or interfere with their functions

pruritic   Itching

pseudomembrane   False membrane

psoriasis   A common, chronic disease of the skin consisting of erythematous papules that coalesce to form plaques with distinct borders; if the disease progresses and is untreated, a silvery, yellow-white scale develops; new lesions tend to appear at sites of trauma; they may be in any location but are frequently located on the scalp, knees, elbows, umbilicus, and genitalia

psychoneuroimmunology   New field of scientific inquiry that studies the system of communication between the mind and the body; the link between the nervous system and the immune system is of particular interest

psychosomatic factors   Mental and emotional processes that can originate or aggravate an actual physiologic disease

Purkinje   Bohemian anatomist and physiologist, 1787–1869

purulent exudate   Also called pus, occurs in a severe injury

pustule   Visible collection of pus within or beneath the epidermis, often in a hair follicle or sweat pore

pyloric sphincter   Lower valve of the stomach

pyogenic   Pus producing

R

Raynaud's disease   A peripheral vascular disorder found most frequently in women between eighteen and thirty years of age; it is marked by abnormal vasoconstriction of the extremities on exposure to cold or with emotional stress

reflux   Abnormal backflow of fluid as when stomach acid flows back into the esophagus

regeneration   Natural renewal of lost tissue as it is replaced by tissue of the same type

rehydration   Administration of fluids to combat dehydration

repair   Replacement of lost tissue by granulation tissue, which becomes a fibrous connective tissue scar

reservoir   "Home" of pathogenic organisms; humans, plants, animals, and organic matter are all reservoirs for various pathogenic organisms, allowing them to live and reproduce

resolution   When an injury is mild and heals without pus forming

respiratory system   The parts of the body involved in respiration, including the nose, pharynx, larynx, bronchial tubes, and lungs

retina   The most essential structure of the eye, which receives the image formed by the lens

retinoic acid   A metabolite of vitamin A used in the treatment of cystic acne

rice water stools   White flecks in the stools, a symptom of cholera

rifampin   Antibacterial drug used to treat tuberculosis

risk factors   Or predisposing factors, the hereditary or lifestyle factors that help determine the likelihood of disease

risus sardonicus   A grinning expression caused by acute spasm of facial muscles as in tetanus

S

sclera   Dense white fibrous protective coat of the eye, connected to the cornea

scoliosis   A lateral curvature of the spine; usually consists of two curves, the original abnormal curve and a compensatory curve in the opposite direction

sebaceous gland   Gland found mainly in the face, center of chest, upper back, shoulders, and neck that secretes sebum

seborrheic   Afflicted with seborrhea

sebum   Fatty secretion of the sebaceous glands that can obstruct hair follicles causing acne spots

secondary healing   *See* repair

secondary prevention   Measures taken to diagnose a disease that may already be present

senescence   The state of being old

sequela   Condition following or caused by an attack of disease

serous   Watery, as exudate produced in the inflammation response

sinoatrial   Pertaining to the sinus venosus and atrium

slow virus   Virus that may remain dormant for years before causing signs and symptoms of illness

sphygmomanometer   Instrument for measuring blood pressure consisting of an inflatable cuff, inflating bulb, and gauge

spirilla   Spiral-shaped bacteria, such as the spirillum that causes syphilis

splenomegaly   Enlargement of the spleen

staging   System used to quantify the extent of a cancer; allows for individualized therapy according to the characteristics of the patient and the case

stapes   Small bones in the middle ear vibrated by the tympanic membrane that relay these vibrations to the fluid in the inner ear

stoma   Mouthlike opening

streptomycin   The first effective drug treatment for tuberculosis

subcutaneous tissue   *See* hypodermis

sulfathiazole   Antibacterial drug

surfactant   Chemical that prevents alveoli from collapsing during exhalation

synaptic gap   Minute space between the axons of one neuron and the dendrites of another

systolic pressure   Maximum blood pressure resulting from contraction of the left ventricle

T

T cell   Cell produced in the thymus that is active in the immune response; helper T cells enhance the production of antibodies; killer T cells kill foreign cells; suppressor T cells suppress the immune response

tachycardia   Excessive rapidity in the action of the heart, usually applied to a heart rate above 100 beats per minute

taeniasis   The condition of being infested with tapeworms of the genus *Taenia*

tamoxifen   Anticancer drug

telomere   The distal extremities of a chromosome arm

tender points   Areas of the body that are painful when pressure is applied; used in the diagnosis of fibromyalgia

tenesmus   Painful and often ineffectual straining at stool or in urination

tertiary prevention   Measures taken to return an individual to a healthy state or to keep the victim alive

tetanus immune globulin (TIG)   Specific immune globulin derived from blood of human donors hyperimmunized with tetanus toxoid and used prophylactically in treating tetanus

tetracycline   Antibiotic used in the treatment of many bacterial diseases

tetralogy of Fallot   An anomaly of the heart consisting of pulmonary stenosis, interventricular septal defect, dextroposed aorta that receives blood from both ventricles, and hypertrophy of the right ventricle

thrombophlebitis   Inflammation of a vein accompanied by the formation of a thrombus

thrombus   Stationary clot, developed in a coronary artery or aorta because of plaque buildup

tinea   A fungus infection of the hair, skin, or nails

tinea barbae   Tinea of the beard, occurring as a follicular infection or as a granulomatous lesion; the primary lesions are papules and pustules; also called ringworm of beard

tinea capitis   Ringworm of scalp; a common form of fungus infection of the scalp caused by various species of *Microsporum* and *Trichophyton,* occurring almost exclusively in children and characterized by irregularly placed and variously sized patches of apparent baldness because of hairs breaking off at the surface of the scalp

tinea corporis   Ringworm of body; a well-defined, scaling, macular eruption that frequently forms annular lesions and may appear on any part of the body

tinea pedis   Athlete's foot; ringworm of foot; dermatophytosis of the feet, especially of the skin between the toes and the nails, caused by one of the dermatophytes; the disease consists of small vesicles, fissures, scaling, maceration, and eroded areas between the toes and on the plantar surface of the foot; other skin areas may be involved *tinea unguium*   Onychomycosis

tinnitus   Ringing in the ears

tophi   Deposits of urate in the joints, as in gout

toxin   Poison

toxoid   Toxin that is no longer toxic but is still capable of inducing formation of antibodies upon injection

Toxoplasma gondii   The causative agent of toxoplasmosis

toxoplasmosis   A disease caused by infection with the protozoan *Toxoplasma gondii*. The organism is found in mammals and birds; symptoms may be so mild as to be barely noticeable or may be more severe with lymphadenopathy, malaise, muscle pain, and little if any fever

trachea   The tube through which air passes from the larynx to the bronchial tubes

tracheostomy   Operation in which an opening is made in the trachea and a tube is inserted to maintain an effective airway

transient ischemic attack (TIA)   Decrease of blood flow in arteries supplying the brain; produces strokelike symptoms lasting less than twenty-four hours and/or dizziness

trichinosis   A disease caused by the ingestion of *Trichinella spiralis* when raw or insufficiently cooked infected pork or wild game is eaten

triglyceride   Fatty substance (lipid) circulating in the blood

TRNG   Tetracycline resistant *Neisseria gonorrhoeae*

tularensis   Transmitted to humans from rodents through the bite of a deer fly and other blood-sucking insects; causes tularemia

tumor   Swelling

tympanic membrane   Thin membrane inside the ear that vibrates when struck by sound waves

U

umbilicus   Navel

undulant   Rising and falling like waves, or moving like them

ureter   Fibromuscular tube conveying urine from kidney to bladder

urticaria   An eruption of itching wheals, usually of systemic origin; it may be due to a state of hypersensitivity to foods or drugs, foci of infection, physical agents (heat, cold, light, friction), or psychic stimuli

uvea   Middle pigmented and vascular layer of the eye, consisting of the iris, ciliary body, and choroid

V

vaccine   Suspension of attenuated or killed microorganisms (bacteria, viruses, rickettsiae) administered for the prevention, amelioration, or treatment of infectious diseases

vacuoles   The clear space in the substance of a cell, sometimes degenerative in character, sometimes surrounding an englobed foreign body and serving as a temporary cell stomach for the digestion of the body

valvuloplasty   Surgical reconstruction of a deformed cardiac valve

vasodilator   A nerve or drug that dilates blood vessels

vector   That which transports a pathogenic organism to a host

ventricular fibrillation   Quivering or spontaneous contraction of individual muscle fibers in ventricles

very-low-density lipoprotein (VLDL)   Lipid with unknown atherogenic effects

vesicle   Small bladder or sac containing liquid

virulent   Exceedingly pathogenic, noxious, or deleterious

virus   Smallest disease-causing organism; made up of DNA or RNA; not technically alive but can penetrate cells and use the cells' nucleic acid to produce more viruses

Y

Yersinestis   A species causing plague in humans, rodents, and many other mammalian species, and transmitted from rat to rat and from rat to man by the rat flea, *Xenopsylla*

Z

zidovudine   *See* azidothymidine (AZT)

zoonosis   Disease of animals that may be transmitted to humans under natural conditions

CREDITS

courtesy Centers for Disease Control and Prevention; Figures 9.10, 9.12, from Habif, TP, *Clinical Dermatology,* ed 2, Mosby, 1990; Figures 9.11, 9.13, from Price-Wilson, *Pathophysiology,* ed 4, Mosby, 1992; Figure 9.14, from McCance/Huether, *Pathophysiology,* Mosby, 1990; Figure 9.19, courtesy World Health Organization.

Chapter 10

Figure 10.1, courtesy Centers for Disease Control and Prevention; Figure 10.4, from McCance/Huether, *Pathophysiology,* Mosby, 1990; Figures 10.5, 10.6, courtesy University of Utah, Department of Dermatology.

Chapter 11

Figures 11.1, 11.6, courtesy Visuals Unlimited; Figures 11.2, 11.5, 11.7, 11.9, 11.10, 11.11, 11.13, from Nester et al., *Microbiology,* ed 2, McGraw-Hill, 1998; Figures 11.4, 11.8, courtesy Centers for Disease Control and Prevention; Figure 11.12, from Price-Wilson, *Pathphysiology,* ed 4, Mosby, 1992; Figure 11.13, from Schmidt/Roberts, *Foundations of Parasitology,* ed 4, Mosby, 1989.

Unit Opener 3

From Raven, *Understanding Biology,* Mosby.

Chapter 12

Figure 12.1, from McCance/Huether, *Pathophysiology,* Mosby, 1990; Figures 12.2, 12.4, 12.5, 12.9B, from Canobbio, *Cardiovascular Disorders,* Mosby, 1990; Figures 12.3, 12.7, 12.9A, 12.10, 12.12, from Christiansen, *Biology of Aging,* Mosby, 1993; Figure 12.6, from McCance/Huether, *Pathophysiology,* ed 2, Mosby, 1990; Figure 12.11, from Thompson, *Mosby's Clinical Nursing,* ed 3, Mosby, 1993.

Chapter 13

Figure 13.1, from Price-Wilson, *Pathophysiology,* ed 4, Mosby, 1992; Figures 13.6, 13.9, 13.12, 13.17, 13.19, from McCance/Huether, *Pathophysiology,* Mosby, 1990; Figure 13.10, from Christiansen, *Biology of Aging,* Mosby, 1993; Figure 13.13, courtesy American Cancer Society.

Chapter 15

Figures 15.1, 15.2, 15.3, 15.5, 15.6, 15.7, 15.8, 15.9, 15.10, 15.11, from McCance/Huether, *Pathophysiology,* Mosby, 1990; Figures 15.4, 15.12, from Christiansen, *Biology of Aging,* Mosby, 1993.

Chapter 16

Figures 16.2, 16.6, from Christiansen, *Biology of Aging,* Mosby, 1993; Figure 16.3, courtesy Arthritis Foundation; Figures 16.4, 16.5, from Booher, *Athletic Injury Assessment,* ed 2, Mosby, 1989.

Chapter 17

Figures 17.1, 17.2, 17.3, 17.4, 17.6, 17.7, 17.8, from Christiansen, *Biology of Aging,* Mosby, 1993; Figure 17.9, from Seeley/Stephens/Tate, *Essentials of Anatomy & Physiology,* p. 190, Mosby, 1991; Figure 17.5, from Christiansen, *Biology of Aging,* McGraw-Hill, 1993.

Chapter 18

Figures 18.1, 18.2, from Moffett, *Human Physiology,* ed 2, Mosby, 1993; Figure 18.3, courtesy Corbis; Figure 18.4, courtesy March of Dimes Birth Defects Foundation; Figure 18.5, from Payne/Hahn, *Understanding Your Health,* McGraw-Hill, ed 3, 1992.

INDEX

Note: Page numbers followed by f indicate figures; those followed by t indicate tables.

443